The Harrie

A Manual for
Thirteenth Edi

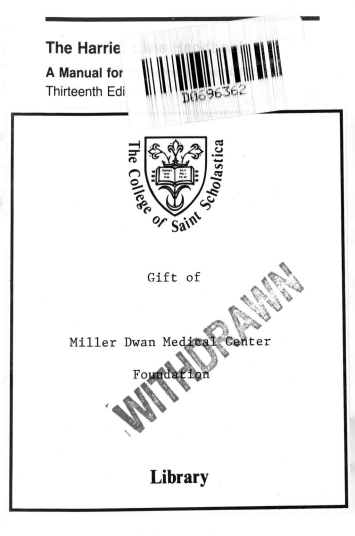

The Harriet Lane Handbook
A Manual for Pediatric House Officers

Thirteenth Edition

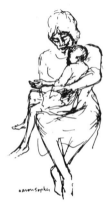

**The Harriet Lane Service
Children's Medical and Surgical Center
of
The Johns Hopkins Hospital**

**Editor
Kevin B. Johnson, M.D.**

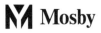 **Mosby**

St. Louis Baltimore Boston Chicago London Philadelphia Sydney Toronto

Mosby

Dedicated to Publishing Excellence

RJ
48
.H35
1993

Sponsoring Editor: Laurel Craven
Assistant Editor: Lauranne Billus
Project Manager: Nancy C. Baker
Project Supervisor: Deborah Thorp
Proofroom Manager: Barbara M. Kelly

2   3   4   5   6   7   8   9   0   CL/MA/UN   97   96   95   94

Library of Congress Cataloging-in-Publication Data
The Harriet Lane handbook : a manual for pediatric house officers / the Harriet Lane Service, Children's Medical and Surgical Center of the Johns Hopkins Hospital. — 13th ed. / Kevin B. Johnson.
   p.   cm.
   Includes bibliographical references and index.
   ISBN 0-8016-8000-X
   1. Pediatrics—Handbooks, manuals, etc.   I. Johnson, Kevin B., M.D.   II. Johns Hopkins Hospital. Children's Medical and Surgical Center.
   [DNLM: 1. Pediatrics—handbooks.   WS 29 H297 1993]
RJ48.H35   1993
DNLM/DLC
for Library of Congress   93-10312
                                                  CIP

NOTICE

Every effort has been made to ensure that the drug dosage schedules herein are accurate and in accord with the standards accepted at the time of publication. However, as new research and experience broaden our knowledge, changes in treatment and drug therapy occur. Therefore, the reader is advised to check the product information sheet included in the package of each drug he or she plans to administer to be certain that changes have not been made in the recommended dosage or in the contraindications. This is of particular importance in regard to new or infrequently used drugs.

We would like to express our gratitude to our "teachers": physicians, nurses, social workers, clerks, technicians, child life volunteers, other Harriet Lane residents, medical students, and countless others who care for children.

Most important, however, we dedicate this edition to our patients and their families, who during times of illness, health, fear, peace, isolation, and friendship, offer us inspiring courage, vast love, and unfailing hope.

FOREWORD

The Harriet Lane Handbook first appeared in 1950. Styles have changed, house staff dress has changed, even the sex of most Pediatric house officers has changed, but the utility of and need for the Handbook have remained constant. The thirteenth edition is no exception; in fact, this edition, with its revised format, is even better than its predecessors. Under the supervision of Chief Resident Kevin Johnson and another group of talented and energetic house officers, a book has been produced that should prove of value to you and ultimately benefit your patients—the children who depend on you.

Frank A. Oski, M.D.
Given Professor and Chairman of Pediatrics
Pediatrician-in-Chief
The Johns Hopkins Hospital
Baltimore, Maryland

PREFACE

As in past years, the thirteenth edition of *The Harriet Lane Handbook* represents the tireless efforts of the senior residents in The Harriet Lane Service at The Johns Hopkins Hospital. Each senior resident revised the Handbook while also performing clinical duties and formulating career plans. Their job was facilitated by 43 years of previous house officer input into the Handbook, as well as by advice from the faculty in the Children's Center.

Readers familiar with the organization of previous editions of the Handbook will be struck, at first, by two major changes:

- Improve readability of the text in this *professionally typeset edition*
- Reorganization of the contents of this edition

The Handbook begins with a section on pediatric acute care, with a revised emergency management chapter, an expanded procedures chapter, and updated chapters on poisonings and burns.

The next section contains the contents of the Diagnostic Tests and Therapeutic Data sections, now alphabetically organized into one section called Diagnostic and Therapeutic Information. The many changes in these chapters should make information easier to both find and use. These include an expanded gastroenterology chapter, with more information about the management of common gastrointestinal symptoms; completely revised genetics, infectious disease, nephrology, neurology, and radiology chapters; a new chapter on immunoprophylaxis; and a revision of the former perinatology chapter that incorporates more reference material for the management of neonates, hence the change of the chapter's name to Neonatology. HIV, CAT/CLAMS, indications for obtaining a karyotype, newborn screen information, and the management of PCA are just a few of the new topics scattered throughout the text. This edition also includes the first **color** illustrations to be included in the Handbook; we have replaced the graphic depiction of urine sediment with photographs. All in all, quite a lot of effort has been put into this edition to make it more useful for the busy house officer or health care professional.

It has been a pleasure to work with the 22 outstanding contribut-

Resident	Advisor	Chapter
Dr. Teresa T. Anderson	Dr. Carlton K. K. Lee, Pharm.D.	Formulary
Dr. Virginia B. Campion	Dr. George Dover	Hematology
Dr. Conrad J. Clemens	Dr. Barbara Fivush	Nephrology
Dr. Karen B. Dewling	Dr. Estelle Gauda	Neonatology
Dr. Laura R. Duncan	Dr. Howard Lederman	Immunology
Dr. Michael C. Engel	Dr. Fred Palmer	Development,
	Dr. Julius Goepp	Poisonings
Dr. Margaret Flowers	Dr. Myron Yaster	Pain and Sedation
Dr. James E. Fragetta	Dr. Carlton K. K. Lee	Formulary
Dr. Patricia R. Hannon	Dr. Thomas Crawford	Neurology
Dr. Sheryl L. Henderson	Dr. Mark Steinhoff	Immunoprophylaxis,
	Dr. Nancy Hutton	Infectious Diseases, Microbiology
Dr. Margaret R. Moon	Dr. Allen Walker	Emergency Management
Dr. William H. Orman	Dr. Mathu Santosham	Fluid and Electrolytes
Dr. Nancy E. Owens	Dr. Julius Goepp	Procedures, Body Fluids
Dr. Colin Phoon	Dr. Barry Byrne	Cardiology
Dr. Paul A. Rufo	Dr. Jerry Loughlin	Pulmonology
Dr. Julia A. Schillinger	Dr. George Taylor	Radiology
Dr. Eric A. Simone	Dr. Leslie Plotnick	Endocrinology, Blood Chemistries
Dr. Robert D. Stapleton	Dr. Leslie Plotnick	Endocrinology, Blood Chemistries
Dr. Corinne Wong	Dr. Karen Hofman	Genetics
	Dr. Carlton, K. K. Lee	Formulary
Dr. Donna K. Zeiter	Dr. Jose M. Saavedra Amy Kovar, R.D., L.D.	Gastroenterology, Nutrition

General Pediatric
Surgery: Dr. Francisco Cigarroa — Burns
Pediatric Pharmacist: Carlton K. K. Lee, (Pharm.D.) — Formulary

Pediatric Oncology: Dr. Daniel Wechsler — Special Drug Topics (Chemotherapeutic Agents)

ing editors of this edition. As I look over this version of the Handbook, I see only a small representation of the exceptional contributions that this group will make to the field of Pediatrics.

I thank the members of the Departments of Pediatrics, Pediatric Surgery, Pediatric Pharmacy, and Nutrition Support Services for their helpful suggestions and review of this edition. I especially appreciate the guidance and support that Dr. Frank A. Oski and Dr. Julia A. McMillan have given me throughout the year.

We are indebted to The Harriet Lane Service house staff and chief residents who have contributed to this Handbook since its inception in 1950. We appreciate the commitment of the previous editors: Drs. Harrison Spencer, Henry Seidel, Herbert Zwick, William Friedman, Robert Haslam, Jerry Winkelstein, Dennis Headings, Kenneth Schuberth, Basil Zitelli, Jeffrey Biller, Andrew Yeager, Cynthia Cole; and especially Peter Rowe and Mary Greene for advice in structuring this revision.

We also thank Vanessa Bradley, Vanassa Ross, and Michelle Carras for their support and stamina; and Clevetta Wells and Kathy Woods for administrative assistance and hand-holding. One other major change in this edition is a new and improved binding. We thank Laurel Craven and Lauranne Billus of Mosby–Year Book for their invaluable assistance and cooperation. As a result of these efforts, Mosby–Year Book has selected a binding of superb quality for this edition.

Finally, I thank my wife, Charlmain, and our families for their support, love, and patience throughout this year. After giving me 10 reasons to stop drinking milk, a wise chairman then proceeded to say that a marriage that survives a chief residency will survive anything!

Kevin B. Johnson, M.D.

CONTENTS

PART III: FORMULARY

PART I

Pediatric Acute Care

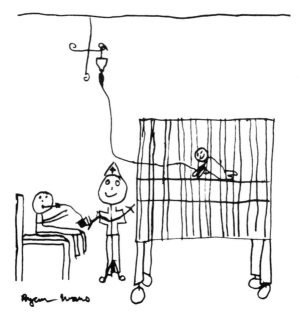

BURNS

1

I. **EPIDEMIOLOGY:** Trauma is the leading cause of death in children. In the United States, burns are the second most common cause of accidental death in children less than 5 years of age. In certain patterns of burns, child abuse must be considered.

II. **INITIAL ASSESSMENT**
A. **Vital Signs**
   1. Assess and establish adequate airway, breathing, and circulation. Intubate if necessary for pulmonary toilet, or if evidence of inhalation injury is present:

   - History of fire in enclosed space
   - Singed nares
   - Facial burns
   - Charring of lips
   - Carbonaceous secretions
   - Edema of posterior pharynx
   - Hoarseness
   - Cough
   - Wheezing

   Neuromuscular blockade with succinylcholine for intubation is contraindicated because of risk of worsening hyperkalemia. Assess and maintain an adequate core temperature; patients with extensive burns are at risk for hypothermia.

   2. Inhalation injury is present in ≈30% of victims of major burns. All patients with large burns should be assumed to have carbon monoxide poisoning until examination and evaluation of blood carboxyhemoglobin is undertaken. Humidified 100% O_2 should be administered during the initial assessment. The presence of inhalation injury increases the risk of mortality.

B. **Pulmonary Status**
   1. Monitor pulmonary status with serial ABGs.
   2. Increasing tachypnea may be seen in patients with pulmonary insufficiency caused by acute asphyxia and CO toxicity, upper airway obstruction secondary to edema, or overwhelming parenchymal damage.

    3. Delivery of 100% O_2 counteracts the effects of CO and speeds its clearance. Chest x-ray may not show changes for 24–72 hours. Carboxyhemoglobin falsely elevates oxygen saturation as determined by pulse oximetry.

C. Other Injuries: One must always remember to maintain the basic principles of any trauma evaluation. Always do a primary and secondary survey to avoid missing associated injuries. Include ECG. Electrical injuries, for example, can produce extensive deep tissue damage, intravascular thrombosis, cardiac and respiratory arrest, fractures due to muscle contractions, and cardiac arrhythmias. Motor vehicle accidents, falls, or explosions may result in associated head, visceral, or bone injuries.

D. Intravenous Access: Establish IV access and begin fluid resuscitation immediately on infants with burns greater than 10% of body surface area (BSA), children with greater than 15% BSA burned, or children with evidence of smoke inhalation. Begin with Ringer's lactate at approximately 500 m^2 of total BSA per hour (enough to maintain a urine output of 0.5–2.0 mL/kg/hr).

E. Stomach and Bladder Decompression: Insert nasogastric (NG) tube (ileus common in major burns) and Foley catheter (monitor urine output). Make NPO initially. Use sucralfate or H_2-blockers/antacids for stress ulcer prophylaxis.

F. Tetanus Toxoid: Give tetanus toxoid if last vaccine was in excess of 5 years. If patient has not received a tetanus vaccine, then administer tetanus immunoglobulin and begin a series of tetanus immunizations. See Chapter 16, Immunoprophylaxis, for details.

G. Analgesia: IV analgesia is often necessary to treat pain. Do not attribute combativeness or anxiety to pain until adequate perfusion and oxygenation are established. The use of subcutaneous (SC) or intramuscular (IM) narcotics is not recommended, because their absorption is unpredictable.

III. BURN ASSESSMENT: Calculate body surface area. See BSA nomogram in Chapter 13, Growth Charts.

A. **Burn Depth**
   1. **First degree**—Only epidermis involved, painful and erythematous.
   2. **Second degree**—Epidermis and dermis involved, but dermal appendages spared. Superficial second-degree burns are blistered and painful. Deep second-degree burns may be white and painless, may require grafting, and may progress to full-thickness burns with wound sepsis.
   3. **Third degree**—Full-thickness burns involve epidermis and all of dermis (including dermal appendages), are painless, and require grafting. **NOTE: The extent and severity of burn injury may change over the first several days after injury; therefore, be cautious in discussing prognosis with the victim's family.**

B. **Burn Assessment Chart:** Use burn assessment chart to map areas of second- and third-degree burn and to calculate the total BSA burned. Extent of tissue damage with electrical burns may not be apparent initially.
   1. The rule of nines: See Figure 1.1. Not accurate for children younger than 10 years. Modify % BSA burned using Lund-Browder chart, below.
   2. Lund-Browder chart: Use to modify % BSA estimates according to age.

Area	Age (yr)					2°	3°	Total
	0–1	1–4	4–9	10–15	Adult			
Head	19	17	13	10	—			
Neck	2	2	2	2	2			
Trunk	13	13	13	13	13			
Buttock (R/L)	2.5	2.5	2.5	2.5	2.5			
Genitalia	1	1	1	1	1			
Upper arm (R/L)	4	4	4	4	4			
Lower arm (R/L)	3	3	3	3	3			
Hand (R/L)	2.5	2.5	2.5	2.5	2.5			
Thigh (R/L)	5.5	6.5	8.5	8.5	9.5			
Leg (R/L)	5	5	5	6	7			
Foot (R/L)	3.5	3.5	3.5	3.5	3.5			

Total_____

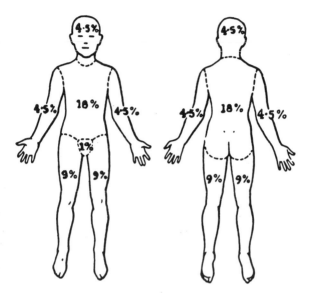

FIG 1.1.
The Rule of Nines

C. **Types of Burns**
1. **Flame:** Approximately 75% of those patients treated in a burn care facility have injuries secondary to fire. When clothing burns, the exposure to heat is prolonged and the severity of the burn is worse.
2. **Scald:** Mortality is similar to that in flame burns when total BSA involved is equal. When scald burns involve the perineum and lower portion of the body, there must be concern about child abuse.
3. **Chemical:** Tissue is damaged by protein coagulation or liquefaction rather than hyperthermic activity. The extent of injury depends on the chemical, its concentration, du-

ration of contact, penetrability into tissues, and systemic effect.

4. **Electrical:** Injury is often extensive, involving skeletal muscle and other tissues in excess to the skin damage. The tissues that have the least resistance are the most heat sensitive. Bone has the greatest resistance and nerve tissue has the least. A cardiac arrest may occur from passage of the current through the heart.

5. **Cold Injury:** Freezing results in direct tissue injury. Excision of tissue should not be done until complete demarcation of nonviable tissue has occurred.

IV. TREATMENT

A. First-Aid

If burn is < 10% of BSA, apply clean towels soaked in cold water to help prevent burn progression. If burn is greater than 10% of BSA, use clean dry towels to avoid heat loss. Do not use grease, butter, etc. In regard to chemical burns, it is important to either wash the chemical away or neutralize it. Except in rare circumstances, the most efficacious first aid treatment for chemical burns is lavaging with copious volumes of water for approximately 20 minutes.

B. Triage

1. If burn is <10% (infants) or <15% (children) and involves no full-thickness areas, may treat as outpatient.
2. Consider inpatient management for the following:
   a. More extensive burn
   b. Electrical or chemical burns (full extent of burn may not be apparent initially)
   c. Burns of critical areas such as face, hands, feet, perineum, or joint surfaces
   d. Suspected child abuse or home situation inadequate to assure good care and follow-up
   e. Child with underlying chronic illness
3. After stabilization, consider transfer to a burn center if any of the following conditions are satisfied:
   a. Burns of at least 20%–30% BSA
   b. Major burns to hand, face, joints, or perineum
   c. Electrical burns
   d. Burns with associated injuries

C. **Outpatient Management**
  1. Cleanse with warm saline or synthetic detergent removing exudate, necrotic skin, etc.
  2. Apply sulfadiazine (Silvadene) in thin layer over burn, then cover with bulky gauze dressing.
  3. Follow patient daily or every other day.
  4. Have patient cleanse burn at home twice daily with mild soap followed with sulfadiazine and sterile dressing as above. Once epithelialization is under way, may be reduced to daily dressing change.
  5. Consider tetanus immunoprophylaxis. See Chapter 16, Immunoprophylaxis, for details.

D. **Inpatient Management: Fluid Therapy: Goal** is to provide sufficient fluid to prevent shock and renal failure from excessive fluid losses and "third spacing." The two formulas listed below are only guidelines. Assess adequacy of perfusion using urine output (0.5–1.5 cc/kg/hr), BP, peripheral circulation, and sensorium. Check electrolytes and ABGs to monitor acidosis.
  1. Galveston formula
      a. Based on BSA, since weight and surface area relationships are not constant in a growing child.
      b. **First 24 hours:** Give 5000 mL/m^2 of burned area (burn losses) plus 2000 mL/m^2 of total BSA (maintenance fluids) over the first 24 hours; infuse half over the first 8 hours post burn injury. Include fluid already given enroute to referral center. For children older than 1 year, use LR + 12.5 g of 25% albumin/L. For infants younger than 1 year, prepare a 1 L solution of 930 mL of $\frac{1}{3}$ NS, 20 mL NaHCO$_3$ (1 mEq/mL) and 50 mL of 25% albumin.
      c. **Second and subsequent days:** Give 3750 mL/m^2 burned area/24 hr (burn losses) plus 1500 mL/m^2 of total BSA/24 hr (maintenance fluids). Since sodium requirements after the first 24 hours are less, use D$_5$ $\frac{1}{3}$ NS with 20–30 mEq/L of potassium phosphate (phosphate is used because of frequent hypophosphatemia).
      d. **Reevaluate fluid requirements as wounds heal.** Map wounds weekly.

2. Parkland formula

   This is a simple formula. It is useful for replacement of deficits and ongoing losses; however, it does not provide maintenance fluids.

   a. **First 24 hours:** Give Ringer's lactate 3 mL/kg/% BSA burned (if less than 30% BSA) or 4 mL/kg/% BSA burned (if greater than 30% BSA) over the first 24 hours; give half of total over the first 8 hours calculated from the time of injury. Give the remaining half over the next 16 hours.

   b. **Second 24 hours:** Fluid requirements average 50% to 75% of first day's requirement. Determine concentrations and rates by monitoring weight, serum electrolytes, urine output, NG losses, etc.

   c. **Consider adding colloid after 18–24 hours** (1g/kg/day of albumin) to maintain serum albumin greater 2 g/100 mL.

   d. **Withhold potassium generally for the first 48 hours** because of large release of potassium from damaged tissues. To most effectively manage electrolytes monitor urine electrolytes biweekly and replace urine losses accordingly.

E. **Inpatient Management: Wound Care**

   1. **Initial care:** Debridement, cleansing with mild Betadine solution, and application of silver sulfadiazine with dry dressing wrap. Escharotomies for vascular, respiratory, or joint impairments may be needed with full-thickness burns.

   2. **Daily care:** Bed bath or hydrotherapy with 1:120 or 1:240 Clorox solution, application of silver sulfadiazine and dry wrap. The active component of silver sulfadiazine is the silver ion, which binds with bacterial DNA to release the sulfonamide compound. Its major side effect is neutropenia, which is reversible. Other topical chemotherapeutic agents for burn wound care are mafenide acetate and silver nitrate.

   3. **Surveillance:** Urine, wound, and respiratory tract cultures. Quantitative wound cultures may better differentiate between infection and colonization. When the concentration of microorganisms exceeds 100,000 per gram of tissue, bacterial invasion and devitalization of tissue occurs. Prophylactic parenteral antibiotics are not recommended.

4. **"Burn Fever":** Postburn hypermetabolism represents a true resetting of central temperature control mediated by interleukins released from burned tissues. For this reason, physical findings are more reliable indicators of sepsis or wound infection than temperature alone.

5. **Debridement:** Early excision of burn wounds is the standard practice as soon as the child's medical condition is stable for surgery. Excision should be accomplished within the first 3–5 days after burn injury. When burns are extensive and an autograft is not sufficient to cover the wound initially, there are temporary biologic dressings that may be utilized. Human or porcine allografts can be used for temporary coverage. Adherence of the biological dressing ensures a favorable wound for subsequent autografting.

6. **Splinting:** Early splinting of upper and lower extremities and mobilization with range-of-motion exercise are critical to restoration of function after a major burn. Patients with severe burns are at increased risk of developing contractures. Emphasis must be placed on their prevention.

7. **With electrical burns, monitor for signs of intracranial and cardiac injuries.** Bone fractures are not infrequent. Muscle necrosis may be extensive; therefore, one must watch for early evidence of compartment syndrome. In addition, rhabdomyolysis and myoglobinuria may occur. Therefore, a brisk urine output must be initiated, often with mannitol. The urine should be alkalinized to help prevent precipitation of myoglobin within the renal tubules.

F. **Inpatient Management: Nutrition**
   1. Increase in metabolic rate may be as high as 100% in a major burn.
   2. Approximate daily caloric requirements:

Age (yr)	Caloric Requirements	Protein Requirements
<2	80 cal/kg + 30 cal/ % burn	3–6 g protein/kg/day
≥2	60 cal/kg + 30 cal/ % burn	2–8 g protein/kg/day

3. Zinc deficiency is common. Supplement feeds with iron-fortified multivitamins, zinc acetate, and ascorbic acid. Monitor weekly Ca, Phos, total protein, albumin, transferrin, cholesterol, and triglycerides as a measure of sufficient nutrition. Check weights and electrolytes daily.
4. Early introduction of enteral feeds provides nutritional support with a decreased risk of line sepsis, upper GI hemorrhage, and bacterial translocation.

G. Inpatient Management: Prognosis

1. Early and effective cardiopulmonary and fluid resuscitation, topical antimicrobial therapy, early wound excision, and adequate nutritional support have improved the LD_{50} of burn wounds from 35% to 90% BSA.
2. Early surgical consultation is recommended in the management of burned children.

V. PREVENTION: The best treatment is prevention! Measures include child-proofing the home, installing smoke detectors, turning hot water tap temperature down to 49–52° C (it takes 2 minutes of immersion at 52° C to cause a full-thickness burn, compared to 5 seconds of immersion at 60° C).

Ref: Agarwal N, Petro J, and Salisbury RE: Physiologic profile monitoring in burned patients, J. Trauma 23: 577, 1983. Aulick, L.H., Hander, E.H., Wilmore, D.W., et al.: The relative significance of thermal and metabolic demands on burn hypermetabolism, J.Trauma 19: 559, 1979. Baxter, C.R.: Present concepts in the management of major electrical injury, Surg. Clin. North Am 50: 1401, 1970. Baxter, C.R.: Fluid volume and electrolyte changes in the early postburn period, Clin. Plast. Surg. 1: 693, 1974. Jackson, B.M., and Stone, P.A.: Tangential excision and grafting of burns; the method and report of 50 consecutive cases, Br. J. Plast. Surg. 25: 416, 1972. Pruitt, B.A., Jr.: Advances in fluid therapy and the early care of the burn patient, World J. Surg. 2: 139, 1978. Wilmore, DW.: Nutrition and metabolism following thermal injury, Clin. Plast. Surg. 1: 603, 1979.

EMERGENCY MANAGEMENT 2

I. AIRWAY
A. Assessment
1. Establish airway.
2. Rule out obstruction: foreign body or anatomic obstruction.

B. Management
1. Equipment
   a. Oral airway
      1) Poorly tolerated in conscious patient.
      2) Size: with flange at teeth, tip reaches angle of jaw.
   b. Nasopharyngeal airway: relatively well tolerated in conscious patient.
      1) Rarely provokes vomiting, laryngospasm.
      2) Size: length = tip of nose to angle of jaw.
      3) Diameter: 12–36 French.
2. Intubation: Sedation and paralysis recommended unless patient is unconscious or a newborn.
   a. Equipment
      1) Endotracheal tube (ETT)
         Uncuffed ET tube in patients less than 8 years.
      2) Laryngoscope blade
         Generally, a straight blade is used <6–10 years; straight or curved blades in older patients

	ETT	Laryngoscope blade
Premie	2.5–3.0	0
Newborn	3.0–3.5	1
Infant	3.5–4.0	1
1 y/o	4.0–4.5	1 1/2
3 y/o	4.5–5.0	2
6 y/o	5.0–5.5	2
10 y/o	6.0–6.5	2
Adol	7.0–7.5	3
Adult	7.5–8.0	3

      3) Bag and mask attached to 100% oxygen

      4) ET tube stylets

      5) Suction with large bore (Yankhauer) suction catheter or 14–18 French suction catheters.

      6) Nasogastric or orogastric tube

      7) Monitoring equipment for ECG, pulse oximetry, blood pressure

   b. Procedure

      1) Preoxygenate with 100% O_2 via bag and mask

      2) Administer intubation meds (table following).

      3) Have assistant apply cricoid pressure to prevent regurgitation.

      4) With patient lying supine on a firm surface, head midline and slightly extended, open mouth with right thumb and index finger.

      5) Hold laryngoscope blade in left hand. Insert blade into right side of mouth, sweeping tongue to the left out of the line of vision.

      6) Advance blade to epiglottis. Lift laryngoscope straight up, gently raising epiglottis until cords are visible.

      7) While maintaining direct visualization, pass the ETT from the right corner of the mouth through the cords.

      8) Verify correct ETT placement by listening for breath sounds in both axillae that are equal and are louder than those heard over the stomach. Attach oxygen source and confirm position by x-ray.

C. Rapid sequence intubation
Note: Titrate drug doses to achieve desired effect.

Drug	Dose	Comments
1. Atropine	0.01–0.02 mg/kg IV min: 0.1 mg, max: 0.5 mg	Blocks vagal reflexes.
2. Pancuronium (defasciculating dose)	0.01 mg/kg IV	Not usually necessary in patients < 4 y/o. May cause complete paralysis.
3. Preoxygenate	Bag and mask, 100% O_2	
4. Thiopental or	4–6 mg/kg IV	Sedating. May cause hypotension in hemodynamically unstable patients; should be used at 25%–50% dose.
Ketamine or	1–2 mg/kg IV	Sedating. May exacerbate increased ICP. Should be used cautiously with alpha and beta blockers.
Midazolam	0.05 mg/kg IV	May cause hypotension, bradycardia.
5. Succinylcholine or	1–2 mg/kg IV	Provides muscle relaxation. Succinylcholine is contraindicated in burns, massive trauma, neuromuscular disease, and eye injuries
Pancuronium (paralyzing dose)	0.04–0.1 mg/kg IV	Provides muscle relaxation. Reverse with: atropine, neostigmine. Not possibe to reverse for 40 min after drug given.

II. BREATHING
A. Assessment: Once airway is established, evaluate air exchange. Examine for evidence of abnormal chest wall dynamics such as tension pneumothorax.

B.   **Management: Methods to Augment Ventilation (application of 100% oxygen is never contraindicated in resuscitation situations).**
1. Mouth-to-mouth, or nose-to-mouth breathing
2. Bag-mask ventilation
3. Endotracheal intubation (see above)

III.   CIRCULATION
A.   **Assessment**
1. Assess pulse (central and peripheral), capillary refill, and blood pressure.
2. Blood pressure is one of the least sensitive measures of adequate circulation in children. For normal values, refer to Cardiology, Chapter 6.

B.   **Management**
1. Chest compressions

	Location	Depth (in.)	Rate (per min)
Infants	1 finger breadth below intermammary line	0.5–1.0	100
Children	2 finger breadths above lower end of sternum	1.0–1.5	80

2. Fluid resuscitation:
   a. Intravenous or intraosseous access required. See Chapter 4, Procedures, for details.
   b. Initial fluid administered should be lactated Ringers or normal saline. Bolus with 20 ml/kg over 2–5 min. If no response, or if patient has suffered acute blood loss, consider plasma or blood, 10 ml/kg. See Chapter 10, Fluids and Electrolytes, for further resuscitation guidelines.
3. Drugs: See front cover for arrest drug guidelines.
   Note: Consider early administration of antibiotics/corticosteriods if clinically indicated.
   Ref: CPR Issue, JAMA 1992; 268(16):2131–2334.

IV. RESPIRATORY EMERGENCIES
A. Asthma
1. Initial Management:
   a. Give inhaled beta agonist with O_2; repeat every 20 minutes. See Formulary for dosing details.

	Onset Peak (min)	Duration (hr)
Albuterol	15–30	4–6
Terbutaline	30	3–4
Metaproterenol	30–60	4–6

   b. If inhaled beta agonists are not tolerated, consider parenteral terbutaline. Nebulized inhalation is usually more effective.
   c. Monitor HR, BP, O_2 saturation.
2. Further Management:
   a. Continue nebulization therapy every 20–30 min.
   b. Consider steroids: Equivalent of 2 mg/kg prednisone.
   c. Consider inhaled anticholinergics with O_2:
      1) Atropine sulfate
      2) Ipratropium
      Note: Safety and efficacy of ipratropium in children less than 12 years old have not been established.
   d. Consider theophylline in the following patients:
      1) Theophylline-dependent patients (check theophylline level, noting time of most recent dose).
      2) Severe obstructive disease unresponsive to adrenergic agents.
B. Upper Airway Obstruction: Most commonly caused by foreign body aspiration or infection.
1. **Croup**
   a. Ensure adequate airway.
   b. Differentiate from epiglottis.
   c. Offer humidified air via face mask or via oxygen tubing held near child's face.
   d. Consider racemic epinephrine.
   e. Consider dexamethasone. See Formulary for dosing information. Useful in children who have persistence of symptoms after mist therapy and in children who may need admission.

    f. If child fails to respond adequately to the above therapy, urgent evaluation by otolaryngology and anesthesia is necessary. (See epiglottitis protocol, below).

2. **Epiglottitis:** Epiglottitis is a true emergency requiring immediate intubation. Any manipulation, including aggressive physical exam, attempt to visualize the epiglottis, venipuncture, or IV placement may precipitate complete obstruction. If epiglottitis is suspected, definitive airway placement should precede all diagnostic procedures. A prototypic "epiglottitis protocol" may include:

    a. Unobtrusively give O_2 (blow-by). Make NPO.

    b. Have parent accompany child to allay anxiety.

    c. Have physician accompany patient at all times.

    d. Summon predetermined "epiglottitis team": Most senior pediatrician, anesthesiologist, and otorhinolaryngologist in hospital.

    e. Unless emergency intubation is indicated, escort patient with team to OR where intubation done under anesthesia (using O_2 and inhaled halothane alone).

    f. Place intravenous catheter in OR before induction of anesthesia, with patient fully monitored and ENT standing by with tracheostomy set ready.

    g. After airway is secured, draw cultures and administer IV antibiotics and fluids.

3. **Foreign Body Aspiration**

    a. Occurs most often in children <5 years old. Involves small toys, objects, or foods such as peanuts, hard candies, nuts, and hot dogs.

    b. If patient is stable (e.g., forcefully coughing, well oxygenated), removal of the foreign body by bronchoscopy or laryngoscopy should be attempted in a controlled environment.

    c. If patient is unable to speak, moves air poorly, or is cyanotic, intervene immediately:

        1) Infant: Straddle infant over arm or rest on lap. Give four back blows between the scapulae. If unsuccessful, turn infant over and give four chest thrusts (in same location as external chest compressions)

        2) Child: Perform four abdominal thrusts (Heimlich maneuver) from behind a sitting or standing child,

      or straddled over a child lying supine. Direct thrusts upward in the midline and not to either side of abdomen.

  d. If back, chest, and/or abdominal thrusts have failed, open mouth and remove foreign body if visualized. Blind finger sweeps are not recommended. Magill forceps may allow removal of foreign bodies in the posterior pharynx.

  e. If the patient is unconscious, give 100% O_2 by face mask. Remove foreign body by direct visualization (use Magill forceps, if necessary), or laryngoscopy. If mask bagging and laryngoscopy are unsuccessful, consider an emergent cricothyrotomy.

V. CARDIOVASCULAR EMERGENCIES

A. **Tachyarrhythmias:** See Table 2.1

B. **Bradyarrhythmias:** See Table 2.2

TABLE 2.1.   Tachyarrhythmias

	Initial Therapy	Secondary Therapy	Remarks
Supraventricular tachycardia	Vagotonic maneuvers (e.g., diving reflex [ice to face], Valsalva, carotid massage)	Adenosine: 0.1 mg/kg IV push. If no effect, double dose. Maximum single dose = 12 mg. Digoxin (see Formulary) Synchronous cardioversion 0.25–1.0 joules/kg Atrial esophageal overdrive pacing	Do not delay cardioversion to establish IV access for adenosine in an unstable patient. Avoid verapamil in infants
Atrial flutter	Atrial esophageal overdrive pacing Synchronous cardioversion 0.25–1.0 joules/kg Digoxin (see Formulary)	Quinidine— see Formulary	
Premature ventricular contractions	Observe in most cases Lidocaine 1 mg/kg IV bolus, then 20–50 mcg/kg/min	Procainamide or Quinidine— see Formulary	Treat asymptomatic patients only in specific situations (e.g. immediately post-op or with myocarditis)
Ventricular tachycardia Hemodynamically stable	Lidocaine: 1 mg/kg bolus IV, then 20–50 mcg/kg/min	Bretylium: 5 mg/kg rapid IV infusion	
Hemodynamically unstable	Synchronous cardioversion: 1–2 joules/kg Treat underlying illness	Lidocaine: 1 mg/kg bolus IV	
Ventricular fibrillation or pulseless ventricular tachycardia	Defibrillation: 2.0 joules/kg; double and repeat × 2 if necessary	Lidocaine: 1 mg/kg bolus IV	

TABLE 2.2.
Bradyarrhythmias

	Initial Therapy	Secondary Therapy	Remarks
Complete heart block			
Congenital	Observe	Atropine: 0.01–0.02 mg/kg; max = 1 mg Isoproterenol: 0.1–0.3 mcg/kg/min Transvenous ventricular pacing	
Acquired, nonsurgical	Observe	Atropine: 0.01–0.02 mg/kg; max = 1 mg Isoproterenol: 0.1–0.3 mcg/kg/min Transvenous ventricular pacing	
Acquired, surgical	Observe	Transvenous ventricular pacing	

(Continued.)

TABLE 2.2 (cont.).

	Initial Therapy	Secondary Therapy	Remarks
Sinus bradycardia	Treat underlying condition (e.g. hypoxemia, hypercapnea, acidosis, increased ICP) Epinephrine: 0.01 mg/kg bolus IV/IO or 0.1 mg/kg per ETT (0.2 mg/kg per ETT may be effective); repeat every 3–5 minutes at the same dose. Atropine: 0.02 mg/kg IV bolus. Minimum dose: 0.1 mg. Maximum single dose: 0.5 mg for child; 1.0 mg for adolescent	Pacemaker	Treatment usually indicated only in symptomatic patients. Prognosis is influenced by underlying etiology.
Sick sinus syndrome	Observe	Pacemaker	
Asystole	CPR. **See inside front cover.**		

C. Hypertensive Crisis
1. **Assessment**
    a. Width of bladder on blood pressure cuff should be at least ⅔ the length of the upper arm.
    b. Evaluate for underlying etiology: iatrogenic, cardiovascular, renovascular, renal parenchymal, endocrine, CNS. Rule out hypertension secondary to increased ICP prior to lowering pressure.
    c. Diagnostic evaluation should include urinalysis, BUN, creatinine, chest x-ray and ECG. Consider obtaining renin level before starting chronic anti-hypertensive therapy.
    d. Patients with blood pressure greater than 95th percentile require further evaluation. Patients with evidence of target organ damage or blood pressure significantly above the 95th percentile require immediate monitoring and treatment.
    e. Secure IV access before beginning therapy.
2. **Management**
    a. Blood pressure should not be decreased by greater than one third of the total goal over the first 4–6 hrs.
    b. Patients with underlying chronic hypertension may have a shifted autoregulatory curve and may require increased blood pressures to maintain normal cerebral perfusion. Therefore, elevated pressures should be lowered more slowly in these patients.
3. Drugs: For dosages, see Formulary (Chapter 25).

Drug	Onset	Duration	Comments
Diazoxide (arteriole vasodilator)	1–5 min	Variable, 2–12h	May be given in ER setting.
Labetalol (alpha, beta blocker)	1–5 min	Variable, about 6h	May require ICU setting. Contraindicated in asthmatics.
Hydralazine (arteriolar vasodilator)	10–20 min	3–6h	
Nifedipine (Ca^{++} channel blocker)	10–15 min	2–3h	May cause headache.
Minoxidil (vasodilator)	1h	8h	May require diuretic.
Nitroprusside (arteriolar and venous vasodilator)	<30 sec	Very short	Requires ICU setting. Allows tight control.

D. Hyperkalemia
1. Assessment
   a. For differential diagnosis, see Fluid and Electrolytes, Chapter 10.
   b. Symptoms: Weakness, parasthesias, tetany.
   c. Progression of ECG changes: T-wave elevation, loss of P wave, widening QRS, S-T depression, further widened QRS, bradycardia, sine-wave QRS-T, 1st degree AV block, ventricular arrhythmia, cardiac arrest.
2. Treatment
   a. Calcium gluconate (10%): 0.2–0.5 mL/kg over 2–5 minutes to correct cardiac defects. Effective for up to 1h.
   b. $NaHCO_3$: 1–3 mEq/kg over 3–5 min (lasts several hours).
   Note: Ca gluconate solution is not compatible with $NaHCO_3$. Flush line between infusions.
   c. Glucose: 0.5 gm/kg with 0.3 units insulin/gm glucose over 2 hr.
   d. Kayexalate (sodium polystyrene resin) 1–2 gm/kg with 3cc sorbitol/gm resin divided q6h PO or with 5cc sorbitol/gm resin as retention enema over 4–6 h. 1 gm/kg of Kayexalate should lower K by 1 mEq/L.
   e. Proceed to dialysis if above measures are unsuccessful.

VI. ENDOCRINE EMERGENCIES
A. Adrenal Crisis
1. Assessment: Characterized by hypoglycemia, hyponatremia, hyperkalemia, metabolic acidosis, and shock.
2. Management
   a. Give D_5 NS to support blood pressure and blood glucose.
   b. Give 4 times the daily maintenance dose of hydrocortisone as IV bolus (4×12.5 mg/M^2). Then give hydrocortisone, 50–100 mg/M^2/24h as a continuous drip or divided q 4–6h. Only hydrocortisone and cortisone have the necessary mineralocorticoid effects. See Special Drug Topics (Chapter 26) for details on steroid replacement therapy.

B. Diabetic Ketoacidosis
1. Assessment: Determine, in known diabetic: usual insulin regimen, last insulin dose, and history of infection or other inciting event.
2. Initial Management
   a. Fluids: Assume 10%–15% dehydration. Give 10–20 cc/kg NS or RL over 1 hr, then start 0.45 NS as follows:
      1) First 8h: Replace ½ the remaining deficit plus insensible losses (40% of maintenance fluids for 8h) plus urine output.
      2) Next 16–24h: Replace remainder of deficit plus maintenance requirements (as hyperglycemia is corrected, urinary losses become minimal).
   b. Insulin:
      1) Insulin drip is preferred over IM or SC injections.
      2) Give 0.1 U/kg regular insulin IV bolus, then 0.1 U/kg/hr regular insulin as continuous drip.
   c. Glucose:
      1) Measure hourly. Rate of glucose fall should not exceed 80–100 mg/dl/hr.
      See note on p. 26.
      2) Increase insulin to 0.14–0.2 U/kg if glucose falls at less than 50 mg/dl/hr. If glucose falls faster than 100 mg/dl/hr, continue insulin infusion (0.1 U/kg/hr) and add D_5W to IV. As glucose approaches 250–300 mg/dl, add D_5W to IV.
   d. Electrolytes:
      1) Potassium: Patients with DKA are potassium depleted. Give maintenance plus deficit over 24h (see Fluid and Electrolytes, Ch. 18). Give no K^+ initially if K^+ is elevated or if patient is not urinating.
      2) Phosphate: Depleted in DKA and will drop further with insulin therapy. PO_4 improves release of oxygen to tissues. Consider replacing K^+ as ½ KCl and ½ KPO_4 for the first 8h, then all as KCl. Excessive PO_4 may induce hypocalcemic tetany.

        3) Bicarbonate: Use of bicarbonate is controversial. Consider in cases with initial pH less than 7.10.

    e. Assessment:

        1) Follow vital signs, dextrostics q1–2h; glucose, pH, pCO_2, electrolytes q3–4h, EKG periodically to follow K^+.

3. Further Management

    a. When blood pH greater than 7.3, ketosis is resolved, HCO_3 greater than 15 mEq/L and enteral nutrition is tolerated, discontinue insulin drip and start subcutaneous insulin.

    b. For previously diagnosed diabetics, begin their usual insulin regimen.

    c. For newly diagnosed diabetics:

        1) For the first 24h after insulin drip is discontinued, give 0.1–0.25 units regular insulin/kg SC q6–8h.

        2) The next 24h, give ⅔ of the previous day's total insulin dose as an intermediate acting form (NPH, Lente); give ⅔ before breakfast and ⅓ before dinner. If needed, give additional regular insulin 0.1 U/kg before each meal.

    d. Usual daily maintenance dose in children: 0.5–1.0 U/kg/24h. In adolescents during growth spurt: 0.8–1.2 U/kg/24h.

    Note: Rapid correction of hyperglycemia may lead to the development of cerebral edema. Actual fluid and electrolyte requirements of patients in DKA may vary according to their clinical and nutritional status. Follow physical examination and laboratory data closely.

Ref: Krane E. Pediatr Clin North Am 1987; 34:933–960. Sperling, M. in Clinical Pediatric Endocrinology, S. Kaplan (ed), Philadelphia, W.B. Saunders, 1990:137–142.

VII. NEUROLOGIC EMERGENCIES

A. **Increased Intracranial Pressure/Coma:** Also see Neurology (Chapter 21) for evaluation and management of hydrocephalus and ventricular shunts.

    1. Assessment

      a. Establish history of trauma, toxin exposure, infection, diabetes, seizure or other neurologic disorder, or other potential etiology.

  b. Obtain laboratory evaluations, including toxicology screen and serum osmolality.
  c. Determine if patient needs immediate surgical (e.g., intracranial mass or bleed) or medical (e.g., hypoglycemia, narcotic overdose, electrolye disturbance, etc.) management.
  d. Increased intracranial pressure may be heralded by headache, nausea, vomiting, altered mental status (including irritability), Cushing's response (abnormal respiratory pattern, hypertension, bradycardia), abnormal posturing or extraocular movements (especially paralysis of upward gaze or abduction), bulging fontanelle, dilated unresponsive pupils. Papilledema is a late finding.
2. Initial Management
  a. See A B C section.
  b. If evidence of increased intracranial pressure exists:
    1) After cervical spine is cleared, place head in midline and elevate 20–30 degrees to maximize venous drainage.
    2) Intubate and hyperventilate to maintain pCO_2 between 20–25 mm Hg. Rapid sequence intubation is recommended. Thiopental is sedating drug of choice. Avoid ketamine.
    3) Give mannitol, 0.5–1 gm/kg over 2 minutes and furosemide, 1 mg/kg/dose IV.
    4) Restrict fluids if patient is not hypovolemic.
    5) Obtain emergent neurosurgical consultation. If patient is stable, obtain head CT.

c. Monitor Glasgow Coma Scale:

Glasgow Coma Scale		Modified Coma Scale for Infants	
Activity	Best Response	Activity	Best Response
Eye Opening			
Spontaneous	4	Spontaneous	4
To speech	3	To speech	3
To pain	2	To pain	2
None	1	None	1
Verbal			
Oriented	5	Coos, babbles	5
Confused	4	Irritable	4
Inappropriate words	3	Cries to pain	3
Nonspecific sounds	2	Moans to pain	2
None	1	None	1
Motor			
Follows commands	6	Normal spontaneous movements	6
Localizes pain	5	Withdraws to touch	5
Withdraws to pain	4	Withdraws to pain	4
Abnormal flexion	3	Abnormal flexion	3
Abnormal extension	2	Abnormal extension	2
None	1	None	1

Ref: Jennet B, Teasdale G. Lancet 1977;1:878, and James HE. Pediatr Ann 1986;15:16.

B. Status Epilepticus

See Neurology (Chapter 21) for non-acute evaluation and management of seizures.

1. Assessment:

Common causes of childhood seizures include: fever, infections, head trauma, metabolic abnormalities, toxic ingestions, withdrawal of anticonvulsant medications.

2. Management:

a. See A B C section.

b. Anticonvulsant therapy—doses are in Formulary (Chapter 14). Note that lorazepam and diazepam may be given rectally.

1) Lorazepam or diazepam

2) Phenytoin

3) Consider intubation

4) Phenobarbital

5) **If the above management fails, consider general anesthesia with neuromuscular blockade or barbiturate coma with EEG monitoring.**

POISONINGS 3

I. SIGNS AND SYMPTOMS OF POISONING
A. Vital Signs
1. **Pulse**
   a. Bradycardia: Gasoline, digoxin, narcotics, organo-phosphates, cyanide, carbon monoxide, plants (lily of the valley, foxglove, oleander), clonidine, beta-blockers
   b. Tachycardia: Alcohol, amphetamines and sympatho-mimetics, atropinics, tricyclic antidepressants, the-ophylline, salicylates, phencyclidine, cocaine
2. **Respirations**
   a. Slow, depressed: Alcohol, barbiturates (late), narcot-ics, clonidine, sedative/hypnotics
   b. Tachypnea: Amphetamines, barbiturates (early), methanol, salicylates, carbon monoxide
3. **Blood pressure**
   a. Hypotension: Methemoglobinemia (nitrates, nitrites, phenacetin), cyanide, carbon monoxide, phenothi-azines, tricyclic antidepressants, barbiturates, iron, theophylline, clonidine, narcotics
   b. Hypertension: Amphetamines/sympathomimetics, (es-pecially phenylpropanolamine in over-the-counter [OTC] cold remedies, diet pills), tricyclic antidepres-sants, phencyclidine, phenothiazines, antihistamines, atropinics, clonidine
4. **Temperature**
   a. Hypothermia: Ethanol, barbiturates, sedative/hypnot-ics, narcotics, phenothiazines, antidepressants, cloni-dine, carbon monoxide
   b. Hyperpyrexia: Atropinics, quinine, salicylates, am-phetamines, phenothiazines, tricyclic antidepressants, theophylline, cocaine

B. Neuromuscular
1. **Coma:** Narcotic depressants, sedative/hypnotics, anti-cholinergics (antihistamines, antidepressants, phenothi-

azines, atropinics, OTC sleep preparations), alcohols, anticonvulsants, carbon monoxide, salicylates, organophosphate insecticides, clonidine

2. **Delirium/Psychosis:** Alcohol, phenothiazines, drugs of abuse (phencyclidine, LSD, peyote, mescaline, marijuana, cocaine, heroin, methaqualone), sympathomimetics and anticholinergics (including prescription and OTC cold remedies), steroids, heavy metals

3. **Convulsions:** Alcohol, amphetamines, cocaine, phenothiazines, antidepressants, antihistamines, camphor, boric acid, lead, organophosphates, isoniazid, salicylates, plants (water hemlock), lindane, lidocaine, phencyclidine

4. **Ataxia:** Alcohol, barbiturates, carbon monoxide, diphenylhydantoin, heavy metals, organic solvents, sedative/hynotics, hydrocarbons

5. **Paralysis:** Botulism, heavy metals, plants (poison hemlock)

C. **Eyes**
   1. **Pupils**
      a. Miosis (constricted pupils): Narcotics, organophosphates, plants (mushrooms of the muscarinic type), ethanol, barbiturates, phenobarbital, phencyclidine, clonidine
      b. Mydriasis (dilated pupils): Amphetamines, atropinics, barbiturates (if comatose), cocaine, methanol, glutethamide, LSD, marijuana, phencyclidine
   2. **Nystagmus:** Diphenylhydantoin, sedative/hypnotics, carbamazepine, glutethamide, phencyclidine (both vertical and horizontal), barbiturates, ethanol

D. **Skin**
   1. **Jaundice:** Carbon tetrachloride, acetaminophen, napthalene, phenothiazines, plants (mushrooms, fava beans), heavy metals (iron, phosphorus, arsenic)
   2. **Cyanosis** (unresponsive to oxygen, as a result of methemoglobinemia): Aniline dyes, nitrites, benzocaine, phenacetin, nitrobenzene, phenazopyridine
   3. **Pinkness to redness:** Atropinics and antihistamines, alcohol, carbon monoxide, cyanide, boric acid
   4. **Dry:** Anticholinergics

E. **Odors**
1. **Acetone:** Acetone, methyl and isopropyl alcohol, phenol and salicylates
2. **Alcohol:** Ethanol
3. **Bitter almond:** Cyanide
4. **Garlic:** Heavy metal (arsenic, phosphorus, and thallium), organophosphates
5. **Oil of wintergreen:** Methyl salicylates
6. **Hydrocarbons:** Hydrocarbons (gasoline, turpentine, etc.)

II. GASTROINTESTINAL DECONTAMINATION
A. **Activated Charcoal:** Activated charcoal is the treatment of choice for gastrointestinal decontamination in the emergency department. Studies in animals, volunteers, and patients with overdoses fail to show a benefit of treatment with ipecac or lavage plus activated charcoal over treatment with charcoal administered without ipecac or lavage.
1. **Mechanism of action:** Effectively adsorbs and prevents systemic absorption of toxins.
2. **Initial dose**
    a. Small children: 15–30 g activated charcoal PO or NG in 70% sorbitol solution.
    b. Children > 12 years old: 50–60 g PO or NG in 70% sorbitol.
    (1 g/kg body weight in a well-mixed slurry diluted at least 1:4.)
    Note: If a patient is obtunded and/or presents within 1 hour of a significant ingestion, orogastric lavage followed by activated charcoal via OG tube may be indicated.
3. **Contraindications:** Ileus, hydrocarbons,* alcohols,* iron,* boric acid, cyanide, caustics.
4. **Serial activated charcoal**
    a. Consider multiple-dose charcoal regimen (alternating with and without cathartic) for severe intoxication with theophylline, phenobarbital, tricyclic antidepressants, digoxin, or tegretol.

    *Activated charcoal is ineffective with these ingested compounds.

b. Give half the initial dose every 4 hours. End point is nontoxic blood levels or lack of signs/symptoms of clinical toxicity after 12–24 hours. Check for bowel sounds and abdominal distention, and watch for hypernatremia.

B. Cathartics
1. Recommended in conjunction with activated charcoal therapy. Give sorbitol administered as 70% solution with appropriate dose of charcoal (preferred) or magnesium citrate 4 mL/kg (**maximum dose** of 200 mL in adults).
2. **Contraindications:** Caustic ingestions, absent bowel sounds, recent bowel surgery. Avoid magnesium-containing cathartics in patients with compromised renal function.

Ref: Rogers GC, et al. Ped Clin North Am 1986, 33:261. Ellenhorn MJ, Barceloux DG, Medical Toxicolgy. New York: Elsevier, 1988.

C. Emesis
1. **Indications and contraindications:** Ipecac remains the drug of choice for home GI decontamination, or for use in children brought to the ER within 1 hour of an ingestion.
   a. Contraindications: Decreased or fluctuating level of consciousness, tricyclic antidepressant ingestions, caustic ingestions, hematemesis, and seizures.
   b. Relative contraindications: <6 months old, severe cardiorespiratory disease, late stage pregnancy, uncontrolled hypertension, bleeding diathesis, and most hydrocarbons.
2. Syrup of ipecac dosages
   a. 6–12 months old: 10 mL with 15 mL clear fluid/kg.
   b. 1–12 years old: 15–30 mL with 240 mL clear fluid.
   c. >12 years old: 30–60 mL with 240–480 mL clear fluid.
   Note: If no emesis occurs in 20 minutes, repeat dose only once and give more fluids.

D. Gastric Lavage
1. **Indications:** Orogastric lavage with a large-bore tube may still be useful in patients who arrive soon after (within 1 hour of) a life-threatening ingestion and/or are ob-

tunded. The decision whether or not to lavage should be made in consultation with a poison control center.

2. **Contraindications:** Caustic or hydrocarbon ingestions, coingestion of sharp objects.

3. **Airway protection:** Insertion and inflation of a cuffed endotracheal tube prior to gastric lavage protects against aspiration of gastric contents, especially in the patient with altered mental status or a depressed gag reflex. **Caution: Aspiration of charcoal/cathartic may cause severe and potentially fatal pneumonitis!**

4. **Method**
   a. Position patient on left side, with the head slightly lower than the body. Insert large-bore orogastric tube.
   b. Lavage with 0.9% normal saline, 15 mL/kg/cycle, to maximum of 200–400 mL/cycle in adults, until gastric contents are clear. This may require several liters. Save initial pass for toxicologic examination. Add activated charcoal to lavage solution to increase amount of poison removed.

III. ANTIDOTES: See table on pp. 34–35.
Note: The table on pp. 34–35 does not include indications or contraindications. Use of these antidotes may prove harmful and should not be initiated without consultation with an AAPCC-certified poison center.

IV. ENHANCED ELIMINATION: Good hydration is recommended in virtually all cases. Use isotonic fluids.
A. Forced Diuresis and pH Alteration
   1. Drugs considered for this method must have low protein binding, limited metabolism, high renal clearance, and primarily extracellular fluid distribution.
   2. May be effective in salicylate or phenobarbital overdoses.
B. Hemodialysis
   1. **Indications:** Indicated in severe ingestions of dialyzable substances (i.e., low volume of distribution, low molecular weight, decreased binding to plasma proteins) that are unresponsive to standard care.

Antidotes

Toxin	Antidote	Comments
Acetaminophen	N-acetylcystiene	See section VI. A.
Anticholinergic agents	Physostigmine	1–2 mg IV over 5 min. **Use only for severe delirium. May be useful to treat seizures or tachydysrhythmias, but strong clinical evidence is lacking.**
Benzodiazepines	Flumazenil	0.2 mg over 30 seconds. If there is no response after 30 seconds, give 0.3 mg over 30 seconds. If there is no response after 30 seconds, give 0.5 mg over 30 seconds at 1-minute intervals up to a total dose of 3 mg. **Should not be given if the patient shows signs of serious overdose from coingestion of tricyclic antidepressants or was taking benzodiazepines for control of seizures. May cause seizures in some patients.**
Beta-blockers	Glucagon	Starting dose 5–10 mg IV. Titrate to response (normalization of vital signs). Maintenance dose of 2–10 mg/hr per hour may be used.
Calcium-channel blockers, hydrofluoric acid, fluorides	Calcium	1 g calcium chloride given over 5 minutes by IV infusion with continuous cardiac monitoring. **May be repeated often in life-threatening situations, but the serum calcium level should be monitored after the third dose.**
Digitalis, glycosides	Digoxin-specific antibody fragments (Digibind)	Equimolar to ingestion: the number of milligrams of digoxin ingested divided by 0.6 is the number of vials required. See formulary (Chapter 25) for details.

Iron	Defuroxamine mesylate	Give in gram-per-gram equivalent doses to what was ingested. If amount ingested is unknown, start with 5 g IV. An overdose of pyridoxine may cause neuropathy.
Isoniazid, hydrazine, monomethylhydrazine (in *gyromitra* species mushrooms)	Pyridoxine (vitamin B$_6$)	
Methanol, ethylene glycol	Ethanol	Loading dose 10 mL of 10% solution/kg/body weight. Maintenance dose 0.15 mL/kg/hr. Double maintenance dose should be used during dialysis. Titrate to a blood ethanol level of 22 mmol/L (100 mg/dL).
Opiates	Naloxone	Starting dose 2 mg. More may be needed for overdoses of some synthetic narcotics; less may be used in addicts to avoid precipitating withdrawal symptoms
Organophosphate or carbamate insecticides	Atropine	Test dose 2 mg IV. Repeat in larger increments until drying of oropharyngeal secretions occurs.
Tricyclic antidepressants	Bicarbonate	1 to 2 mmol/kg IV for substantial cardiac conduction delay or ventricular dysrhythmias. Titrate to response and arterial pH.

2. **Dialyzable poisons (partial list)**

- Ammonia
- Amphetamines
- Anilines
- Antibiotics
- Barbiturates (long acting)
- Boric Acid
- Bromides
- Calcium
- Chloral Hydrate
- Ethylene Glycol
- Fluorides

- Iodides
- Isoniazid
- Meprobamate
- Methanol
- Paraldehyde
- Potassium
- Quinidine
- Quinine
- Salicylates
- Strychnine
- Thiocyanates

Ref: Arena JM, Poisoning. Springfield: Charles C Thomas, 1985. Gellis SS, Kagan BM, Current Pediatric Therapy. Philadelphia: WB Saunders, 1986.

C. **Hemoperfusion**

1. To initiate, must weigh benefits of accelerated toxin clearance against risks of anticoagulation and mechanical problems.
2. Useful with short-acting barbiturates, nonbarbiturate sedative-hypnotics, theophylline, disopyramide, salicylates, phenytoin, and chloramphenicol.

Ref: Peterson RG, Peterson LG, Ped Clin North Amer 1986,33:675–689. Mauer SM, et al., J Peds 1980, 136–139.

D. **Serial Activated Charcoal**

See Activated Charcoal, section II.A.

V. **TOXIC SYNDROMES:** (See table on pp. 37–39.)

VI. **SPECIFIC POISONINGS**

A. **Acetaminophen Poisoning**

1. **Symptoms:** Nausea, vomiting, and malaise for 24 hours, improvement over the next 48 hours, followed by clinical or laboratory evidence of hepatic dysfunction. Death can occur due to fulminant hepatic failure.
2. **Hepatic toxicity:** Likelihood of hepatic toxicity related to:
   a. Dose: 140 mg/kg is considered toxic.
   b. Plasma level: Draw level at 4 hours postingestion and plot on nomogram (see Fig 3–1).

Toxic Syndromes

Syndrome	Manifestations	Examples
Anticholinergic	**Parasympatholytic:** Dry skin/mucous membranes, thirst/dysphagia, blurred vision, (near objects), fixed dilated pupils, tachycardia, hypertension, flushing, scarlatiniform rash, hyperthermia, abdominal distention, urinary urgency and retention	Belladonna alkaloids, atropine, scopolamine
	Central: Lethargy, confusion, delirium, hallucinations, delusions, ataxia, respiratory failure, cardiovascular collapse, extrapyramidal movements	Synthetic: Glycopyrrolate Other: Antihistamines, tricyclic antidepressants
Anticholinesterase	**Muscarinic:** Sweating, constricted pupils, lacrimation, wheezing, cramps, vomiting, diarrhea, tenesmus, bradycardia, hypotension, blurred vision, urinary incontinence, excessive salivation	Organophosphates, carbamate insecticides
	Nicotinic: Striated muscle: fasciculations, cramps, weakness, twitching, paralysis, respiratory compromise, cyanosis, cardiac arrest	
	Sympathetic ganglia: Tachycardia, hypertension	
	Central: Anxiety, restlessness, ataxia, convulsions, insomnia, coma, absent reflexes, Cheyne-Stokes breathing, respiratory/circulatory depression	
Cholinergic	See anticholinesterases: Nicotinic and Muscarinic	Acetylcholine, betel nut, bethanecol, muscarine, pilocarpine

(Continued.)

Toxic Syndromes (cont.).

Syndrome	Manifestations	Examples
Extrapyramidal	**Parkinsonian:** Dysphonia, dysphagia, oculogyric crisis, rigidity, tremor, torticollis, opisthotonos, shrieking, trismus	Chlorpromazine, haloperidol, perphenazine, promazine, thioridazine, trifluoperazine
Hemoglobinopathy	Disorientation, headache, coma, dyspnea, cyanosis, cutaneous bullae, gastroenteritis	Carboxyhemoglobin (carbon monoxide), methemoglobin, sulfhemoglobin
Metal Fume Fever	Chills, fever, nausea, vomiting, muscular pain, throat dryness, headache, fatigue, weakness, leukocytosis, respiratory distress	Fumes of oxides: brass, cadmium, copper, iron, magnesium, mercury, nickel, titanium, tungsten, and zinc
Narcotic	CNS depression, pinpoint pupils, slowed respirations, hypotension. Response to naloxone: pupils may dilate and excitement may predominate.	Codeine diphenoxylate (Lomotil), fentanyl, heroin, morphine, opium, oxycodone
Sympathomimetic	CNS excitation, convulsions, hypertension, tachycardia	Aminophylline, amphetamines, caffeine, cocaine, dopamine, ephedrine, epinephrine, fenfluramine, levarterenol, methylphenidate, pemoline, phencyclidine
Narcotic withdrawal	Diarrhea, mydriasis, goose bumps, hypertension, tachycardia, insomnia, lacrimation, muscle cramps, restlessness, yawning, hallucinosis	Cessation of: alcohol, barbiturates, benzodiazepines, chloral hydrate, glutethimide, meprobamate, methaqualone, narcotics, opioids, paraldehyde

Ref: Adapted from Done AK: Poisoning–A Systematic Approach for the Emergency Department Physician in *Emergency Medicine*, Tintinhalli et. al. eds., McGraw-Hill 1985.

c. Delay in treatment: *N*-acetylcysteine (NAC) is most effective if administered within 10 hours of ingestion. Efficacy is lower between 10–16 hours postingestion. Few deaths have been reported when NAC is used within 24 hours.

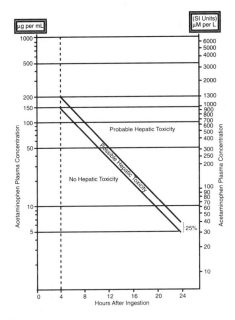

FIG 3.1.
Semilogarithmic plot of plasma acetaminophen levels vs. time, for use following single ingestions of acetaminophen.

Ref: Adapted from Pediatrics 1975, 55:871–6 and Micromedex, Inc. with permission.

3. Therapy
   a. Treatment in <1 hour of ingestion: Lavage or give ipecac; after emesis give charcoal; draw plasma level at 4 hours.

    b. Treatment 1–4 hours after ingestion: Give charcoal and draw acetaminophen level at 4 hours.

    c. Treatment in >4 hours after ingestion: Draw level and treat with NAC orally or IV if level is in toxic range. **Note: Charcoal adsorbs oral NAC; avoid simultaneous administration.**

      1) Oral NAC regimen (PO or NG): Give 20% NAC diluted 1:4 in a carbonated beverage as a loading dose of 140 mg/kg, then 70 mg/kg q4h for 17 doses.

      2) IV NAC regimen (approved in Canada and UK, but not by USFDA; to use IV NAC in US, contact local Poison Center): Indicated when patient is unable to take PO or requires repeated charcoal. Use 20% NAC solution: Give 150 mg/kg in 200 mL of D_5W over 15 minutes. Then 50 mg/kg in 500 mL of D_5W over 4 hours. Then 100 mg/kg in 1000 mL of D_5W over next 16 hours. Check plasma level at 24 hours. Small risk of anaphylaxis with IV NAC. **Note: Do not use oral preparation of NAC IV.**

      Ref: Rumack, BH. Ped Clin North Am 1986,33:691–701, Tenenbein M, Curr Probl Pediatr 1986, 16:185–233, Prescott LF, Drugs 1983, 25:290–314, Peterson RG, Personal Communication, 1988.

B. Anticholinergic Toxicity

  1. **Agents:** Tricyclics, antihistamines, antiparkinsonians, scopolamine, belladonna, plants (jimson weed, nightshade, mushrooms, Jerusalem cherries), ophthalmic mydriatics, atropine, phenothiazines.

  2. **Symptoms:** "Mad as a hatter, red as a beet, blind as a bat, hot as a hare, dry as a bone": oral dryness and burning, speech and swallowing difficulties, thirst, blurred vision, photophobia, mydriasis, skin flushing, tachycardia, fever, urinary urgency, delirium, hallucinations, cardiovascular collapse.

  3. **Treatment**

    a. Activated charcoal and cathartic as above.

    b. Observation is all that is necessary in mild cases.

    c. In life-threatening emergencies (arrhythmias, hypertension, myoclonic seizures, severe hallucinations), physostigmine will reverse symptoms.

Note: Neostigmine and pyridostigmine will not affect the CNS symptoms. Do not use physostigmine simply to maintain an alert state in an otherwise stable patient in coma.

1) Dose: In children <5 years, give physostigmine 0.5 mg IV every 5 minutes until a therapeutic effect is seen or until a **total dose** of 2.0 mg is achieved. In those >5 years, give 1–2 mg IV. Repeat in 10 minutes if ineffective. **Maximum dose:** 4 mg in 30 minutes.

2) Rate: Infuse at 1 mg/min. Faster rates can cause seizures or precipitate a cholinergic crisis. Effective within 3–5 minutes.

3) Reversal: Atropine should be available to reverse excess cholinergic side effects. Give 0.5 mg for each 1 mg of physostigmine just given.

Ref: Rumack BH. Pediatrics 1973, 52:449. Rogers M. Textbook of Pediatric Intensive Care, Baltimore, 1993.

C. **Barbiturates**
1. **Agents:** Pentobarbital, phenobarbital, methylqualone, secobarbital, street "downers"
2. **Diagnosis**
   a. Symptoms: CNS: ataxia, lethargy, headache, vertigo, coma. Respiratory: Pulmonary edema, respiratory depression. CVS: Shock, hypothermia. Skin: Bullae.
   b. Blood levels not required for management.
   c. EEG may correlate with progression of coma.
3. **Treatment**
   a. Assure ventilation.
   b. Give 10 times ingested dose or 1 gm/kg of body weight of charcoal followed by a cathartic. May use serial activated charcoal.
4. **Urinary alkalinization**
   Can increase phenobarbital and metharbital excretion.
5. **Hemodialysis and hemoperfusion may be considered.**
6. **Withdrawal:** If withdrawal symptoms develop, reinstitute usual phenobarbital dose; reduce dose gradually.

Ref: Ellenhorn MJ, Barceloux DG, Medical Toxicology. New York:Elsevier,1988. Smith DE, Wesson DR, JAMA 1970, 213:294–5.

D. Carbamazepine (Tegretol)
1. **Diagnosis**
   a. Symptoms: Bradycardia, AV block, hypotension or hypertension, respiratory depression, lethargy, coma, dystonic posturing, anticholinergic symptoms, SIADH, abnormal DTRs.
   b. Toxic serum level is >20 μg/mL.
2. **Treatment**
   a. Maintain airway and cardiovascular status.
   b. Ipecac or gastric lavage if less than 1 hour.
   c. Activated charcoal and cathartics.
   d. With prolonged coma, charcoal hemoperfusion.
   e. Limited use of physostigmine for dystonic/athetoid posturing.

   Ref: Leslie PJ, et al, Br Med J 1983, 286:545–7. O'Neal W Jr, et al, Clin Pharm 1984, 3:545–7.

E. Carbon Monoxide Poisoning
1. **Diagnosis**
   a. Symptoms: Headache, cyanosis, confusion, dizziness, nausea, gastroenteritis, weakness, syncope, seizures, or coma.
   b. Sources: Fire, automobile exhaust, gasoline or propane engines operating in enclosed spaces, faulty furnaces or gas stoves, charcoal burners, paint remover with methylene chloride.
   c. Obtain carboxyhemoglobin (COHb) level in blood.
   d. Pulse oximetry for decreased saturation (may be normal even with significant exposure).
2. **Treatment**
   a. Administer 100% O_2.
   b. Ensure adequate airway, prevent hypercapnea.
   c. Proceed to hyperbaric O_2 therapy if COHb level >40%, patient exhibits cardiovascular instability or impaired mentation, or patient is pregnant with COHb >20% or has fetal distress. If hyperbaric O_2 is unavailable, administer 100% O_2 until COHb level decreases below 10%.
   d. Complications of severe CO poisoning include cardiac dysrhythmias, pulmonary edema, myoglobinuria with

acute renal failure, temporary blindness, encephalopathy, and cerebral edema.

Ref: Zimmerman SS, Truxal B. Pediatrics 1981, 68:215–24, Gozal D, et al. Clin Pediatr 1985, 24:132–6. Noncool DM. Ann Emerg Med 1985, 14:1168–71.

F. Caustic Ingestions (Strong Acids and Alkalis)

1. All patients with a history of caustic ingestion should be hospitalized for possible endoscopy. Absence of oropharyngeal damage does **not** exclude esophageal burns.

2. Maintain NPO. Attempts to "neutralize" the burn are ineffective and obscure and delay endoscopy. Ipecac or lavage is contraindicated.

3. Begin IV fluid therapy.

4. Begin IV ampicillin l00–200 mg/kg/day.

5. Consider IV steroid therapy—may be of benefit for some patients.

6. Provide tetanus prophylaxis as indicated.

7. Obtain blood count, chest x-ray, blood type, and cross-match. Chest X-ray may demonstrate esophageal perforation.

8. Proceed to endoscopy. Do **not** pass NG tube. Discontinue endoscopy immediately if esophageal burn identified.

9. In the **absence** of esophageal burn, antibiotics and steroids may be discontinued. Provide care for local burns.

10. In the **presence** of esophageal burns, continue antibiotics for at least 5–7 days and steroids for 3 weeks. Advance diet slowly after patient is able to handle own secretions well. Steroids may be changed to oral prednisone 2 mg/kg/day if tolerated. Taper prednisone slowly after full 3-week course.

11. Provide close follow-up and further surgical therapy for esophageal or antral/pyloric strictures, as required. Risk of developing esophageal carcinoma after caustic ingestion is markedly increased.

    Note: Ingestion of alkaline button batteries can lead to esophageal and gastric burns. If initial X-ray shows battery to be lodged in esophagus, immediate endoscopic retrieval is indicated. If the disc is beyond the esophagus, patient is discharged and follow up X-rays performed only if battery has not passed in 4–7 days.

For batteries >23 mm diameter a 48 hour X-ray should be performed to exclude persistent gastric position and need for endoscopic retrieval.

Ref: Rothstein FC. Ped Clin North Am 1986, 33:665–74. Moore WR. Clin Pediatr 1986, 25:192–6. Wason S. Emerg Med, 1985, 2:175–182.

G. **Digoxin Intoxication**
  1. **Symptoms:** Major manifestations include the following: GI: anorexia, nausea, vomiting; CNS: headache, disorientation, somnolence, seizures, and cardiac: any new rhythm, especially those combining increased automaticity of ectopic pacemakers and impaired conduction. Most cases result in GI symptoms with mild CNS and cardiac disturbances.
  2. **Diagnosis**
     a. Determine serum digoxin level and electrolytes (including Mg and Ca) stat. (Their imbalance enhances digoxin toxicity.)
     b. Doses of >0.07 mg/kg (or 2–3 mg in adolescent) are associated with toxicity.
     c. Signs and symptoms predict digoxin level >2 ng/ml; however, absence of symptoms when level >2 ng/ml cannot predict potential for toxicity.
     d. Quinidine, amiodarone, or poor renal function will increase the digoxin level. Low K, Mg, or T_4 will increase digoxin toxicity at a given level, as will high Ca.
     e. Initial hyperkalemia results from release of intracellular potassium and indicates serious toxicity.
  3. **Treatment**
     a. Give ipecac, charcoal (even several hours after ingestion), and cathartic.
     b. Start continuous ECG monitoring.
     c. In cardiac rhythm disturbances:
        1) AV block: **Atropine** alone 0.01 mg/kg IV may reverse sinus bradycardia or AV block. Repeated doses may be necessary. Avoid propranolol, quinidine, procainamide, or disopyramide if AV block is present. **Phenytoin** improves AV conduction. Dose is 1–2 mg/kg, no faster than 50 mg/min. Repeat every 5 minutes until arrhythmia is controlled

or maximum dose is reached. **Transvenous ventricular pacing** is usually effective if atropine and phenytoin fail.

2) Ventricular tachycardia, PVCs: Phenytoin and lidocaine are effective.

d. In severe poisonings with uncontrollable dysrhythmia and/or hyperkalemia, administer purified digoxin specific Fab fragments. Since this therapy can be lifesaving, continue CPR for prolonged periods if Fab fragments are available. Dose (based on total body load of digoxin): Digoxin immune Fab (Digibind) is available in 40 mg vial. Each vial will bind approximately 0.6 mg of digoxin. Estimate **body load** in milligrams using either of the following 2 methods:

1) Use the known acutely ingested dose in milligrams. (If taken PO, multiply dose by 0.8 to correct for incomplete absorption of tablets or elixir. If ingested as liquid-filled capsules or given IV, do not multiply by 0.8.) **OR**

2) [Serum drug concentration (ng/ml) $\times$ 5.6 $\times$ wt. in kg]/1000. (The volume of distribution of digoxin is 5.6 L/kg.)

Then, **number of vials to be given = body load (mg)/0.6 mg of digoxin neutralized per vial.** Administer IV over 30 minutes. Give as bolus injection if cardiac arrest is imminent.

Note: If digitoxin, rather than digoxin, is ingested, the total body load can be estimated either using the mg dose of drug ingested acutely (without any correction factor) OR using the equation: [serum drug concentration (ng/ml) $\times$ 0.56 $\times$ wt. in kg]/1000, where 0.56 L/kg is the volume of distribution of digitoxin.

Ref: Smith TW, et al. N Engl J Med 1982, 307:1357, Tenenbein M. Curr Probl Pediatr 1986, 16:185, Lewander WJ, et al. Am J Dis Child 1986, 140:770, Murphy DJ, et al. Pediatr 1982, 70:472, McEvoy G, editor. Drug Information 90, American Hospital Formulary Service, 1990:1885.

H. Hydrocarbon Ingestions

1. **Symptoms:** Pulmonary: tachypnea, dyspnea, tachycardia, cyanosis, grunting, cough. CNS: lethargy, seizures, coma.

2. **Evaluation**
   a. Aliphatic hydrocarbons have the greatest aspiration hazard and pulmonary toxicity. They include: gasoline, kerosene, mineral seal oil, lighter fluid, tar, mineral oil, lubricating oils, turpentine.
   b. Aromatic hydrocarbons (benzene, toluene, xylene) and halogenated hydrocarbons (carbon tetrachloride) have mainly CNS and hepatic toxicity.

3. **Therapy**
   a. Remove toxin.
      1) Avoid emesis or lavage if possible as these increase the risk of aspiration.
      2) If the hydrocarbon contains a potentially toxic substance (insecticide, heavy metal, camphor) and a toxic amount has been ingested, induce emesis with ipecac in the fully conscious patient. In lethargic patients, consider intubation with a cuffed ETT, followed by lavage.
      3) **Avoid charcoal.** It does not bind aliphatics and will increase the risk of aspiration.
   b. Obtain CXR and arterial blood gases on patients with pulmonary symptoms.
   c. Observe patient for 6 hours.
      1) If child asymptomatic for 6 hours and CXR normal—discharge home.
      2) If child becomes symptomatic in 6 hour period—admit.
      3) If asymptomatic but CXR abnormal—consider admission for further observation. Discharge only if close follow up can be ensured.
   d. Treat pneumonitis with oxygen and PEEP. Antibiotics and steroids are not routinely warranted.

   Ref: Tenenbein M. Curr Probl Pediatr 1986, 16:185–233. Klein BL. Ped Clin North Am 1986, 33:411–19.

I. Iron Poisoning

1. **Diagnosis**
   a. Symptoms
      1) First phase: GI toxicity (30 min − 12 hrs after ingestion): nausea, vomiting, diarrhea, abdominal pain, hematemesis, melena. Rarely, this phase may progress to shock, seizures, coma.

2) Second phase: Latent period (8–36 hrs after ingestion): improvement in clinical symptoms.
3) Third phase: Systemic toxicity (12–48 hrs after ingestion): hepatic injury or failure, hypoglycemia, metabolic acidosis, bleeding, shock, coma, convulsions, death.
4) Fourth phase: Late complications (4–8 wks after ingestion): pyloric or antral stenosis, CNS sequelae. Postintoxication liver cirrhosis not seen in children.

b. Determination of estimated dose (for children less than 5 years old):

Elemental Fe	Therapy
>20 mg/kg	None
20–60 mg/kg	Syrup of ipecac, home management
>60 mg/kg	Physician evaluation

c. Deferoxamine challenge test: give 1 gm IM. Presence of "vin rose" color to urine indicates significant ingestion of iron.
d. Determine serum iron concentration 4–6 hrs post ingestion.
1) Level of 300–500 mcg/dl: Begin chelation if iron concentration exceeds TIBC or if patient showing signs/symptoms of toxicity.
2) Level of >500 mcg/dl: 20% risk of shock. Institute chelation therapy immediately.
Note: Serum iron levels obtained beyond 6 hours after ingestion may not be elevated, even in the presence of severe poisoning.

2. **Treatment**
a. Induce emesis if patient awake, alert.
b. Obtain abdominal x-ray.
c. Give deferoxamine IV at 15 mg/kg/hr in all cases of serious poisoning. If serum iron concentration >500

mcg/dl continue chelation until serum iron <300 mcg/dl. When traditional "vin rose" urine does occur, continue chelation until 24 hours after the child is producing an adequate volume of normally colored urine.

d. Above all, supportive care is the most important therapy. Large IV fluid volumes may be needed in first 24 hours to avoid hypovolemic shock and acidemia. Urine output should be maintained at >2 ml/kg/hr.

Ref: Banner W Jr, Tong TG. Ped Clin North Am 1986, 33:393–409. Gellis SS, Kagan BM. Current Pediatric Therapy. WB Saunders, 1986.

J. Lead Poisoning: See Chapter 14, Hematology, for risk classification and diagnostic criteria.

1. **Treatment of symptomatic cases:** Children with one or more of following: persistent vomiting, ataxic gait, gross irritability, severe anemia, seizures, or alteration in state of consciousness are treated as potential cases of acute encephalopathy. Therapy:

a. Establish urine output with 10–20 ml/kg IV if necessary. Then adjust fluid therapy to maintain urine output of 350–500 ml/M^2/24h.

b. Control seizures initially with diazepam. Phenobarbital and/or phenytoin may be necessary for long term seizure control.

c. Chelate with BAL-CaEDTA in combination.

1) Dosage: BAL 83 mg/M^2/dose IM q4h, CaEDTA 250 mg/M^2/dose IM q4h

2) Administration: For first dose inject BAL (IM) only. Beginning 4 hours later and every 4 hours thereafter for 5 days inject BAL and CaEDTA simultaneously at separate and deep IM sites, rotate injection sites.

d. Supplement second course of EDTA with 5 mg oral elemental zinc acetate tid and 0.5 mg oral copper acetate tid.

Note: Usual 5 day course may be extended to 7 days cautiously if clinical evidence of encephalopathy persists beyond 4 days.

e. Serial lead measurements should be made after the last doses of BAL and CaEDTA and at day 4, 11, and 18 thereafter. If lead rebounds to 35 mcg/dl or more, additional 5 day courses of CaEDTA are indicated. Rebound is minimized if the initial course of BAL/CaEDTA is followed by oral D-penicillamine.

Note: BAL contraindicated in acute hepatocellular injury and G6PD deficiency. Medicinal iron should not be given concomitantly with BAL.

Ref: Revisions recommended by Chisholm JJ, Gellis SS, Kagen BM. Current Pediatric Therapy. 12th Edition. Philadelphia: WB Saunders, 1986. See also Piomelli S, et al. J Pediatr 1984,105: 523–32.

K. Narcotics, Opiates, and Morphine Analogs

1. **Diagnosis:** Suspect in any patient with depressed mental status of unknown etiology.

2. **Withdrawal response:** Nausea, vomiting, hyperactive BS, yawning, piloerection, pupillary dilatation (may vary, e.g., present with demerol and propoxyphene).

3. **Treatment**

   a. Administer IV naloxone (Narcan) 0.01 mg/kg. If this is ineffective, administer 0.1 mg/kg. Improvement in mental status indicates a clinical response.

   b. Careful inpatient monitoring is required due to the short half life of naloxone compared to most opiates.

   c. Indications for continuous naloxone infusion include:
      1) Requirement for repeat bolus therapy
      2) Requirement of large initial bolus
      3) Ingestion of large amount of opiate or long-acting opiate
      4) Decreased opiate metabolism.

   d. Suggested regimen is as follows:
      1) Administer as loading dose the previously successful bolus.
      2) Administer 75%– 100% of the above loading dose as an hourly infusion dose.
      3) Wean naloxone drip in 50% increments as tolerated over 6– 12h depending on the half-life of the narcotic ingested. For methadone, may require infusion up to 48 hours.

      Ref: Moore R, et al. Am J Dis Child 1980, 134:156. Tenebein M, J Pediatr 1984, 105:645.

4. **Neonatal abstinence syndrome**
   a. **Symptoms:** Hyperactivity, restlessness, excessive crying, tremor, hyperreflexia, vomiting, hypertonia, sweating, hyperphagia, rhinorrhea, seizures, and tearing.
   b. Treatment
      1) Paregoric (anhydrous morphine 0.4 mg/ml): 0.2–0.5 ml/dose q3–4h.
      2) Diazepam: 1–2 mg IM q8h.
      3) Phenobarbital: 15–20 mg/kg loading dose, then 2–8 mg/kg/24h.
      Ref: Chasnoff J. Peds Rev 1988, 9:273.

L. **Phenothiazine and Butyrophenone Intoxication**
   1. **Agents:** Chlorpromazine (Thorazine), thioridazine (Mellaril), trifluoperazine (Stelazine), perphenazine (Trilafon), prochlorperazine (Compazine), fluphenazine (Prolixin), haloperidol (Haldol)
   2. **Diagnosis**
      a. Symptoms: (may be delayed 6–24 hours postingestion): Depressed neurologic status, meiosis, hypotension, dysrhythmias, extrapyramidal signs or neuroleptic malignant syndrome (fever, diaphoresis, rigidity, tachycardia, coma), anticholinergic symptoms.
      b. Blood levels confirm ingestion but do not correlate with clinical effects.
   3. **Treatment**
      a. Support and monitoring of respiratory and cardiovascular status.
      b. Ipecac followed by activated charcoal if patient awake and cooperative. Dialysis is contraindicated.
      c. Extrapyramidal Signs: IV diphenhydramine 2 mg/kg (up to 50 mg) slowly over 2–5 minutes, **OR** IV benztropine mesylate 0.5 mg/kg.
      d. Dysrhythmias:
         1) Ventricular: Phenytoin 10–15 mg/kg IV slowly or lidocaine 1 mg/kg IV push.
         2) Supraventricular: Supportive, however, if hemodynamically unstable proceed to cardioversion.
         3) AV dissociation: Pacemaker.

    e. Neuroleptic malignant syndrome: (hyperthermia, muscle rigidity, autonomic disturbances of heart rate and blood pressure, and altered consciousness).

      1) Reduce hyperthermia with lavage and cooling blankets. Antipyretics not helpful.

      2) Support respiratory and cardiovascular status— monitor neurologic and fluid status.

      3) Use of dantrolene (0.5 mg/kg PO q12h) to reduce muscle rigidity and oxygen consumption is experimental.

        Ref: Knight ME, et al. Pediatr Clin North Am, 1986, 33:299–309.

M. Phenytoin (Dilantin)

  1. **Diagnosis**

    a. Symptoms include ataxia, drowsiness, tremor, seizures, hyperglycemic nonketotic coma.

    b. Symptoms seen with blood levels $>>20$ mcg/ml.

  2. **Treatment**

    a. Supportive care. If seizures, discontinue phenytoin and use diazepam. Use insulin for hyperglycemic nonketotic coma. Give fluids and monitor glucose.

    b. Ipecac if no evidence of obtundation, seizures.

    c. Use charcoal and cathartics via OG tube if indicated

    d. Other methods not helpful. Plasmapharesis is investigational.

        Ref: Larsen LS, et al. Clin Toxicol 1986, 24:37–49.

N. Salicylate Poisoning

  1. **Symptoms:** Hyperpnea, hyperthermia, lethargy, nausea, vomiting, tinnitus, dehydration, metabolic acidosis, coma.

  2. **Dosages:** Establish the severity of ingestion:

    a. The acute toxic dose (single-dose ingestion): 150 mg/kg.

    b. Chronic overdosage can produce toxicity at much lower doses.

    c. Preparations (mg of salicylate):

      1) Children's aspirin: 1.25 grain (81 mg) tablets (36 tablets per bottle).

      2) Adult aspirin: 5 grain (325 mg) tablets.

      3) Methyl salicylate (oil of wintergreen): 1.4 gm/ml.

      4) Pepto Bismol: 8.77 mg/ml.

3. **Evaluation**
   a. Urine ferric chloride: Mix 1 ml of urine with 1 ml 10% FeCl$_3$ solution. Purple color change indicates a positive test. However, even an insignificant amount of salicylate will produce a positive test. Urinary ketones also will produce a false positive test; these can be removed by first boiling the urine.
   b. Serum salicylate level: Therapy must be based upon quantitative serum level and not upon the above presumptive tests. At least two levels obtained several hours apart are necessary to determine the severity of ingestion, as continued slow absorption may increase the serum level for up to 24 hours. See Done nomogram, Figure 3–2.

4. **Treatment**
   a. Institute therapy immediately. Do not wait for the salicylate level to return.
   b. Empty the stomach by emesis. Administer activated charcoal and cathartic via OG tube if indicated.
   c. Monitor serum electrolytes, calcium, arterial blood gases, glucose, urine pH and SG, and coagulation studies as needed.
   d. Treat fluid and solute deficits
      1) Replenish intravascular volume with D$_5$ Ringer's lactate at 20 ml/kg/hr for 1–2 hrs until adequate urine output is established.
      2) Then begin infusing D$_5$W with 50 mEq Na HCO$_3$/L and 20–40 mEq K/L at rates of 3–6 L/M^2/24h (i.e., 2–4 times maintenance fluids). Aim for a urine output of 2 ml/kg/hr, as this will enhance salicylate excretion. Adjust concentrations of the electrolytes as needed to correct serum electrolyte abnormalities (especially hypokalemia, which inhibits salicylate excretion), and to maintain a urinary pH > 7.0.
   e. Administer parenteral vitamin K as indicated by coagulation studies (especially in chronic intoxications).
   f. Continue fluid therapy until the patient is asymptomatic for several hours, regardless of the serum salicylate level.

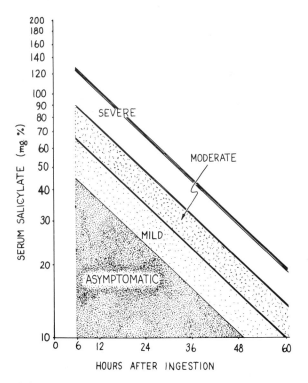

FIG 3.2.
Done nomogram. The nomogram relates serum salicylate and expected severity of intoxication at varying intervals following ingestion of a **single** dose of salicylate, starting six hours after the ingestion.

g. Proceed to hemodialysis in the presence of unresponsive acidosis (pH < 7.10), renal failure, seizures unresponsive to calcium gluconate and anticonvulsants, or progressive deterioration when all other methods have been carried out appropriately.

Ref: Snodgrass WR, Ped Clin North Am 1986, 33:381–91. Temple AR, Arch Intern Med, 1981, 141:364–9.

O. Theophylline Toxicity

1. **Symptoms:** GI: vomiting, hematemesis, abdominal pain, bloody diarrhea. CV: tachycardia, arrhythmia, cardiac arrest. CNS: seizures, agitation, coma, hallucinations.

2. **Evaluation**
   a. Obtain a theophylline level stat and again in 1–4 hours to see the pattern of absorption. Peak absorption has been reported to be delayed as long as 13–17 hr after ingestion.
   b. Levels >20 µg/ml are associated with increasing toxicity, especially if >40 µg/ml.
   c. Levels >40 g/ml or patients with neurotoxicity require admission and careful monitoring.
   d. Hypokalemia, hypotension, and low serum bicarbonate may occur with acute ingestion.

3. **Therapy**
   a. Cardiac monitor until level falls below 20 µg/ml. Treat arrhythmias.
   b. Ipecac.
   c. Charcoal followed by cathartic, regardless of the length of time after ingestion. For severe intoxication begin multiple dose charcoal regimen as outlined earlier.
   d. Consider theophylline bezoar if level continues to rise after adequate lavage and patient deteriorates.
   e. Establish IV access and treat dehydration.
   f. Monitor serum K, Mg, P, Ca, acid base balance in moderate to severe intoxication until peak levels are confirmed.
   g. Charcoal hemoperfusion: An effective and safe method of rapidly lowering theophylline levels. Start hemoperfusion whenever signs of neurotoxicity (seizures, coma) are present. Whether a high theophyl-

line level alone is an indication for hemoperfusion is controversial.

Ref: Ellenhorn MJ, Barceloux DG, Medical Toxicology. New York: Elsevier, 1988. Sahney S, et al. Pediatrics 1983, 71:615.

P. Tricyclic Antidepressant Overdose

1. **Agents:** Imipramine, desipramine, amitriptyline, nortriptyline, doxepin, maprotiline

2. **Symptoms:** Symptoms of anticholinergic toxicity. CNS: agitation, seizures, myoclonus, lethargy, coma, choreoathetosis, cardiovascular: hypo- or hypertension, conduction abnormalities, dysrhythmias, respiratory depression.

3. **Evaluation**
   a. Signs of toxicity usually appear within 4 hrs of ingestion. Any ingestion should be observed at least 6 hrs.
   b. Toxicity associated with doses >10 mg/kg. A dose of >30 mg/kg can be lethal.
   c. ECG (acute overdose): QRS duration >0.10 sec predicts risk of seizures and QRS duration >0.16 sec predicts ventricular dysrhythmia in acute overdose. ECG must be monitored for at least 24 hrs.
   d. Serum drug levels are not of predictive value.

4. **Therapy**
   a. If ingestion is more than 10–20 mg/kg, start IV and cardiac monitoring.
   b. Assess adequate ventilation.
   c. If altered mental status, stabilize with oxygen, naloxone, and glucose.
   d. Treat seizures with diazepam, then phenytoin if seizures persist.
   e. For cardiac symptoms, correct acidosis with $NaHCO_3$ 1–2 mEq/kg to keep pH >7.45 (lessens risk of arrhythmia) and a loading dose of phenytoin 10–15 mg/kg slowly. May repeat phenytoin once. Monitor alkalinization by following electrolytes and ABG.
   f. Give charcoal and cathartic. For severe intoxication begin multiple dose charcoal regimen as outlined earlier.

g. Reserve physostigmine for pure anticholinergic symptoms or for life-threatening symptoms unresponsive to above modalities.

h. Admit if any signs of major toxicity; cardiac monitor until symptom-free for 24 hours.

Ref: Boehnert MT, Lovejoy FH: N Engl J Med 1985, 313:474–9.
Braden NJ. Pediatr Clin North Am 1986, 33:287–97.

PROCEDURES 4

I. **LOCAL ANESTHETIC:** For many procedures, local anesthetic is indicated for control of pain. However, lidocaine preparations are buffered to an acid pH, and are therefore painful when injected. To reduce this pain, mix 0.5% or 1.0% lidocaine with 8.4% sodium bicarbonate in a 9 to 1 lidocaine to bicarbonate dilution. Use this solution within 24 hours of mixing.

Ref Bartfield JM, Homer PJ, Ford DT, Sternklar P: Buffered Lidocaine as a Local Anesthetic: An Investigation of Shelf Life. Ann Emerg. Med. 1992;21:16–19.

II. **VENIPUNCTURE**
A. **Heel or Finger Stick**
1. Warm extremity in order to provide optimal blood flow and more accurate samples. To prevent burns, do not use a warming towel that is >40° C.
2. Lance either lateral or medial side of heel; avoid the heel pad. For digital artery sampling use medial surface of the distal phalanx of second, third, or fourth finger.
3. Use a 2.5 mm lancet or an Autolet for optimal skin penetration.
4. Wipe away first drop of blood with dry gauze. Alcohol used in cleaning skin may produce hemolysis.
5. Massage (but do not squeeze) finger or heel.
6. Samples may be inaccurate if patient is poorly perfused or polycythemic.

   Ref: Blumenfeld TA, et. al. Lancet 1979;1:230; Morgan EJ. Am Rev Resp Dis 1979;120:795.

B. **External Jugular Puncture**
1. Restrain infant securely.
2. Extend neck, and turn head slightly to one side. This accentuates the posterior margin of contralateral sternocleidomastoid muscle. This may be facilitated by positioning infant so that head falls over the side of the table or by placing a rolled towel under the infant's shoulders.

3. Prepare area carefully with povidone-iodine and 20% alcohol.

4. To distend the external jugular vein, occlude its most proximal segment, or provoke child to cry. The vein runs from angle of mandible to posterior border of lower third of sternocleidomastoid muscle.

5. While continually providing negative suction on the syringe, insert the needle at about a 30° angle to the skin. Continue as with any peripheral venipuncture.

C. **Femoral Puncture:** Careful skin antisepsis is needed to prevent septic arthritis. Femoral puncture is particularly hazardous in neonates and is not recommended in this age group. Avoid femoral punctures in children who are thrombocytopenic, have coagulation disorders, or are scheduled for cardiac catheterization.

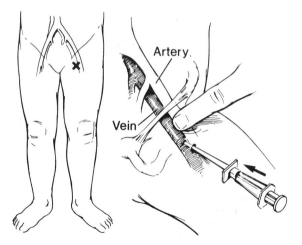

FIG 4.1.
Femoral puncture technique.
Ref: Nichols: Golden Hour, St Louis, Mosby, 1991, p 123.

1. Have an assistant hold child securely with the hips flexed and abducted (in a frog-leg position).
2. Prepare area as for blood culture with providone-iodine and 70% alcohol.
3. Locate femoral pulse, then insert needle 2.0 cm distal to inguinal ligament and 0.5 to 0.75 cm. into the groin. Continually aspirate while maneuvering the needle until blood is obtained.

   Ref: Asnes RS, et. al. Pediatrics 1966;38:837.

D.   Internal Jugular Puncture

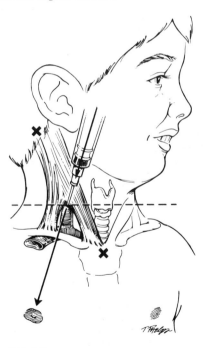

FIG 4.2.
Internal jugular puncture technique.
Ref: Nichols: *Golden Hour,* St Louis, Mosby, 1991, p 124.

1. Securely restrain the infant.
2. Extend neck, and turn head slightly to one side. This accentuates the posterior margin of the sternocleidomastoid muscle. This may be facilitated by positioning the infant so that the head falls over side of the table, or by placing a rolled towel under the infant's shoulders.
3. Prepare area as for blood culture with povidone-iodine and 70% alcohol.
4. Insert needle just deep to and behind posterior margin of sternocleidomastoid muscle, approximately halfway between its origin and insertion. Then advance needle under the muscle, parallel to skin surface in direction of suprasternal notch. Advance for a distance equal to width of sternocleidomastoid muscle.
5. While exerting suction, slowly withdraw needle until blood is withdrawn.
6. After obtaining blood, hold child upright and apply pressure to puncture site.

III.   INTRAOSSEOUS INFUSION

A.   Indication: Use as an alternative mode of intravenous access in children less than 5 years old when peripheral IV access is unobtainable or unacceptably delayed.

B.   Technique

1. Use the tibia, approximately 2 cm below the tibial tuberosity on the anteromedial surface. Alternatively, use the femur in the midline, 2–3 cm superior to the lateral condyle. Finally, consider using the medial surface of the distal tibia, proximal to the medial malleolus.
2. Prepare and drape the patient for a sterile procedure.
3. Anesthetize the puncture site down to the periosteum.
4. Use an intraosseus needle, a 16- or 18-gauge bone marrow needle or an 18-gauge spinal needle.
5. Insert the needle perpendicular to the skin and advance to the periosteum. Then, with a boring motion, penetrate into the marrow.

6. Remove the stylet, and aspirate some marrow into a saline-filled syringe. Next, infuse some saline to insure location and remove any clotted material from the needle. Make sure the needle is firmly embedded in bone.

7. Attach standard IV tubing. Any crystalloid, blood product or drug that may be infused into a peripheral vein, also may be infused into the intraosseus space.

Ref: Rosetti VA, et. al. Ann Emerg Med 1985; 14:885-88.

IV. RADIAL ARTERY CATHETERIZATION: Use the right radial artery because it is more representative of preductal blood flow.

A. **Allen Test:** Assesses the adequacy of ulnar blood flow to the entire hand.

1. Passively clench the hand and simultaneously compress the ulnar and radial arteries.

2. Release the ulnar artery and note the degree of flushing of the blanched hand. Catheterization may be performed if the entire hand flushes while the radial artery is still compressed.

3. Avoid inadvertent compression of the ulnar artery while compressing the radial vessel.

B. **Technique**

1. Secure the hand to an arm board with the wrist extended. Leave the fingers exposed to observe any color changes.

2. Under sterile conditions, palpate the radial artery at the wrist and note the point of maximum impulse. After infiltrating the area with 1% lidocaine, use a 20-gauge needle to make a small skin puncture at the point of maximal impulse.

3. Place a 22-gauge intravenous catheter through the puncture site at a 30° angle to the horizontal and pass the needle through the artery to transfix it. Withdraw the inner needle. Very slowly withdraw the catheter until free flow of blood is noted, then advance the catheter.

4. Apply an antibiotic ointment and pressure dressing over the puncture site and secure the catheter with adhesive tape or suture.

5. Firmly attach the catheter to a T-connector. Continuously infuse heparinized isotonic saline (1 unit heparin/ml saline) at a rate of 1 ml/hour using a constant infusion pump. Connect a pressure transducer to monitor blood pressure.

C. **Blood Sampling**

1. Occlude the distal end of the T-connector with a clamp, and clean the rubber end of the T-connector with antiseptic solution.

2. Insert a 22- or 25-gauge needle into the rubber end of the T-connector. Withdraw 0.3–0.5 ml of blood and fluid to clear the line. Attach a 1 ml syringe and withdraw 0.3–0.5 ml of blood.

3. Flush the line with 2 cc normal saline.
   Note: Do not infuse any fluids (other than the flushing fluid), medications, or blood products through the arterial line.
   Ref: Todres ID, et. al. J Pediatr 1975; 87:273.

V. **UMBILICAL ARTERY CATHETERIZATION**

A. **Catheter Position:** Umbilical artery catheters may be placed in either of two positions: low-line position, between lumbar vertebrae 3 and 5; or high-line position, between thoracic vertebrae 6 and 9. The tip of a low line is below the renal and mesenteric arteries, perhaps decreasing the incidence of clots. However, a high line may be recommended in less than 750 gm infants when a low line could easily slip out. The length of catheter required to achieve either position may be determined using a standardized graph or a regression formula. Catheter length is about ⅓ the crown heel length.

1. **Graphical representation**
   a. Determine the shoulder-umbilical length by measuring the perpendicular line dropped from the tip of the shoulder to the level of the umbilicus.
   b. Use the graph on p. 63 (Fig 4.3) to determine the catheter length to be inserted for either a high or low line. For a low line, the tip of the catheter should lie just above the aortic bifurcation (avoid renal artery orifice, around L_1). With a high line, the tip should be above the diaphragm.

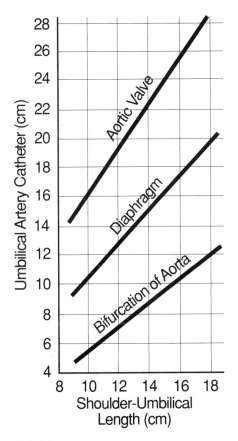

FIG 4.3.
Umbilical Artery Catheter Length.

2. **Birthweight (BW) regression formula**
   a. High-line: UA catheter length (cm) = [3 × BW (kg)] + 9
   b. Low-line: Catheter length (cm) approximates birth weight plus 7.
      Note: Formula may not be appropriate for SGA or LGA infants.

B. **Catheter Placement**
   1. Restrain infant. Prepare and drape umbilical cord and adjacent skin using sterile technique. Place sterile drapes sparingly to expose infant to the radiant warmer.
   2. Determine the length of catheter to be inserted for either high (T_6 to T_9) or low (L_3 to L_5) position (see Figure 4.3).
   3. Flush catheter with sterile saline solution prior to insertion.
   4. Place sterile umbilical tape around base of cord. Cut through cord horizontally approximately 1.5–2.0 cm from skin; tighten umbilical tape to prevent bleeding.
   5. Identify large, thin-walled umbilical vein and smaller, thick-walled arteries. Use one tip of open curved iris forceps to gently probe and dilate one artery. Then gently probe with both points of closed forceps and dilate artery by allowing forceps to open gently.
   6. Grasp catheter 1 cm from tip with toothless forceps and insert catheter into lumen of artery. Aim the tip toward the feet, and gently advance catheter to desired distance. **DO NOT FORCE.** If resistance is encountered, try loosening umbilical tape, applying steady gentle pressure, or manipulating angle of umbilical cord to skin.
   7. Secure catheter with both a suture through the cord and marker tape, and a tape bridge. Confirm the position of the catheter tip radiologically.
   8. Look for complications of catheter placement: blanching or cyanosis of lower extremities, perforation, thrombosis, embolism, and infection.

Ref: Mokrohisky ST, et. al. New Engl J Med 1978; 299:561. May H. Emergency Medicine 2nd Edition, Vol. II; Little Brown & Company; Boston, Mass.;1992. Shukla H, et. al. Am J Dis Child 1986; 140:786.

VI. UMBILICAL VEIN CATHETERIZATION: See umbilical artery catheterization above.

A. Catheter Position: Umbilical vein catheter should be placed in the inferior vena cava above the level of the ductus venosus and the hepatic veins. The length of the catheter necessary to achieve the position can be determined using the graph or regression formula below.

1. **Graphical representation**
   a. Determine the shoulder-umbilical length by measuring the perpendicular line dropped from the tip of the shoulder to the level of the umbilicus.
   b. Using Figure 4.4, determine the catheter length needed to place the tip between the diaphragm and left atrium. Add length for the height of the umbilical stump.

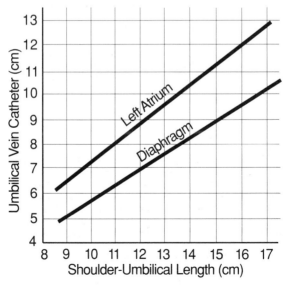

FIG 4.4.
Umbilical Vein Catheter Length.

2. **Birthweight regression formula**
   UV catheter length (cm) = [0.5 × UA catheter length (cm)] + 1
   Note: May not be appropriate for SGA or LGA infants.
   Ref: Shukla H, et. al. Am J Dis Child 1986; 140:786. Adapted from Dunn P. Arch Dis Child 1966; 41:69.

B. Catheter Placement
1. After restraining infant, clean, drape, and cut umbilical stump as for umbilical artery catheterization described above.
2. Determine the length of the catheter needed to place the catheter tip in the inferior vena cava above the level of the ductus venosus or hepatic veins. Place marker (sterile bandage or tape) on catheter at desired length.
3. Flush catheter with sterile saline solution prior to insertion.
4. Isolate thin-walled umbilical vein, clear thrombi with forceps, and insert catheter, aiming the tip toward the right shoulder. Gently advance catheter to desired distance. **DO NOT FORCE.** If resistance is encountered, try loosening umbilical tape, applying steady gentle pressure, or manipulating angle of umbilical cord to skin.
5. Secure catheter as described for umbilical artery catheter. Confirm position of the catheter tip radiologically.

VII. NEONATAL EXCHANGE TRANSFUSION: (See Chapter 14, Hematology, for volume calculations.)
Note: CBC, reticulocyte count, peripheral smear, bilirubin, Ca, glucose total protein, infant blood type, and Coombs test should be performed on pre-exchange sample of blood since they are of no diagnostic value on post-exchange blood. If indicated, save pre-exchange blood for serologic or chromosome studies.
A. Sensitized Cells or Hyperbilirubinemia
1. Cross match donor blood against maternal serum for first exchange and against post-exchange blood for subsequent exchanges.

2. Use Type O-negative (low titer), irradiated blood; may use infant's type if no chance of maternal-infant incompatibility. Blood should be stored at room temperature, either fresh or up to 48 hours old, and anticoagulated with ACD or CPD unless infant is acidotic or hypocalcemic.

3. Make infant NPO during, and at least 4 hours after exchange. Empty stomach if infant was fed within 4 hours of procedure.

4. Follow vital signs, blood sugar, and temperature closely; have resuscitation equipment ready.

5. Prepare and drape patient for sterile procedure.

6. Insert umbilical artery and vein catheters as per sections IV and V above. During the exchange, blood is removed through the umbilical artery catheter and infused through the venous catheter. If unable to pass an arterial catheter, use a single venous catheter.

7. Prewarm blood in quality-controlled blood warmer if available; do not improvise with a water bath!

8. Exchange 15 ml increments in vigorous full-term infants, smaller volumes for smaller, less stable infants. Do not allow cells in donor unit to form sediment.

9. Withdraw and infuse blood 2–3 ml/kg/min to avoid mechanical trauma to patient and donor cells.

10. Give 1–2 ml of 10% calcium gluconate solution IV slowly for ECG evidence of hypocalcemia (prolonged Q-Tc intervals). Flush tubing with NaCl before and after calcium infusion. Observe for bradycardia during infusion.

11. To complete double volume exchange, transfuse 160 ml/kg for full-term infant and 160-200 ml/kg for preterm infant.

12. Send last aliquot withdrawn for Hct, smear, glucose, bilirubin, potassium, Ca^{2+}, and type and match.

Ref: Kitterman JA, et. al. Pediatr Clin North Am 1970; 17:895.

B. **Anemic Heart Failure**

Have O-negative concentrated RBCs in the delivery room. Perform a partial exchange transfusion with packed RBCs to correct anemia and failure (30–50 ml/kg).

C.   **Complications**
1. **Cardiovascular:** Thromboemboli or air emboli, thromboses, dysrhythmias, volume overload, and cardiorespiratory arrest.
2. **Metabolic:** Hyperkalemia, hypernatremia, hypocalcemia, hypoglycemia, and acidosis.
3. **Hematologic:** Thrombocytopenia, D.I.C., over-heparinization (may use 3 μg of protamine for each unit of heparin in donor unit), and transfusion reaction.
4. **Infectious:** Hepatitis, HIV, and bacteremia.
5. **Mechanical:** Injury to donor cells (especially from overheating), vascular or cardiac perforation, and blood loss.

VIII.   **BONE MARROW ASPIRATION**
A.   **General Comments**
1. Always use sterile surgical technique for bone marrow aspirations.
2. In children from birth to 3 months of age, the tibia is the preferred site for aspiration.
3. In children over 3 months of age, the posterior iliac crest is a technically superior site.
4. Anesthetize skin, soft tissue, and periosteum with local anesthetic.
5. Insert needle with a boring motion and steady but not excessive pressure; direct needle perpendicular to the surface of the bone.
6. When the needle enters the marrow space, decreased resistance may be felt. The needle becomes anchored in place.
7. Do not aspirate more than 0.2 ml of marrow to prevent dilution with sinusoidal blood.

B.   **Iliac Crest Marrow Technique**
1. Position patient on a firm table in the lateral recumbent position (with neck, knees, and hips flexed), or prone with a pillow under the pelvis to elevate it slightly.

2. Enter the ileum at the posterior superior iliac spine, which is a visible and palpable bony prominence superior and lateral to the intergluteal cleft. It is inferior and medial to the crest.

C. **Smear Technique**
   1. Eject marrow from syringe onto clean slide.
   2. With another syringe and needle, aspirate excessive blood and plasma from marrow to concentrate it.
   3. Use remaining marrow to make multiple smears in usual way.

IX. **CHEST TUBE: PNEUMOTHORAX/HEMOTHORAX**
A. **Technique**

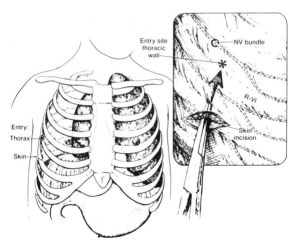

FIG 4.5.
Chest tube placement.

Ref: Nichols: *Golden Hour,* St Louis, Mosby, 1991, p 317.

1. For infants, position with the affected side up. For seriously ill children position supine. Preferably, chest tubes are placed in the third to fifth intercostal space in the midaxillary line, avoiding breast tissue.
2. If necessary, temporarily decompress pneumothorax by inserting a "butterfly" or angiocatheter in the same location or in the ipsilateral anterior 2nd intercostal space.
3. After cleaning and anesthetizing the area locally with 0.5% lidocaine, make an 0.5 cm incision directly over the rib below the desired interspace. Insert a small curved hemostat to bluntly dissect a track over the superior margin of the rib through the intercostal muscles and into the pleural cavity.
4. Place clamp 0.5–1.0 cm from tip of chest tube and pass through previously punctured space into pleural cavity. Angle tube anteriorly and superiorly and insert tube desired distance.
5. Secure tube to chest wall with suture through skin incision and then around tube. Cover incision with petroleum gauze and a sterile dressing.
6. Confirm position and function with chest x-ray.

B. **Complications:** Lung perforation, hemorrhage, scarring, and tube malposition.

Ref: Henderson R. Pediatrics 1976; 58:861.

X. **THORACENTESIS**
A. **Indications:** Diagnosis or relief of an abnormal collection of fluid within the pleural space.

B. **Technique**

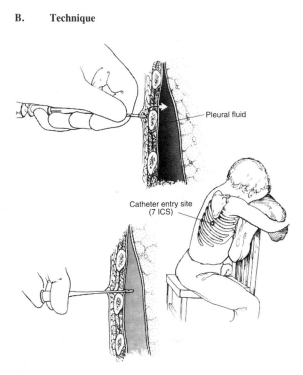

FIG 4.6.
Thoracentesis.

1. Ideally, perform procedure with the patient sitting on the side of the bed, and with an assistant standing in front to support the patient.

2. Select the interspace to be tapped on the basis of dullness to percussion and the level of effusion on the erect chest x-ray. In the event of a small effusion the patient may be tilted laterally toward the affected side to maximize yield.
3. Clean and drape chest.
4. Use of local anesthetic to infiltrate the skin, the underlying tissue and the pleura in the interspace above the rib.
5. Attach a large bore needle or intravenous catheter to a 3-way stopcock and syringe. With needle bevel down, insert needle directly on the rib below the desired interspace, and "walk" needle over superior edge of the rib. Gradually advance the needle; a "pop" is felt upon entering the pleural space. Advance the catheter 2–3 mm, and remove the stylet.
6. Attach syringe with a stopcock to the hub of the catheter and slowly withdraw the desired volume of fluid.
7. At the end of the procedure, withdraw the needle or catheter and place dressing over the thoracentesis site.
8. Obtain follow-up chest x-ray after thoracentesis to rule out pneumothorax.
9. Send pleural fluid for routine lab studies (see below, Paracentesis).

XI. PERICARDIOCENTESIS
A. **Indications:** To remove effusion fluid, purulent material, or blood for diagnostic or therapeutic purposes.
B. **Technique: See Fig 4.7 on p. 73.**
1. Unless contraindicated, sedate the patient. Monitor ECG during procedure.
2. Seat patient at a 30° angle. Have an assistant secure patient.
3. Prepare and drape puncture site. A drape across the upper chest is unnecessary and may obscure important landmarks.
4. Anesthetize the puncture site with 1% lidocaine.
5. Insert an 18 or 20 gauge needle just to the left of the xiphoid process, 1.0 cm inferior to the bottom rib at approximately a 60° angle to the skin.

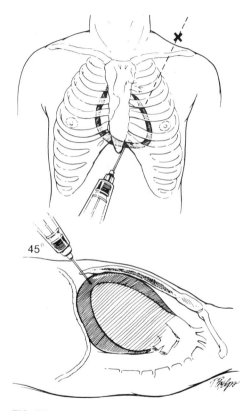

FIG 4.7.
Pericardiocentesis.

Ref: Nichols: *Golden Hour,* St Louis, Mosby, 1991, p 325.

6. While gently aspirating, advance needle toward the patient's left shoulder until pericardial fluid is obtained.

7. Upon entering the pericardial space clamp the needle at the skin edge to prevent further penetration. Attach a 30 ml syringe with a stopcock.

8. Gently and slowly remove the fluid. Too rapid a withdrawal of the pericardial fluid can result in shock or myocardial insufficiency.

XII.   PARACENTESIS

A.   Indications: Diagnosis or relief of abnormal collection of fluid within the peritoneal cavity.

B.   Precautions

1. In performing a paracentesis for therapeutic measures, do not remove a large amount of fluid too rapidly because hypovolemia and hypotension may result from rapid fluid shifts.

2. Avoid scars from previous surgery; localized bowel adhesions increase the chances of entering a viscus in these areas.

3. The bladder should be empty to avoid perforation.

C.   Technique

1. Prepare and drape the abdomen as for a surgical procedure. Anesthetize puncture site.

2. With patient in supine position, insert intravenous catheter just lateral to the rectus muscle in either the right or left lower quadrants, a few centimeters above the inguinal ligament. If patient is placed in semi-Fowler or cardiac position, place needle midline approximately midway between the umbilicus and pubis.

3. Apply negative pressure as catheter is inserted into the peritoneal cavity. Use a "Z" tract technique in most instances.

4. Once fluid appears in the syringe, remove intoducer needle and leave catheter in place. Continue to aspirate slowly until an adequate amount of fluid has been obtained for diagnostic studies.

5. If, upon entering the peritoneal cavity, air is aspirated, withdraw the needle immediately. Aspirated air indicates entrance into a hollow viscus. (In general, penetration of a hollow viscus during paracentesis does not lead to complications.) Then repeat paracentesis with sterile equipment.

6. Send fluid for lab studies, including electrolytes, glucose, protein, cell count, differential, Gram stain, culture (AFB, if suspected), and cytospin (if malignancy suspected).

XIII. EVALUATION OF PLEURAL, PERICARDIAL, ASCITIC FLUID
A. Transudate vs. Exudate

Measurement†	Transudate	Exudate
Specific gravity	< 1.016	> 1.016
Protein (gm/dL)	< 3.0	> 3.0
Fluid:serum ratio	< 0.5	> 0.5
LDH (IU)	< 200	> 200
Fluid:serum ratio (isoenzymes not useful)	< 0.6	> 0.6
WBC	< 1000/mm³ (lymphs)	> 10,000/mm³
RBC	< 10,000	Variable (> 100,000 is suspicious)
Glucose	Same as serum	Decreased
pH*	> 7.2	< 7.0

*Collect anaerobically in a heparinized syringe.
†Always get serum for glucose, LDH, protein, amylase, etc.

B. Other Information

1. For pleural fluid, amylase >500 U/ml or fluid: serum ratio >1 suggests pancreatitis.
2. For ascitic fluid, WBC >800 cells/mm³ suggests peritonitis.

Ref: Fleisher G, et al. Textbook of Pediatric Emergency Medicine, Second Edition, Baltimore: Williams and Wilkins, 1988. Wallach J. Interpretation of Pediatric Tests. Boston: Little Brown and Co, 1983.

XIV. LUMBAR PUNCTURE
A. **Indications:** Examination of spinal fluid for suspected infection or malignancy, or instillation of intrathecal chemotherapy.
B. **Precautions**
1. **Increased intracranial pressure:** Prior to lumbar puncture, perform funduscopic examination. The presence of papilledema, retinal hemorrhage, or clinical suspicion of increased intracranial pressure may be contraindications to the procedure. A sudden drop in intraspinal pressure by rapid release of CSF may cause fatal herniation. If LP is to be performed, proceed with extreme caution.
2. **Bleeding diathesis:** A platelet count of 50,000/mm^3 is desirable prior to LP. Correct any clotting factor deficiencies.
3. **Overlying skin infection:** May result in inoculation of CSF with organisms.
C. **Technique**
1. Position the child in either the sitting position or lateral recumbent position with hips, knees, and neck flexed. Ensure that small infants' cardiorespiratory status is not compromised by positioning.
2. Locate the desired interspace (either L_3-L_4 or L_4-L_5) by drawing a line between the top of the iliac crests.
3. Clean the skin with providone-iodine and 70% alcohol. Drape conservatively so as to be able to monitor the infant. Use a spinal needle with stylet. (Epidermoid tumors from introduced epithelial tissue have been reported.)
4. Anesthetize overlying skin with 0.5% lidocaine.
5. Puncture skin in midline just below palpated spinous process, angling slightly cephalad. Advance several millimeters at a time and withdraw stylet frequently to check for CSF flow. In small infants, one may not feel a change in resistance or "pop" as the dura is penetrated.
6. If resistance is met, withdraw needle to skin surface and redirect angle slightly.

7. Send CSF for appropriate studies: cultures, glucose, protein, cell count and differential, antigen detection tests, and cytospin (if suspected malignancy).

D.   Evaluation of Cerebrospinal Fluid

1. **Cerebrospinal fluid pressure**
   a. Accurate measurement of CSF pressure can only be made with the patient lying quietly on his side. Once free flow of spinal fluid is obtained, attach the manometer and measure CSF.
   b. A recent study has suggested that in quiet patients who are in a lateral recumbent position, CSF pressure may be estimated by the number of drops of CSF that are produced in a fixed amount of time:

Needle Size	Counting Period (sec), With Patient's Temperature	
	<40° C	≥40° C
22 G 1.5 inch	21	20
22 G 3.5 inch	39	37
20 G 3.5 inch	12	11

Ref: Ellis RW, et al. A Simple Method of Estimating Cerebrospinal Fluid Pressure During Lumbar Puncture. Pediatrics 1992;89:895-897.

2. **Cerebrospinal fluid collection:** Collect 3 tubes of spinal fluid under sterile conditions (save a fourth tube if possible for additional studies). Send first tube for culture, second for chemistries, and third for cell count. About 1–2 ml per tube is adequate, although cell count and Gram stain can be done on less than 1 ml. Larger amounts of fluids are needed for special studies (i.e. IgG, myelin basic protein, LDH, antigen studies, cytology).

3. **Appearance:** Record color and clarity. Note presence of coagulae, pellicles, or sediment. Time required for their formation will vary with different diseases; coagulae may form in a short time in suppurative meningitis, whereas tuberculosis meningitis may take 12–24 hours to produce a pellicle.

4. **Microbiology**
   a. Culture: If a hospital laboratory is not readily available, refer to staining and culture techniques described in Microbiology, Chapter 18.

     b. Gram and acid-fast stain (bacteria): If pellicle forms, remove and crush it between 2 clean slides. Pull the slides apart, giving 2 smears. Stain one with Gram stain and the other for acid-fast bacilli. Spin uncontaminated CSF, smear the sediment on a slide and Gram stain it.

     c. India ink (fungi): Place one drop of CSF and one of India ink on a slide and mix well. Cover with coverslip and press out excess fluid. Ring with petroleum jelly. Examine for round organisms with large halos. If the index of suspicion for fungi is high, incubate the preparation at 37° C and reexamine at 24 and 48 hours.

   5. **Hematology, chemistry, and serology:** Send CSF to laboratory immediately for cell count, WBC differential, cell morphology, glucose, protein, and relevant antigen detection studies.

E.   **Normal Laboratory Values**

Cell Count		
Preterm mean	9.0 (0–25.4 WBC/mm^3)	57% PMNs
Term mean	8.2 (0–22.4 WBC/mm^3)	61% PMNs
< 1 mo	0–7 WBC/mm^3	0% PMNs
Glucose		
Preterm	24–63 mg/dl (mean 50)	
Term	34–119 mg/dl (mean 52)	
Child	40–80 mg/dl	
CSF Glucose/Blood Glucose		
Preterm	55–105%	
Term	44–128%	
Child	50%	
Lactic Acid Dehydrogenase		
Mean	20 (5–30 U/L), or about 10% of serum value	
Myelin Basic Protein	<4 ng/ml	
Opening Pressure		
Newborn	80–110 (<110 mm H_2O)	
Infant/Child	<200 mm H_2O (lateral recumbent)	
Respirations	5–10 mm H_2O	

(Continued.)

Normal Laboratory Values (cont.).

Protein

Preterm	mean 115 (65–150 mg/dl)
Term	mean 90 (20–170 mg/dl)
Child	
ventricular	5–15 mg/dl
cisternal	5–25 mg/dl
lumbar	5–40 mg/dl

XV. **TYMPANOCENTESIS**
A. **Indications:** Diagnosis or relief of middle ear fluid.
B. **Technique**
  1. Restrain patient in standard fashion.
  2. Sedation is not usually necessary in infants and toddlers. An anxiolytic may be used with larger child.
  3. If necessary, gently remove cerumen with a wire curette.
  4. Attach 1 ml plastic syringe (containing approximately 0.2 ml non-bacteriostatic saline) to a 22-gauge, 3 inch spinal needle that has a double bend to permit visualization of needle point.
  5. Visualize the posterior inferior quadrant of tympanic membrane using an otoscope with operating head.
  6. Perforate the tympanic membrane and apply negative pressure for 1–2 seconds. Then remove needle quickly.
  7. Send first drop for culture, the next drop for Gram stain. Place one drop each on blood and chocolate agar plates and the rest into thioglycollate broth.

XVI. **URINARY BLADDER CATHETERIZATION**
A. **Indications:** To obtain urine for culture in suspected urinary tract infection or sepsis.
B. **Technique**
  1. Prepare the urethral opening using sterile technique.
  2. In the male, apply gentle traction to the penis in a caudal direction to straighten the urethra.
  3. Gently insert a lubricated catheter into the urethra. Slowly advance the catheter until resistance is met at the external sphincter. Continued pressure will over-

come this resistance and the catheter will enter the bladder. In the female only a few centimeters of advancement is required to reach the bladder.

4. Carefully remove the catheter once the specimen is obtained.

XVII.   SUPRAPUBIC BLADDER ASPIRATION

A.   **Indications:** To obtain urine for culture in suspected urinary tract infection or sepsis. Avoid in children with genitourinary tract anomalies.

B.   **Technique**

1. The infant's diaper should be dry and the infant should not have voided in the 30–60 minutes before the procedure. Anterior rectal pressure in females, or gentle penile pressure in males may be used to prevent urination during the procedure.

2. Restrain the infant in the supine, frog-leg position. Clean the suprapubic area with providone-iodine and 70% alcohol.

3. The site for puncture is 1–2 cm above the symphysis pubis in the midline. Use a syringe with a 22-gauge 1 inch needle and puncture at 10–20 angle to the perpendicular, aiming slightly caudad.

4. Exert suction gently as the needle is advanced until urine enters syringe. The needle should not be advanced more than 2.5 cm. Aspirate the urine with gentle suction.

XVIII. KNEE JOINT ASPIRATION
A.   Indications
Removal of joint effusion causing severe pain or limitations of function. To obtain fluid for diagnosis of systemic illness (collagen vascular disease) or septic arthritis.

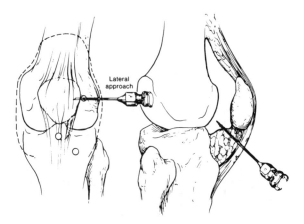

FIG 4.8.
Knee joint aspiration.

Ref: Fleisher G, Ludwig S, Textbook of Pediatric Emergency Medicine, 2nd edition. Baltimore; Williams and Wilkins, 1988:1318.

B.   Technique
1. Secure the child.
2. Prepare and drape for a sterile procedure.
3. Use a lateral approach to avoid neuro-vascular structures. Needle should go under the patella in superior aspect (note that the patella is 1–2 cm in thickness). See Figure 4.8.
4. Anesthetize the aspiration site with 1% lidocaine/bicarbonate. Anesthetize the subcutaneous tissue down to the joint capsule.

5. Localize the under surface of patella. You may flex the knee *slightly* to create space for the injection. Insert an 18 gauge or larger bore needle into the joint space at a 60° angle to the skin. See Figure 4.8.

6. Aspiration of joint contents confirms an intraarticular placement.

7. Collect fluid for microbiologic, chemistry and other studies. See Section VIII.C. Place a dry, sterile dressing over aspiration site when done.

Refs: Fleisher G., et al. Textbook of Pediatric Emergency Medicine. Baltimore; Williams and Wilkins, 1993. Schwartz G.R. et al. Principles and Practice of Emergency Medicine, 1986. W.B. Saunders, Inc. Philadelphia, PA.

C. **Evaluation of Synovial Fluid**

1. **Appearance:** Note quantity, turbidity, pH, clot formation, viscosity, and presence of icterus.

2. **Microscopy:** Examine undiluted specimen for total RBC and WBC count; differential and crystals. Dilute with saline to obtain WBC if necessary. The use of acidic WBC diluting fluids may produce clotting. **Note: A portion of the fluid may be placed in a heparinized tube to prevent clotting. Any cell count >50,000/mm³ must be assumed to represent septic arthritis until proven otherwise. Crystal-induced synovitis is rare in children, with the exception of acute gout in Lesch-Nyhan syndrome or glycogen storage disease.**

3. **Chemistry:** Obtain sugar and protein determinations. Sugar should be within 10 mg/dl of blood sugar. Be sure to obtain sugar before procedure. Normal joint fluid contains little protein.

4. **Mucin:** A qualitative test for hyaluronic acid. To 1 ml of synovial fluid, from which the cells have been centrifuged, add 4 ml water, then 2–3 drops glacial acetic acid, and stir. A tight rope of mucin is normal. In infection and rheumatoid arthritis no precipitate or a loose fibrillar precipitate is formed.

5. **Microbiology:** Gram stain sediment; culture aerobically, anaerobically, and for AFB.

6. **Icterus:** May indicate trauma. Send sample to chemistry lab for bilirubin.

7. **Inflammatory vs. infectious effusions**

Etiology	Appearance	WBC/mm^3 (% polys)	Mucin	Serum Glucose/ Synovial Glucose
Normal	Clear, straw	< 200 (<40)	good	< 2
Inflammatory	Clear to turbid	2–10,000 (~50)	loose friable	≥2
Infectious	Turbid	>50,000 (~75)	loose friable	≥2

8. **Differential Diagnosis**

Disease	WBC	Complement	Rheum. Factor	Other
Gout	↑	↑	Absent	
Pseudogout	↑	↑	Absent	Pyrophosphate crystals
Reiter's	Markedly ↑	Markedly ↑	Absent	Macrophages with ingested WBCs
SLE	Markedly ↓	Low or absent	Variable	LE cells
JRA	↑	Low	Absent	

Adapted from: Hoekelman RA, et al. (eds): Principles of Pediatrics. New York: McGraw Hill, 1978, 1099.

XIX. BASIC LACERATION REPAIR
Note: Lacerations of the hands, genitalia, mouth, or periorbital area may require consultation with a specialist.

A. **Technique**
1. Securely restrain child.
2. Irrigate wound with copious amounts of sterile normal saline. Use at least 60 cc for smaller, superficial wounds; more for larger wounds. This is the most important step in preventing infection.
3. Prep and drape the patient for a sterile procedure.
4. Anesthetize the wound with lidocaine/bicarbonate by infusing the anesthetic into the subcutaneous tissues.
5. Debride the wound and probe for foreign bodies. Consider x-ray if a foreign body was involved in injury.

6. Select suture type for percutaneous closure

Guidelines for Suture Material, Size, and Removal

Body Region	Monofilament* (for Superficial Lacerations)	Absorbable† (for Deep Lacerations)	Duration Time‡ (Days)
Scalp	5–0/4-0	4–0	5–7
Face	6–0	5–0	3–5
Eyelid	7–0/6–0	—	3–5
Eyebrow	6–0/5–0	5–0	3–5
Trunk	5–0/4–0	3–0	5–7
Extremities	5–0/4–0	4–0	7
Joint Surface	4–0	—	10–14
Hand	5–0	5–0	7
Foot/Sole	4–0/3–0	4–0	7–10

*Examples of monofilament nonabsorable sutures: nylon, polypropylene
†Examples of absorbable sutures: polyglycolic acid and polyglactin 910 (Vicryl)
‡As a general rule, the longer sutures are left in place, the more scarring and potential for infection. Sutures in cosmetically sensitive areas should be removed as soon as possible, while sutures in high-tension areas such as exterior surfaces should stay in longer.

7. There are a variety of suture techniques used to close wounds, including (see Figure 4.9)

   • Simple interrupted (for deep or percutaneous closure)
   • Horizontal mattress (for percutaneous closure)
   • Running intradermal ("subcuticular"—for better approximation of deep lacerations)

8. When suturing is complete, apply topical antibiotic and sterile dressing.

9. Check wounds at 48–72 hours for patients with wounds of questionable viability, if wound was packed, or for patients prescribed prophylactic antibiotics. Change dressings at check.

10. For hand lacerations, close skin only, do not use subcutaneous stitches. Elevate and immobilize the hand.

11. Consider the child's need for tetanus prophylaxis.

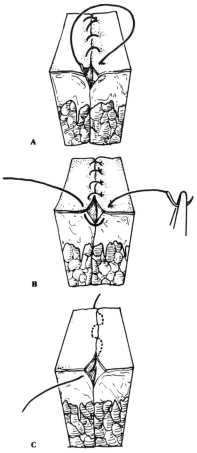

FIG 4.9. Basic skin-closure techniques. **A**, running percutaneous sutures. **B**, interrupted percutaneous sutures. **C**, running intradermal ("subcuticular") sutures.

Ref: Adapted from Trott A, et al. Wounds and Lacerations: Emergency Care and Closure, 1991. Mosby-Year Book, St. Louis. Used with permission.

PART II

Diagnostic and Therapeutic Information

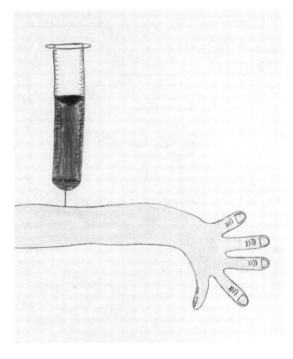

BLOOD CHEMISTRIES

5

These values are compiled from the published literature and from the Johns Hopkins Hospital Department of Laboratory Medicine. Normal values vary with the analytic method used. If any doubt exists, consult your laboratory for its analytical method and range of normal values. The values between the parentheses are normal values according to the International System (SI) of measurement. Hematologic values may be found at the end of Chapter 3, Hematology, and endocrine values may be found in Chapter 10, Endocrinology.

Ref: Meites S, ed. Pediatric Clinical Chemistry, 2nd and 3rd Editions. The American Association for Clinical Chemistry, 1981; Tietz NW. Textbook of Clinical Chemistry, 1986; Lundberg GD, et al. JAMA 1988; 260:73.

	Conventional Units	SI Units
Acid Phosphatase		
Newborn	7.4–19.4 U/L	(7.4–19.4 U/L)
2–13 yr	6.4–15.2 U/L	(6.4–15.2 U/L)
Adult male	0.5–11.0 U/L	(0.5–11.0 U/L)
Adult female	0.2–9.5 U/L	(0.2–9.5 U/L)
Alanine Aminotransferase		
(ALT):		
Infants	<54 U/L	(<54 U/L)
Children/Adults	1–30 U/L	(1–30 U/L)
Aldolase:		
Adult	<8 U/L	(<8 U/L)
Children	<16 U/L	(<16 U/L)
Newborn	<32 U/L	(<32 U/L)
Alkaline Phosphatase		
Infant	150–420 U/L	(150–420 U/L)
2-10 yr	100–320 U/L	(100–320 U/L)
11–18 yr male	100–390 U/L	(100–390 U/L)

(Continued.)

	Conventional Units	SI Units
11–18 yr female	100–320 U/L	(100–320 U/L)
Adult	30–120 U/L	(30–100 U/L)
Alpha-1 Antitrypsin	150–350 mg/dl	(1.5–3.5 g/L)
Alpha Fetoprotein		
Fetal (1st trimester)	200–400 mg/dl	(Peak 2–4 g/L)
Cord	<5 mg/dl	(<0.05 g/L)
>1 yr–adult	<30 ng/ml	(<30 µg/L)
Tumor marker	0–10 mg/ml	
Ammonia Nitrogen		
(Heparinized venous		
specimen in ice water,		
analyzed within 30 min)		
Newborn	90–150 µg/dl	(64–107 µmol N/L)
0–2 wk	79–129 µg/dl	(56–92 µmol N/L)
>1 mo	29–70 µg/dl	(21–50 µmol N/L)
Adult	15–45 µg/dl	(11–32 µmol N/L)
Amylase		
Newborn	0–44 U/L	(5–65 U/L)
Adult	0–88 U/L	(0–130 U/L)
Anti-Hyaluronidase Antibody	<1:256	
Antinuclear Antibody	<1:160	
Anti-Streptolysin O Titer	(4× rise at weekly	
	interval is significant)	
Preschool	<1:85	
School age and adults	<1:170	
Older adults	<1:85	
Note: Alternatively, values		
up to 200 Todd units is		
normal.		
Arsenic		
Normal	0.2–6.2 µg/dl	(0.03–0.83 µmol/L)
Acute poisoning	60–930 µg/dl	(7.98–124 µmol/L)
Chronic poisoning	10–50 µg/dl	(1.33–6.65 µmol/L)
Aspartate Aminotransferase		
(AST)		
Newborn/Infant	20–65 U/L	(20–65 U/L)
Child/Adult	0–35 U/L	(0–4350 U/L)
Bicarbonate		
Premature	18–26 mEq/L	(18–26 mmol/L)
Full term	20–25 mEq/L	(20–25 mmol/L)
>2 yrs	22–26 mEq/L	(22–26 mmol/L)

		Conventional Units	SI Units
Bilirubin (Total)			
Cord	Preterm	<1.8 mg/dl	(<30 μmol/L)
	Term	<1.8 mg/dl	(<30 μmol/L)
0–1 day	Preterm	<8 mg/dl	(<137 μmol/L)
	Term	<6 mg/dl	(<103 μmol/L)
1–2 days	Preterm	<12 mg/dl	(<205 μmol/L)
	Term	<8 mg/dl	(<137 μmol/L)
3–7 days	Preterm	<16 mg/dl	(<274 μmol/L)
	Term	<12 mg/dl	(<205 μmol/L)
7–30 days	Preterm	<12 mg/dl	(<205 μmol/L)
	Term	<7 mg/dl	(<120 μmol/L)
Thereafter	Preterm	<2 mg/dl	(<34 μmol/L)
	Term	<1 mg/dl	(<17 μmol/L)
Adult		0.1–1.0 mg/dl	(2–18 μmol/L)
Bilirubin (Conjugated)		0–0.4 mg/dl	(0–8 μmol/L)
Calcium (Total)			
Premature <1 wk		6–10 mg/dl	(1.5–2.5 mmol/L)
Full term <1 wk		7.0–12.0 mg/dl	(1.75–3.0 mmol/L)
Child		8–l0.5 mg/dl	(2–2.6 mmol/L)
Adult		8.5–10.5 mg/dl	(2.1–2.6 mmol/L)
Calcium (Ionized)			
Newborn <48 hr		4.0–4.7 mg/dl	(1.00–1.18 mmol/L)
Adult		4.52–5.28 mg/dl	(1.13–1.32 mmol/L)
Carbon Dioxide (CO_2 Content):			
Cord blood		14–22 mEq/L	(14–22 mmol/L)
Infant/Child		20–24 mEq/L	(20–24 mmol/L)
Adult		24–30 mEq/L	(24–30 mmol/L)
Carbon Monoxide (Carboxyhemoglobin)			
Nonsmoker		0–2% of total hemoglobin	
Smoker		2–10% of total hemoglobin	
Toxic		20–60% of total hemoglobin	
Lethal		>60% of total hemoglobin	
Carotenoids (Carotenes)			
Infant		20–70 μg/dl	(0.37–1.30 μmol/L)
Child		40–130 μg/dl	(0.74–2.42 μmol/L)
Adult		50–250 μg/dl	(0.95–4.69 μmol/L)

(Continued.)

	Conventional Units	SI Units
Ceruloplasmin		
Newborn	1–30 mg/dl	(10–300 μmol/L)
6 mo–1 yr	5–50 mg/dl	(150–500 μmol/L)
1–12 yrs	30–65 mg/dl	(300–650 μmol/L)
>12 yrs	15–60 mg/dl	(150–600 μmol/L)
Chloride	96–109 mEq/L	(96–109 mmol/L)
Cholesterol	(See Lipids)	
Copper		
0–6 mo	20–70 μg/dl	(3.1–11 μmol/L)
6 yr	90–190 μg/dl	(14–30 μmol/L)
12 yr	80–160 μg/dl	(12.6–25 μmol/L)
Adult male	70–140 μg/dl	(11–22 μmol/L)
Adult female	80–155 μg/dl	
C-Reactive Protein	Negative	
Creatine Kinase (Creatine Phosphokinase)		
Newborn	10–200 U/L	(10–200 U/L)
Adult male	0–175 U/L	(12–80 U/L)
Adult female	10–55 U/L	(10–55 U/L)
Creatinine (Serum)		
Cord	0.6–1.2 mg/dl	(53–106 μmol/L)
Newborn	0.3–1.0 mg/dl	(27–88 μmol/L)
Infant	0.2–0.4 mg/dl	(18–35 μmol/L)
Child	0.3–0.7 mg/dl	(27–62 μmol/L)
Adolescent	0.5–1.0 mg/dl	(44–88 μmol/L)
Adult male	0.6–1.3 mg/dl	(53–115 μmol/L)
Adult female	0.5–1.2 mg/dl	(44–106 μmol/L)
Ferritin		
Newborn	25–200 ng/ml	(25–200 μg/L)
1 mo	200–600 ng/ml	(200–600 μg/L)
<6 mo	50–200 ng/ml	(50–200 μg/L)
<6 mo–15 yr	7–140 ng/ml	(7–140 μg/L)
Adult male	15–200 ng/ml	(15–200 μg/L)
Adult female	12–150 ng/ml	(12–150 μg/L)
Fibrinogen	200–400 mg/dl	(2–4 g/L)
Folic Acid (Folate)	>3ng/ml	(4.0–20.0 nmol/L)
Folic Acid (RBCs)	153–605 μg/ml RBC	
Galactose		
Newborn	0–20 mg/dl	(0–1.11 mmol/L)
Thereafter	<5 mg/dl	(<0.28 mmol/L)

	Conventional Units	SI Units
Gamma-glutamyl Transferase (GGT)		
Cord	19–270 U/L	(19–270 U/L)
Premature	56–233 U/L	(56–233 U/L)
0–3 wk	0–130 U/L	(0–130 U/L)
3 wk–3 mo	4–120 U/L	(4–120 U/L)
>3 mo males	5–65 U/L	(5–65 U/L)
>3 mo females	5–35 U/L	(5–35 U/L)
1–15 yr	0–23 U/L	(0–23 U/L)
16 yr-adult	0–35 U/L	(0–35 U/L)
Gastrin	<100 pg/ml	(100 ng/L)
Glucose (Serum)		
Premature	20–65 mg/dl	(1.1–3.6 mmol/L)
Full term	20–110 mg/dl	(1.1–6.4 mmol/L)
1 wk–16 yr	60–105 mg/dl	(3.3–5.8 mmol/L)
>16 yr	70–115 mg/dl	(3.9–6.4 mmol/L)
Iron:		
Newborn	100–250 μg/dl	(18–45 μmol/L)
Infant	40–100 μg/dl	(7–18 μmol/L)
Child	50–120 μg/dl	(9–22 μmol/L)
Adult male	65–170 μg/dl	(12–30 μmol/L)
Adult female	50–170 μg/dl	(9–30 μmol/L)
Ketones		
Qualitative	Negative	
Quantitative	0.5–3.0 mg/dl	(5–30 mg/L)
Lactate		
Capillary blood		
Newborn	<27 mg/dl	(0.0–3.0 mmol/L)
Child	5–20 mg/dl	(0.56–2.25 mmol/L)
Venous	5–18 mg/dl	(0.5–2.0 mmol/L)
Arterial	3–7 mg/dl	(0.3–0.8 mmol/L)
Lactate Dehydrogenase (37° C)		
Neonate	160–1500 U/L	(160-1500 U/L)
Infant	150–360 U/L	(150–360 U/L)
Child	150–300 U/L	(150–300 U/L)
Adult	100–250 U/L	(100–250 U/L)
Lactate Dehydrogenase Isoenzymes (% Total)		
LD_1 Heart	24–34%	
LD_2 Heart, Erythrocytes	35–45%	
LD_3 Muscle	l5–25%	

(Continued.)

	Conventional Units	SI Units
LD₄ Liver, Trace Muscle	4–10%	
LD₅ Liver, Muscle	i–9%	
Lead (see Poisonings, Chapter 19)		
Child	<10 μg/dl	(<48 μmol/L)
Lipase	20–180 U/L	(20–180 U/L)
Lipids		

Age (yr)	Normal Upper Limits			
	Total Serum Cholesterol, mg/dl (mmol/L)		Serum Triglycerides, mg/dl (mmol/L)	
	M	F*	M	F*
0–4	203 (5.28)	200 (5.2)	99 (0.99)	112 (1.12)
5–9	203 (5.28)	205 (5.33)	101 (1.01)	105 (1.05)
10–14	202 (5.25)	201 (5.22)	125 (1.25)	131 (1.31)
15–19	197 (5.12)	200 (5.2)	148 (1.48)	124 (1.24)
20–24	218 (5.67)	216 (5.62)	201 (2.01)	131 (1.31)
25–29	244 (6.34)	222 (5.77)	249 (2.49)	144 (1.44)
30–34	254 (6.60)	230 (5.98)	266 (2.66)	150 (1.50)
35–39	270 (7.02)	242 (6.24)	321 (3.21)	176 (1.76)
40–44	268 (6.97)	252 (6.55)	320 (3.20)	191 (1.91)
45–49	276 (7.18)	265 (6.89)	327 (3.27)	214 (2.14)

Age (yr)	Normal Upper Limits, mg/dl (mmol/L)*					
	HDL-Cholesterol		LDL		VLDL	
	Males	Females	Males	Females	Males	Females
0–4	—	—	—	—	—	—
5–9	74 (1.91)	73 (1.89)	129 (3.34)	140 (3.62)	18 (0.47)	24 (0.62)
10–14	74 (1.91)	70 (1.81)	132 (3.41)	136 (3.52)	22 (0.57)	23 (0.59)
15–19	63 (1.63)	73 (1.89)	130 (3.36)	135 (3.49)	26 (0.67)	24 (0.62)
20–24	63 (1.63)		147 (3.80)	—	28 (0.72)	—
25–29	63 (1.63)	81 (2.09)	165 (4.27)	151 (3.90)	36 (0.93)	24 (0.65)
30–34	63 (1.63)	75 (1.94)	185 (4.78)	150 (3.88)	48 (1.24)	25 (0.65)
35–39	62 (1.60)	82 (2.12)	189 (4.89)	172 (4.45)	56 (1.49)	35 (0.91)
40–44	67 (1.73)	87 (2.25)	186 (4.81)	174 (4.50)	56 (1.49)	29 (0.75)
45–49	64 (1.66)	86 (2.22)	202 (5.22)	187 (4.84)	51 (1.32)	38 (0.98)

*Use of oral contraceptives significantly raises both total serum cholesterol and serum triglyceride levels.

	Conventional Units	SI Units
Magnesium:	1.5–2.0 mEq/L	(0.75-1 mmol/L)
Magnesium:	1.3–3.0 mEq/L	(0.65–1 mmol/L)
Manganese (Blood):		
Newborn	2.4–9.6 µg/dl	(2.44–1.75 µmol/L)
2–18 yrs	0.8–2.1 µg/dl	(0.15–0.38 µmol/L)
Methemoglobin:	(0–1.3% of total hg)	
Osmolality:	285–295 mOsm/kg	(285–295 mmol/kg)
Phenylalanine:		
Premature	2.0–7.5 mg/dl	0.12–0.45 mmol/L)
Newborn	1.2–3.4 mg/dl	(0.07–0.21 mmol/L)
Adult	0.8–1.8 mg/dl	(0.05–0.11 mmol/L)
Phosphorus:		
Newborn	4.2–9.0 mg/dl	(1.36–2.91 mmol/L)
l yr	3.8–6.2 mg/dl	(1.23–2.0 mmol/L)
2–5 yrs	3.5–6.8 mg/dl	(1.13–2.2 mmol/L)
Adult	2.7–4.5 mg/dl	(0.87–1.45 mmol/L)
Porcelain:	10–25 mg/dl	(no SI conversion factor)
Potassium:		
<10 days of age	3.5–6.0 mEq/L	(3.5–6.0 mmol/L)
>10 days of age	3.5–5.0 mEq/L	(3.5–5.0 mmol/L)
Pre-albumin*	mean ± SD µg/ml	
Premature	130 ± 54 µg/ml	
Full term	189 ± 73 µg/ml	
3 mo	182 ± 11 µg/ml	
6 mo	207 ± 25 µg/ml	
6 mo–2 yrs	192 ± 22 µg/ml	
2–8 yrs	179 ± 37 µg/ml	
8–12 yrs	205 ± 30 µg/ml	
12–18 yrs	219 ± 26 µg/ml	
Adult male	325 ± 54 µg/ml	
Adult female	248 ± 45 µg/ml	

*Ref: Adapted from Valquist A, et al. Scand J Clin Lab Invest 1975; 35:569.

Proteins: (g/L)

Age	Total Protein	Albumin	Alpha$_1$-Globulin	Alpha$_2$-Globulin	Beta-Globulin	Gamma-Globulin
Birth	46–70	32–48	1–3	2–6	3–6	6–12
<1 wk	44–76	29–55	0.9–25	3–4.6	1.6–6	3.5–13
3 mo	45–65	32–48	1–3	3–7	3–7	2–7
3–4 mo	42–74	28–50	0.7–3.9	3.1–8.3	3.1–8.3	1.1–7.5
4 mo–1 yr	56–72	39–51	1–3.4	2.8–8.0	3.8–8.6	3.5–7.5
1–2 yr	54–75	37–57	1–3	5–11	4–10	2–9
2 yr–adult	53–80	33–58	1–3	4–10	3–12	4–14

(Continued.)

	Conventional Units	SI Units
Pyruvate:	0.3–0.9 mg/dl	(0.03–0.10 mmol/L)
Rheumatoid Factor:	<20	
Rheumaton Titer (Modified Waaler-Rose slide test)		
Normal	Negative	
Significant	>10	
Sodium:		
Premature	130–140 mEq/L	(130–140 mmol/L)
Older	135–145 mEq/L	(135–145 mmol/L)
Transaminase (SGOT):		
See AST (Aspartate Aminotransferase)		
Transaminase (SGPT):		
See ALT (Alanine Aminotransferase)		
Transferrin:		
Newborn	130–275 mg/dl	(1.3–2.75 g/L)
Adult	220–400 mg/dl	(2.2–4.0 g/L)
Triglycerides: See Lipids		
Urea Nitrogen:	5–25 mg/dl	(1.8–9.0 mmol/L)
Uric Acid:		
0–2 yrs	2.0–7.0 mg/dl	(0.12–0.42 mmol/L)
2–12 yrs	2.0–6.5 mg/dl	(0.12–0.39 mmol/L)
12–14 yrs	2.0–7.0 mg/dl	(0.12–0.42 mmol/L)
14 yrs–Adult male	3.0–8.0 mg/dl	(0.18–0.48 mmol/L)
Adult female	2.0–7.0 mg/dl	(0.12–0.42 mmol/L)
Vitamin A (Retinol):		
Newborn	35–75 µg/dl	(1.22–2.62 µmol/L)
Child	30–80 µg/dl	(1.05–2.79 µmol/L)
Adult	30–65 µg/dl	(1.05–2.27 µmol/L)
Vitamin B_1(Thiamine):	5.3–7.9 µg/dl	(0.16–0.23 µmol/L)
Vitamin B_2 (Riboflavin):	3.7–13.7 µg/dl	(98–363 mmol/L)
Vitamin B_{12} (Cobalamin):	130–785 pg/ml	(96–579 pmol/L)
Vitamin C (Ascorbic Acid):	0.2–2.0 mg/dl	(11.4–113.6 µmol/L)
Vitamin D_3 (1,25 Dihydroxy):	25–45 pg/ml	(60–108 pmol/L)
Vitamin E:	5–20 mg/dl	(11.6–46.4 µmol/L)
Zinc:	70–150 µg/dl	(10.7–22.9 µmol/L)

CARDIOLOGY   6

I.   CARDIAC CYCLE

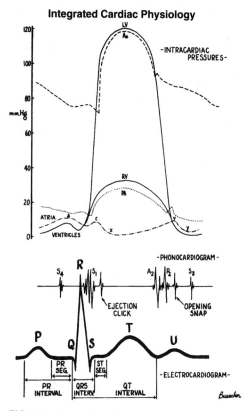

FIG 6.1. The Cardiac Cycle.

II. USE OF THE CHEST X-RAY
A. Heart
    1. Size
    2. Situs (levocardia, mesocardia, dextrocardia)
    3. Although there are "classic" shapes for several well-known lesions (e.g., the "boot" for tetralogy of Fallot, or the "egg on a shoestring" for transposition of the great arteries), the shapes vary widely enough that they are often not useful.

B. Lung Fields
    1. Pulmonary blood flow: decreased in pulmonary stenosis, tetralogy of Fallot, increased in left-to-right shunting lesions.
    2. Evidence of venous congestion in patients with total anomalous pulmonary venous return, mitral valve stenosis/regurgitation.

C. Airway: The trachea usually bends slightly to the right above the carina in normal patients with a left-sided aortic arch; a perfectly straight or left-bending trachea suggests a right aortic arch (which is usually associated with other defects). Also, asplenia and polysplenia syndromes usually have anomalies of the mainstem bronchial branching and lobation.

D. Abdominal Situs
    1. Asplenia/polysplenia syndromes.
    2. Abnormalities of abdominal situs are usually associated with complex congenital heart disease.

E. Skeletal Anomalies
    1. Rib notching (e.g., coarctation of the aorta)
    2. Sternal abnormalities (e.g., Down's syndrome)
    3. Vertebral anomalies (e.g., VATER association)
    4. Limb anomalies (e.g., Holt-Oram syndrome)

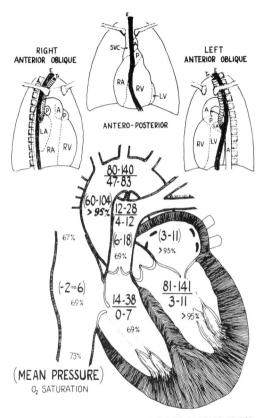

RIGHT ANTERIOR OBLIQUE

LEFT ANTERIOR OBLIQUE

ANTERO-POSTERIOR

$$\frac{80\text{-}140}{47\text{-}83}$$

$\frac{60\text{-}104}{}$ >95%

$\frac{12\text{-}28}{4\text{-}12}$

67%

(6-18)
69%

(3-11) >95%

$\frac{81\text{-}141}{3\text{-}11}$ >95%

(-2 to 6)
69%

$\frac{14\text{-}38}{0\text{-}7}$
69%

73%

(MEAN PRESSURE)
O_2 SATURATION

BASED ON NORMAL PATIENTS 2 MONTHS TO 20 YEARS OF AGE

FIG 6.2.
X-ray contour of the heart, which includes normal pressures and saturations. Plain films of the chest are a valuable part of the initial workup of congenital heart disease.

III. **ELECTROCARDIOGRAPHY**
A. **Lead Placement**
  1. **Bipolar leads**
     a. Lead I: Right arm-left arm.
     b. Lead II: Right arm-left leg.
     c. Lead III: Left arm-left leg.
  2. **Unipolar leads**
     a. aVR: Right arm.
     b. aVL: Left arm.
     c. aVF: Left foot.
  3. **Precordial leads**
     a. V_1: 4th RICS at right sternal border.
     b. V_2: 4th LICS at left sternal border.
     c. V_3: Midway between V_2 and V_4.
     d. V_4: 5th LICS at mid-clavicular line.
     e. V_5: 5th LICS at anterior axillary line.
     f. V_6: 5th LICS at mid-axillary line.
     g. V_3R: V_3 on right chest.
     h. V_4R: V_4 on right chest.
     i. V_7: Posterior axillary line (use if no Q wave in V_6).
B. **Terminology:** (See Figure 6.1.)
  1. **P Wave:** Atrial depolarization.
  2. **QRS complex:** Ventricular depolarization.
     a. Q wave: The first negative deflection before a positive deflection.
     b. R wave: The first positive deflection.
     c. S wave: The negative deflection following the R wave.
     d. QS wave: A monophasic negative complex.
     e. R′ wave: The second positive deflection.
     f. S′ wave: The second negative deflection.
  3. **T wave:** Ventricular repolarization.
  4. **U wave:** May follow the T wave.
C. **Rate**
  1. **Determination**
     a. Standard ECG paper speed is 25 mm/second.
     b. 1 mm = one small square = 0.04 sec; 5 mm = one large square = 0.20 sec
     c. Heart rate = 60 divided by (average R-R interval in seconds)

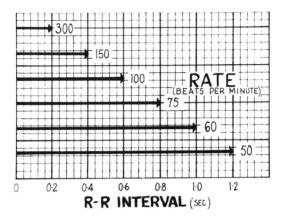

FIG 6.3.
Estimation of the rate based on the R-R interval.

d. Record both atrial and ventricular rates when A-V block is present.
e. Figure 6.3 summarizes the method for estimating the rate based on the R-R interval in 0.20 second increments:

2. **Age-specific heart rates (beats/min)**

Age	2%	Mean	98%
<1 day	93	123	154
1–2 days	91	123	159
3–6 days	91	129	166
1–3 wk	107	148	182
1–2 mo	121	149	179
3–5 mo	106	141	186
6–11 mo	109	134	169
1–2 yr	89	119	151
3–4 yr	73	108	137
5–7 yr	65	100	133
8–11 yr	62	91	130
12–15 yr	60	85	119

D. **Intervals**
   1. **P-R Interval (sec)– Lead II**

Age	2%	Mean	98%
<1 day	0.08	0.11	0.16
1–2 days	0.08	0.11	0.14
3–6 days	0.07	0.10	0.14
1–3 wk	0.07	0.10	0.14
1–2 mo	0.07	0.10	0.13
3–5 mo	0.07	0.11	0.15
6–11 mo	0.07	0.11	0.16
1–2 yr	0.08	0.11	0.15
3–4 yr	0.09	0.12	0.16
5–7 yr	0.09	0.12	0.16
8–11 yr	0.09	0.13	0.17
12–15 yr	0.09	0.14	0.18

   2. **QTc (corrected QT interval)**
      QT interval varies with and should be corrected for rate.
      a. Equation

$$QTc = \frac{\text{measured QT(sec)}}{\sqrt{\text{R-R interval (sec)}}}$$

      b. Normal Values
         QTc should not exceed:
            0.45 in infants < 6 mo,
            0.44 in children,
            0.425 in adolescents and adults.

E. Axis

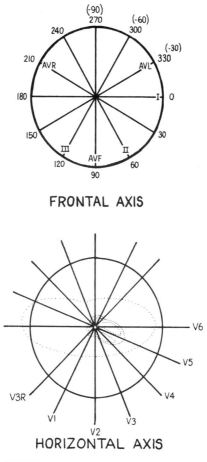

FRONTAL AXIS

HORIZONTAL AXIS

FIG 6.4.

1. **P wave axis:** The normal frontal P wave axis in sinus rhythm is 0–90°.
2. **QRS axis:** The normal frontal QRS axis is age specific:

Age	2%	Mean	98%
<1 day	59	137	−167
1–2 days	64	134	−161
3–6 days	77	132	−167
1–3 wk	65	110	161
1–2 mo	31	74	113
3–5 mo	1	60	104
6–11 mo	1	56	99
1–2 yr	1	55	101
3–4 yr	1	55	104
5–7 yr	1	65	143
8–11 yr	1	61	119
12–15 yr	1	59	130

3. **T wave axis**

Age	V_1, V_2	aVF	I, V_5, V_6
Birth–1 day	±	+	±
1–4 days	±	+	+
4 days-adolescent	−	+	+
Adolescent-adult	+	+	+

+ = T wave positive; − = T wave negative, ± = T wave normally either positive or negative.

F. **Atrial Enlargement**
  1. **Right atrial enlargement (RAE):** Peaked P wave, >2.5 mm (normal standardization = 10 mv/mm) in any lead (best seen in II, III, V_3R, and V_1.)
  2. **Left atrial enlargement (LAE)**
    a. P wave duration >0.08 sec; may have "plateau" or "notched" contour.
    b. Terminal and deep inversion of the P wave in V_3R or V_1.

G.   Ventricular Hypertrophy
1. Normal range for R and S waves
a. Amplitude in V1 (mm at normal [10 mv/mm] standardization):

	R Wave			S Wave		
Age	2%	Mean	98%	2%	Mean	98%
<1 day	5.2	13.8	26.1	0.0	8.5	22.7
1–2 days	5.3	14.4	26.9	0.0	9.1	20.7
3–6 days	2.8	12.9	24.2	0.0	6.6	16.8
1–3 wk	3.2	10.6	20.8	0.0	4.2	10.8
1–2 mo	3.3	9.5	18.4	0.0	5.0	12.4
3–5 mo	2.7	9.8	19.8	0.0	5.7	17.1
6–11 mo	1.4	9.4	20.3	0.4	6.4	18.1
1–2 yr	2.6	8.9	17.7	0.7	8.4	21.0
3–4 yr	1.0	8.1	18.2	1.8	10.2	21.4
5–7 yr	0.5	6.7	13.9	2.9	12.0	23.8
8–11 yr	0.0	5.4	12.1	2.7	11.9	25.4
12–15 yr	0.0	4.1	9.9	2.8	10.8	21.2

b. Amplitude in V_6 (mm at normal [10 mv/mm] standardization):

	R Wave			S Wave		
Age	2%	Mean	98%	2%	Mean	98%
<1 day	0.0	4.2	11.1	0.0	3.2	9.6
1–2 days	0.0	4.5	12.2	0.0	3.0	9.4
3–6 days	0.3	5.2	12.1	0.0	3.5	9.8
1–3 wk	2.6	7.6	16.4	0.0	3.4	9.8
1–2 mo	5.2	11.6	21.4	0.0	2.7	6.4
3–5 mo	6.4	13.1	22.4	0.0	2.9	9.9
6–11 mo	5.8	12.6	22.7	0.0	2.1	7.2
1–2 yr	5.9	13.3	22.6	0.0	1.9	6.6
3–4 yr	8.1	14.8	24.4	0.0	1.5	5.2
5–7 yr	8.4	16.3	26.5	0.0	1.2	4.0
8–11 yr	9.2	16.3	25.4	0.0	1.0	3.9
12–15 yr	6.5	14.3	23.0	0.0	0.8	3.7

2. **Right ventricular hypertrophy—at least one of criteria below:**
   a. R in V_1 above 98th percentile for age.
   b. S in V_6 above 98th percentile for age.
   c. Upright T in V_1 after 4 days.
   d. qR in V_{3R} or V_1.
   e. Normal duration RSR' in V_{3R} or V_1 with R' >15 mm if <1 yr; >10 mm thereafter. (Suggestive of diastolic volume overload–e.g., ASD.)

3. **Left ventricular hypertrophy—at least one of criteria below:**
   a. R in V_6 above 98th percentile for age (suggests volume overload).
   b. Q wave >4 mm in V_5 or V_6 (suggests volume overload).
   c. R in V_1 below 5th percentile for age (suggests pressure overload).
   d. S in V_1 above 98th percentile for age (suggests pressure overload).

4. **Precautions**
   a. In the event of abnormal conduction, abnormal cardiac position, or complex congenital heart disease, these criteria may not be applicable.
   b. There is a gradual progression from LV to RV predominance as an infant approaches term. Therefore, these conventional electrocardiographic criteria for interpretation of ventricular hypertrophy are not reliable in the premature infant.

H. **The ECG and Myocardial Infarction in Children**
   1. **Predisposing conditions:** Myocardial infarction (MI) and ischemia (see below) in children occurs infrequently but can be seen in the setting of such diseases as:
      a. Anomalous origin of the coronary artery from the pulmonary artery
      b. Myocarditis
      c. Kawasaki disease (with coronary artery aneurysms)
      d. Asphyxia
      e. Cocaine ingestion
      f. Adrenergic drugs (e.g., beta-agonists in asthma)

2. **ECG criteria** for MI have not been well-established in children, and adult criteria may not be useful. However, the following criteria have been proposed recently:
   a. New-onset Q waves >35msec in duration
   b. Increased amplitude/duration (>35 msec) of pre-existing Q waves
   c. New-onset Q waves in serial tracings
   d. Notching of Q waves
   e. ST segment elevation (≥2mm) and long QTc (>440 msec) when associated with any other criterion
   Note: These criteria seem to be useful in detecting acute MI but are less useful for diagnosing nonacute MI in children. They may provide a useful adjunct to other tests of myocardial injury, such as CPK/MB fraction and LDH.

   Ref: J.A., Bricker TB, and Garson A. Electrocardiographic criteria for diagnosis of acute myocardial infarction in childhood. Am J Cardiol 1992; 69:1545–1548.

3. **Myocardial ischemia** may be subtle to detect. An ECG may exhibit flat or inverted T waves overlying the ischemic area. In the case of subendocardial ischemia, however, peaked and symmetrical T waves overlie the ischemic area.

   Ref: Garson A Jr. Electrocardiography. In *The Science and Practice of Pediatric Cardiology*, p.742. Philadelphia: Lea and Febiger, 1990.

I. **Conduction and Rhythm Disturbances**
   1. **Sinus arrhythmia:** Normal respiratory variation of the RR interval without morphological changes of the P wave or QRS complex.

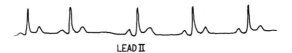

LEAD II

2. **Low right atrial pacemaker ("coronary sinus rhythm"):** Shortened to normal PR interval with negative P in II, III, aVF, and upright in V_6. P wave axis is 180–360°.

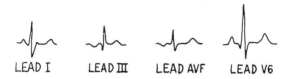

LEAD I   LEAD III   LEAD AVF   LEAD V6

3. **Left atrial rhythm:** Varying P configurations in limb leads depending on site of origin (high, low, mid); however, frequently negative in II, III, aVF, and always negative in V_6. Dome and dart configuration diagnostic of left atrial rhythm with the dome representing the left atrium and the dart the right atrium. Best seen in II and V_1. P wave axis is 90–270°.

LEAD I

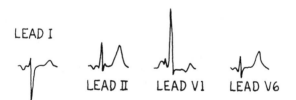

LEAD II   LEAD V1   LEAD V6

4. **Premature atrial contraction (PAC):** Premature beat with abnormal P wave, normal QRS complexes, and usually not followed by a fully compensatory pause.

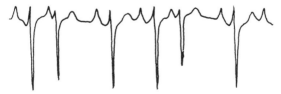

5. **PAC with aberrancy:** Similar to 4, but with wide QRS complex resembling a right bundle branch block (RBBB) or left bundle branch block (LBBB) pattern. The initial vector is often in the same direction as the normal sinus QRS.

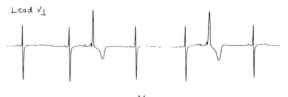

Lead V₁

V₁

6. **Supraventricular tachycardia (PAT or SVT):** Normal QRS complexes at a rapid rate with or without discernible P waves. After the first 10–20 beats, the QRS in SVT almost always has the same morphology as the QRS in sinus rhythm. If after the first 10–20 beats the QRS has a BBB pattern, consider ventricular tachycardia (see Section III.I.18).

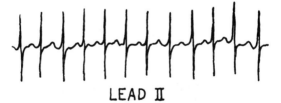

LEAD II

7. **Atrial flutter:** Normal QRS complexes, absent P waves, "flutter waves" between QRS complexes.

LEAD V1

8. **Atrial fibrillation:** Normal QRS complexes, absent P waves, irregularly irregular RR interval.

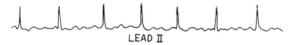

LEAD II

9. **First degree AV block:** PR interval longer than normal for age and rate (see Section III.D.).

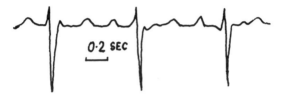

0·2 SEC

10. **Second degree AV block:** Atrial rate greater than ventricular rate with conduction of the atrial impulse at regular intervals, i.e., every other (2:1 block), every third (3:1 block), three atrial for every 2 ventricular (3:2 block).
    a. Type I (Wenckebach): Progressive lengthening of the PR interval until an atrial impulse is not conducted and a ventricular contraction does not occur.

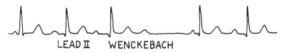

LEAD II   WENCKEBACH

   b. Type II: Paroxysmal skipped ventricular contractions without lengthening of the PR interval.

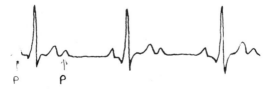

P   P

11. **Complete AV block:** No conducted atrial impulses (complete AV dissociation), with a slow unrelated junctional or ventricular rhythm.

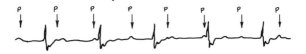

12. **A-V dissociation with junctional tachycardia:** Failed conduction of atrial impulse through A-V node with a faster, independent nodal or ventricular rhythm.

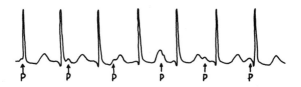

13. **Wolff-Parkinson-White (WPW):** Prolonged QRS duration and shortened PR interval secondary to initial slurring of the upstroke of the QRS (delta wave). Type A has predominantly positive QRS complexes in lead V_1. Type B has predominantly negative QRS complexes in V_1.

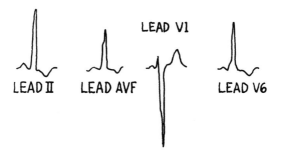

14. **Complete bundle branch block (BBB):** The normal QRS duration is <0.09 for <4 yr, <0.10 for >4 yr. BBB is present when QRS is prolonged.
    a. LBBB: Monophasic R wave in I; absence of Q wave in V_6. (LBBB is rare in children; W-P-W frequently mimics LBBB.)

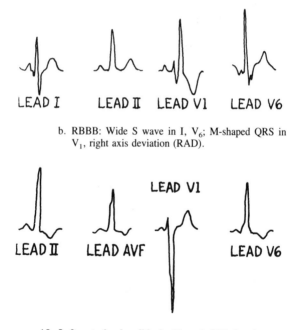

LEAD I   LEAD II   LEAD V1   LEAD V6

    b. RBBB: Wide S wave in I, V_6; M-shaped QRS in V_1, right axis deviation (RAD).

LEAD VI

LEAD II   LEAD AVF   LEAD V6

15. **Left anterior hemiblock:** Normal QRS duration, left axis deviation; qR in I, rS in III.
16. **Premature ventricular contraction (PVC):** Unusually prolonged QRS complexes that always differ morphologically from sinus, ST segments slope away from QRS, and T waves are inverted. PVCs occur before the

expected atrial beat and are usually followed by a compensatory pause. Bigeminy is alternating normal and abnormal ventricular complexes. Couplets are two consecutive PVCs.

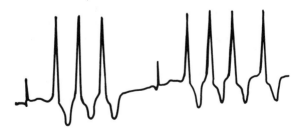

17. **Fusion beat:** Characteristics of both a sinus beat and a PVC. It has the same early activation of a sinus beat and late activation of a PVC. (*arrow* in preceding PVC figure marks fusion beat.)

18. **Ventricular tachycardia (VT):** ≥3 serial PVCs occurring at a rapid rate. P waves, if present, may be dissociated. Usually no Q wave in V_{5-6}. Presence of fusion beats prior to onset or at termination of VT is usually diagnostic. The QRS in VT may not be wide in children. If (after 10–20 beats) morphology of the QRS differs from the sinus QRS, the diagnosis is probably VT (see Section III.I.).

J. Childhood Tachyarryrthmias: Diagnosis: For treatment, refer to chapter on Emergency Management.

	Sinus Tachyarryrthmias	SVT	Atrial Flutter	Ventricular Tachycardia
History	Sepsis, fever, hypovolemia, etc	Usually otherwise normal	92% have abnormal heart	70% have abnormal heart
Rate	Almost always <230/min	60% >230/min. Infants usually 260–300	Atrial 250–500. Ventric. 1:1 to 4:1 conduction	Usual rate <250/min. Infants 200–500
Ventricular rate variation	Over several seconds, may get faster and slower	After first 10–20 beats extremely regular	May have variable block (1:1, 2:1, 3:1) giving different ventricular rates	Slight variation over several beats
P wave axis	Same as sinus almost always visible P waves	60% visible P waves; usually P waves do not look like sinus P waves	Flutter waves (best seen in II, III, aVF, V₁)	May have sinus P waves that are unrelated to V. Tach. (AV dissociation), retrograde P waves, or no visible P waves
QRS	Almost always same as slower sinus rhythm	After first 10–20 beats almost always same as sinus	Usually same as sinus, may have occasional beats different from sinus	Different from sinus (may not be "wide")

Ref: Tables and values for electrocardiography section adapted from: Adams FH, Emmanouilides GC, Riemenschneider TA, eds. Moss, Heart Disease in Infants, Children and Adolescents, 4th Edition. Baltimore: Williams & Wilkins, 1989. Garson A Jr. The Electrocardiogram in Infants and Children: A Systematic Approach. Philadelphia: Lea & Febiger, 1983: 99–118, 396–403. Davignon A, et al. Normal ECG Standards for Infants and Children. Pediatr Cardiol 1979; 1:123–131.

K. Systemic Effects on Electrocardiogram:

	Short QT	Long QT-U	Prolonged QRS	ST-T Changes	Sinus Tach	Sinus Brady	AV Block	V Tach	Miscellaneous
Chemistry									
Hyperkalemia			X	X			X	X	Low voltage Ps; peaked Ts
Hypokalemia		X	X	X					
Hypercalcemia	X							X	
Hypocalcemia		X				X	X		
Hypermagnesemia					X		X		
Hypomagnesemia		X							
Drugs									
Digitalis	X			X		T	X	T	
Phenothiazines		T						T	
Phenytoin	X								
Propranolol	X					X	X		
Quinidine		X	X			T	T	T	
Tricyclics		T	T	T	T		X		
Verapamil						X	T		
Imipramine								T	Atrial flutter
Miscellaneous									
CNS injury		X		X	X	X	X		
Freidreich's ataxia				X	X				Atrial flutter
Duchenne's			X	X	X				Atrial flutter
Myotonic dystrophy			X	X					
Collagen disease				X			X		Low voltage
Hypothyroidism						X	X		
Hyperthyroidism				X	X			X	
Other diseases		Romano-Ward	Lyme disease				X (Holt-Oram, maternal lupus)		

Note: X = present; T = present only with drug toxicity. Ref: Garson A Jr. The Electrocardiogram in Infants and Children: A Systematic Approach. Philadelphia: Lea and Febiger, 1983:172. Walsh EP, Electrocardiography and introduction to electrophysiologic techniques. In: Nadas A, Pediatric Cardiology. Fyler DC, ed. Philadelphia: Hanely and Belfus, 1992:143

IV. ECHOCARDIOGRAPHY

A. 2-D Echocardiogram

1. **Structure and function of heart and vessels:** Useful to examine abnormalities of the great arteries, semilunar valves, A-V valves, atria and atrial septum, ventricles and ventricular septum, the systemic and pulmonary veins, and the proximal coronary arteries. It is also useful for evaluating myocardial function.

2. **Detection of pericardial effusion**

3. **Masses**

4. **Insertion of central catheter**

   Note: Angiography may be superior to ultrasound for detecting defects which are inaccessible to the beam or beyond the resolution of the system, for instance, muscular VSDs (unless combined with color flow mapping); branch pulmonary artery anatomy; aortopulmonary collaterals; anomalous pulmonary veins; distal coronary artery anatomy; and, sometimes, lesions of the descending aorta. Chest and abdominal wall defects, prior chest surgery, certain lung problems, and large patient size may also limit the usefulness of echocardiography because of the poor window afforded.

B. M-Mode Echocardiogram

1. More accurate for calculation of standardized indices and measurement of structures.

2. **Useful for assessing ventricular function.** M-mode echocardiography can be used serially to detect changes (e.g., size of the aortic root in a patient who has the Marfan syndrome).

C. Doppler Echocardiography

Doppler technology includes pulsed wave, continuous wave, and color flow mapping. The Doppler principle is used to convert changes between transmitted and received ultrasound frequencies to *velocity of blood flow.* When coupled with a 2-D echocardiogram, doppler is sensitive for the detection and quantification of valvular stenosis or regurgitation, vascular stenosis, and atrial, ventricular, or arterial shunting.

Ref: Sanders SP. Echocardiography. In Nadas' Pediatric Cardiology, pp.159–186. DC Fyler, ed. Hanley and Belfus, Philadelphia, 1992.

V. OXYGEN CHALLENGE TEST

A. **Technique:** Used to evaluate etiology of cyanosis in neonates. Obtain baseline ABG or pulse oximetry saturation at $FiO_2 = 0.21$, then place infant in oxygen hood at $FiO_2 = 1.00$ for a minimum of 10 min and repeat ABG or pulse oximetry. Pulse oximetry will not be useful for following the change in oxygenation once the saturations reach 100% (approximately $pO_2 \geq 90$).

B. **Interpretation**

	$F_iO_2 = .21$ PaO_2 (% saturation)		$F_iO_2 = 1.00$ PaO_2 (% saturation)	$PaCO_2$
Normal	70 (95)		>200 (100)	35
Pulmonary disease	50 (85)		>150 (100)	50
Neurologic disease	50 (85)		>150 (100)	50
Methemoglobinemia	70 (95)		>200 (100)	35
Cardiac disease				
Separate circulation*	<40 (<75)		<50 (<85)	35
Restricted PBF†	<40 (<75)		<50 (<85)	35
Complete mixing without restricted PBF‡	50 (85)		<150 (<100)	35
Persistent pulmonary hypertension	Preductal	Postductal		
PFO (no R to L shunt)	70 (95)	<40 (<75)	variable	35–50
PFO (with R to L shunt)	<40 (<75)	<40 (<75)	variable	35–50

PBF = pulmonary blood flow.
*D-Transposition of the great arteries (D-TGA) with intact ventricular septum.
†Tricuspid atresia with pulmonary stenosis or atresia; pulmonary atresia or critical pulmonary stenosis with intact ventricular septum; or tetralogy of Fallot.
‡Truncus, total anomalous pulmonary venous return, single ventricle, hypoplastic left heart, D-TGA with ventricular septal defect, tricuspid atresia without pulmonary stenosis or atresia.

Ref: Lees MH, J. Pediatr 1970; 77:484–98. Kitterman JA, Pediatr Rev 1982; 4:13–23. Jones RWA, et al. Arch Dis Child 1976; 51:667–73.

VI. SELECTED CARDIAC PROCEDURES

A. **Cardiac Catheterization Lab Procedures**
   1. **Park:** A knife-tipped cardiac catheter enlarges the intraatrial communication at the foramen ovale.
   2. **Rashkind:** A balloon-tipped cardiac catheter is rapidly pulled across the foramen ovale to create a defect in the atrial septum.

3. **Interventional devices:** Umbrellas, clamshells, and coils are used to close septal defects, PDAs, or collaterals. Stents are used to keep stenotic vessels open.

B. **Closed-heart Procedures**

1. **Shunts** (see Figure 6.5)

   a. **Blalock-Taussig (classic):** Subclavian artery to pulmonary artery anastomosis.

   b. **Blalock-Taussig (modified):** Gore-Tex graft interposed between subclavian artery and pulmonary artery.

   c. **Glenn:** Superior vena cava to right pulmonary artery anastomosis. The original Glenn shunt required ligation of the proximal RPA, while the now more commonly used "bidirectional" Glenn shunt (cavopulmonary anastomosis) allows flow to both the RPA and LPA.

   d. **Potts:** Descending aorta to left pulmonary artery anastomosis.

   e. **Waterston:** Ascending aorta to right pulmonary artery anastomosis.

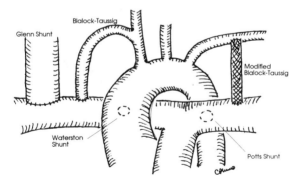

FIG 6.5.
Schematic diagram of cardiac shunts.

2. **Heart**
   a. Blalock-Hanlon: Closed-heart atrial septectomy.
   b. Brock: Closed-heart pulmonary valvulotomy or infundibulotomy.
   c. Waldhausen: Use of left subclavian artery as an onlay patch for repair of coarctation of the aorta.

C. Open-heart Procedures

1. **Mustard:** Intra-atrial baffle (usually pericardium) for repair of simple transposition of the great arteries.
2. **Senning:** Intra-atrial baffle constructed using flaps of native atrial septum and atrial wall as repair for TGA.
3. **Arterial Switch (of Jatene):** Pulmonary artery and aorta transected above valves and switched, for repair of TGA. Coronaries moved from old aortic root to new aorta (former pulmonary root).
4. **Rastelli:**
   a. Placement of valved conduit or graft between right ventricle and pulmonary arteries; used for pulmonary atresia and complex TGA.
   b. Repair of A-V canal by resuspension of mitral and tricuspid valves upon the newly created ventricular septum.
5. **Fontan:** Anastomosis of the right atrium, or the SVC and IVC to the pulmonary artery in order to separate systemic and pulmonary circulations in lesions without two A-V valves and two ventricles (e.g. tricuspid atresia, hypoplastic left heart syndrome).
6. **Norwood** (Palliation for hypoplastic left heart):
   a. Stage 1: Anastomosis of proximal pulmonary artery to aorta, with transection of distal main pulmonary trunk; central shunt between new aorta and distal main pulmonary artery; atrial septectomy.
   b. Stage 2: Modified Fontan. More recently, Stage 2 has been subdivided into two stages: a hemi-Fontan (essentially a Glenn shunt) followed later by completion of Fontan in which the IVC is also directly incorporated into the pulmonary circulation.
7. **Damus-Kaye-Stansel** (For double-outlet right ventricle with subpulmonic VSD): VSD patched to right of PA;

anastomosis of pulmonary artery to aorta; conduit placed between RV and distal main PA.

Refs: Arciniegas E. Pediatric Cardiac Surgery. Chicago: Year Book Medical Publishers, 1985. Fyler DC (ed). Nadas' Pediatric Cardiology. Philadelphia: Hanley and Belfus, 1992.

VII. PAROXYSMAL HYPERPNEA—"Tetralogy Spells":

Emergency management of paroxysmal hyperpnea in cyanotic heart disease. Mechanism is usually infundibular spasm, and may be incited by anything that distresses the infant. The spasm severely reduces pulmonary blood flow and shunts blood right-to-left across the VSD. As with any emergency, the rule **"do what you can do easily first"** applies: oxygen; knee-chest position; morphine; correct underlying abnormalities of volume, anemia, hypoglycemia.

Treatment	Rationale
Oxygen	Reduces hypoxemia (limited value)
Knee-chest position	Decreases venous return and increases systemic resistance
Propranolol	Negative inotropic effect on infundibular myocardium; may block drop in systemic vascular resistance
Morphine	Decreases venous return depresses respiratory center relaxes infundibulum
Phenylephrine HCl	Increases systemic vascular resistance
Methoxamine	Increases systemic vascular resistance
Sodium bicarbonate	Reduces metabolic acidosis
Correct anemia	Increases delivery of oxygen to tissues
Correct pathological tachyarrhythmias	May abort hypoxic spell
Infuse glucose	Avoids hypoglycemia from increased utilization and depletion of glycogen stores

VIII. BACTERIAL ENDOCARDITIS: PROPHYLAXIS
A. Cardiac Conditions
1. **Endocarditis prophylaxis recommended**
   a. Prosthetic cardiac valves, including bioprosthetic and homograft valves
   b. Previous history of bacterial endocarditis
   c. Surgically constructed systemic-pulmonary shunts
   d. Most congenital cardiac malformations
   e. Rheumatic and other acquired valvular dysfunction

      f. Hypertrophic cardiomyopathy
      g. Mitral valve prolapse with valvular regurgitation
  2. **Endocarditis prophylaxis not recommended**
      a. Isolated secundum atrial septal defect
      b. Surgical repair without residua beyond 6 months of secundum atrial septal defect, ventricular septal defect, or patent ductus arteriosus
      c. Previous coronary artery bypass graft surgery
      d. Mitral valve prolapse without valvular regurgitation (thickened or redundant leaflets may be at higher risk for SBE)
      e. Physiologic, functional, or innocent heart murmurs
      f. Previous Kawasaki disease without valvular dysfunction
      g. Previous rheumatic fever without valvular dysfunction
      h. Cardiac pacemakers and implanted defibrillators

B. Procedures
  1. All **dental procedures** likely to cause gingival bleeding, including routine professional cleaning (not simple adjustment of orthodontic appliances or shedding of deciduous teeth)
  2. **Tonsillectomy and/or adenoidectomy**
  3. Surgical procedures involving **intestinal or respiratory mucosa**
  4. Bronchoscopy with a **rigid bronchoscope**
  5. **Incision and drainage of infected tissue** (in addition to prophylactic regimen for genitourinary procedures, antibiotic therapy should be directed against the most likely bacterial pathogens)
  6. Specific **genitourinary and gastrointestinal procedures** including: cystoscopy, urethral dilatation, urethral catheterization if UTI is present, urinary tract surgery if UTI is present, vaginal hysterectomy, vaginal delivery in presence of infection, esophageal dilatation, and gallbladder surgery. In presence of infection, antibiotic therapy should also be directed against likely bacterial pathogens.
  7. In patients with prosthetic heart valves, previous history of endocarditis, or surgically constructed systemic-

pulmonary shunts/conduits, physicians may choose to administer prophylaxis even for low risk procedures involving the lower respiratory, GU, or GI tracts.

8. **Not recommended** in: injection of local intraoral anesthetic (except intraligamentary injections), tympanostomy tube insertion, endotracheal intubation alone, flexible bronchoscopy (with or without biopsy), cardiac catheterization, endoscopy (with or without gastraintestinal biopsy), Cesarean section. In the absence of infection: urethral catheterization, D & C, uncomplicated vaginal delivery, therapeutic abortion, sterilization procedures, or insertion/removal of IUDs.

C. **Antibiotic Regimen**

1. **Dental, oral, or upper respiratory tract procedures**

a. **Standard** regimen: Amoxicillin 50 mg/kg PO 1h before procedure, then half of initial dose 6h after initial dose (**max:** 3.0 gm initial dose, 1.5 gm follow-up dose)

b. **High-risk** regimen (e.g., prosthetic heart valves, history of endocarditis, surgically constructed systemic-pulmonary shunts): Ampicillin 50 mg/kg (**max:** 2.0 gm) plus gentamicin 2 mg/kg (adults 1.5 mg/kg; **max:** 80 mg) IV/IM 30 minutes before procedure; followed by amoxicillin 25 mg/kg PO 6h after initial dose (**max:** 1.5 gm). Alternatively, the parenteral regimen may be repeated 8h after the initial dose.

c. **Penicillin-allergic** patients: Erythromycin (EES or stearate) 20 mg/kg (**max:** EES 800 mg; stearate 1.0 gm) PO 2h before procedure; then half of initial dose 6h after initial dose, or clindamycin 10 mg/kg (**max:** 300 mg) PO 1h before procedure, then half of initial dose 6h after initial dose. For **high-risk** patients: Vancomycin 20 mg/kg (**max:** 1.0 gm) IV over 1h, 1h before procedure. No repeat dose necessary.

d. **Alternate regimens for patients at risk**

1) Patients unable to take PO meds: Ampicillin 50 mg/kg (**max:** 2.0 gm) 30 minutes before procedure IV/IM, then ampicillin at half initial dose

       or amoxicillin 25 mg/kg PO (**max**: 1.5 gm) 6 hours after the initial dose.

2) Penicillin-allergic patients unable to take PO meds: Clindamycin 10 mg/kg (**max**: 300 mg) IV 30 minutes before the procedure; 5 mg/kg IV/PO (**max**: 150 mg) 6 hours after the initial dose.

  2. **Gastrointestinal/genitourinary procedures**

    a. **Standard** regimen: Ampicillin 50 mg/kg (**max:** 2.0 gm) plus gentamicin 2 mg/kg (adults 1.5 mg/kg; **max:** 80 mg) IV/IM 30 minutes before procedure; followed by amoxicillin 25 mg/kg PO 6h after initial dose (**max:** 1.5 gm). Alternatively, the parenteral regimen may be repeated once 8h after the initial dose.

    b. **Penicillin-allergic** patients: Vancomycin IV 20 mg/kg (**max:** 1.0 gm) over 1h plus gentamicin IV/IM 2 mg/kg (adults 1.5 mg/kg, **max:** 80 mg) 1h before procedure. May repeat once 8h after initial dose.

    c. Alternate **low-risk** regimen: Amoxicillin 50 mg/kg PO 1h before procedure, then half of initial dose 6h after initial dose (**max:** 3.0 gm initial dose, 1.5 gm follow-up dose).

D. **Specific Situations and Circumstances**

  1. **Rheumatic Fever:** Antibiotic regimens used to prevent recurrence of acute rheumatic fever are inadequate for the prevention of bacterial endocarditis. Individuals on oral penicillin prophylaxis may have resistant *viridans* streptococci and should be placed on erythromycin or other alternate regimen instead of amoxicillin/penicillin for endocarditis prophylaxis.*

  2. **Patients on anticoagulants:** Avoid IM injections.

  3. **Renal dysfunction:** modify doses in patients with significant renal insufficiency (see Chapter).

  4. Patients undergoing cardiac surgery: Perioperative antibiotics are recommended for patients with cardiac conditions or in whom "hardware" is to be placed. Prophylaxis should be directed against staphylococci and

---

*Editors' note: Children may be on penicillin prophylaxis (e.g., for sickle cell disease) or amoxicillin prophylaxis (e.g., for recurrent otitis media) for conditions other than rheumatic fever; they should placed on an alternate regimen as well.

should be of short duration; modify according to institutional susceptibility patterns.

Adapted from: Committee on Rheumatic Fever, Endocarditis, and Kawasaki Disease of the Council on Cardiovascular Disease in the Young, the American Heart Association; JAMA 1990;264:2919–2922.

IX.   BLOOD PRESSURE NORMS
A.   Blood Pressures, Premature Infants

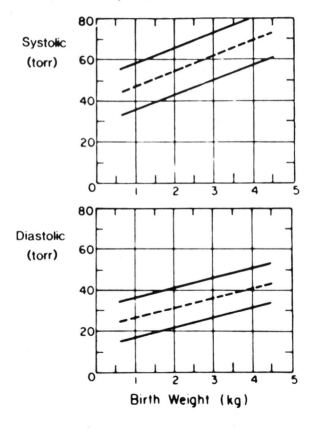

B. Blood Pressures, Ages 0–12 Months

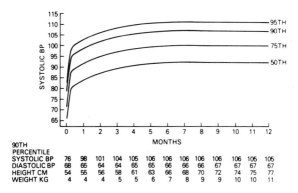

90TH PERCENTILE													
SYSTOLIC BP	76	98	101	104	105	106	106	106	106	106	106	105	105
DIASTOLIC BP	68	65	64	64	65	65	66	66	66	67	67	67	67
HEIGHT CM	54	55	56	58	61	63	66	68	70	72	74	75	77
WEIGHT KG	4	4	4	5	5	6	7	8	9	9	10	10	11

GIRLS

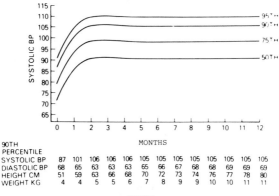

90TH PERCENTILE													
SYSTOLIC BP	87	101	106	106	106	105	105	105	105	105	105	105	105
DIASTOLIC BP	68	65	63	63	63	65	66	67	68	68	69	69	69
HEIGHT CM	51	59	63	66	68	70	72	73	74	76	77	78	80
WEIGHT KG	4	4	5	5	6	7	8	9	9	10	10	11	11

BOYS

Ref: Horan MJ. Pediatrics 1987; 79:1–25 (with permission).

C. Blood Pressures, Ages 1–13 Years

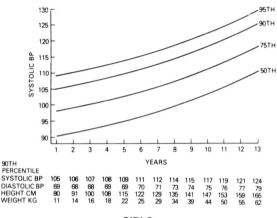

90TH PERCENTILE													
SYSTOLIC BP	105	106	107	108	109	111	112	114	115	117	119	121	124
DIASTOLIC BP	69	68	68	69	69	70	71	73	74	75	76	77	79
HEIGHT CM	80	91	100	108	115	122	129	135	141	147	153	159	165
WEIGHT KG	11	14	16	18	22	25	29	34	39	44	50	55	62

GIRLS

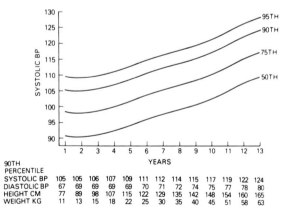

90TH PERCENTILE													
SYSTOLIC BP	105	105	106	107	109	111	112	114	115	117	119	122	124
DIASTOLIC BP	67	69	69	69	69	70	71	72	74	75	77	78	80
HEIGHT CM	77	89	98	107	115	122	129	135	142	148	154	160	165
WEIGHT KG	11	13	15	18	22	25	30	35	40	45	51	58	63

BOYS

Ref: Horan MJ. Pediatrics 1987; 79: 1–25 (with permission).

D. Blood Pressures, Ages 13–18 Years

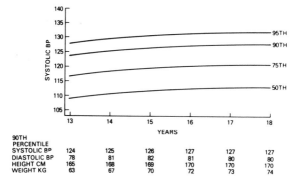

90TH PERCENTILE						
SYSTOLIC BP	124	125	126	127	127	127
DIASTOLIC BP	78	81	82	81	80	80
HEIGHT CM	165	168	169	170	170	170
WEIGHT KG	63	67	70	72	73	74

GIRLS

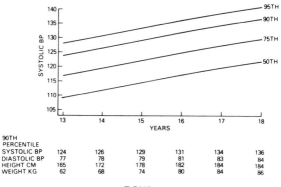

90TH PERCENTILE						
SYSTOLIC BP	124	126	129	131	134	136
DIASTOLIC BP	77	78	79	81	83	84
HEIGHT CM	165	172	178	182	184	184
WEIGHT KG	62	68	74	80	84	86

BOYS

Ref: Horan MJ. Pediatrics 1987; 79:1–25 (with permission).

CONVERSION FORMULAS

7

I. TEMPERATURE
A. Calculation
1. To convert degrees Celsius to degrees Fahrenheit: (9/5 × temperature) + 32.
2. To convert degrees Fahrenheit to degrees Celsius: (temperature − 32) × 5/9.

B. Temperature Equivalents

Centigrade	Fahrenheit	Centigrade	Fahrenheit
34.0	93.2	38.6	101.4
34.2	93.6	38.8	101.8
34.4	93.9	39.0	102.2
34.6	94.3	39.2	102.5
34.8	94.6	39.4	102.9
35.0	95.0	39.6	103.2
35.2	95.4	39.8	103.6
35.4	95.7	40.0	104.0
35.6	96.1	40.2	104.3
35.8	96.4	40.4	104.7
36.0	96.8	40.6	105.1
36.2	97.1	40.8	105.4
36.4	97.5	41.0	105.8
36.6	97.8	41.2	106.1
36.8	98.2	41.4	106.5
37.0	98.6	41.6	106.8
37.2	98.9	41.8	107.2
37.4	99.3	42.0	107.6
37.6	99.6	42.2	108.0
37.8	100.0	42.4	108.3
38.0	100.4	42.6	108.7
38.2	100.7	42.8	109.0
38.4	101.1	43.0	109.4

II. LENGTH AND WEIGHT

A. Length

To convert inches to centimeters, multiply by 2.54.

B. Weight*

Ounces	1 lb	2 lb	3 lb	4 lb	5 lb	6 lb	7 lb	8 lb
0	454 gm	907	1,361	1,814	2,268	2,722	3,175	3,629
1	482	936	1,389	1,843	2,296	2,750	3,204	3,657
2	510	964	1,418	1,871	2,325	2,778	3,232	3,686
3	539	992	1,446	1,899	2,353	2,807	3,260	3,714
4	567	1,021	1,474	1,928	2,381	2,835	3,289	3,742
5	595	1,049	1,503	1,956	2,410	2,863	3,317	3,771
6	624	1,077	1,531	1,985	2,438	2,892	3,345	3,799
7	652	1,106	1,559	2,013	2,466	2,920	3,374	3,827
8	680	1,134	1,588	2,041	2,495	2,948	3,402	3,856
9	709	1,162	1,616	2,070	2,523	2,977	3,430	3,884
10	737	1,191	1,644	2,098	2,552	3,005	3,459	3,912
11	765	1,219	1,673	2,126	2,580	3,033	3,487	3,941
12	794	1,247	1,701	2,155	2,608	3,062	3,515	3,969
13	822	1,276	1,729	2,183	2,637	3,090	3,544	3,997
14	851	1,304	1,758	2,211	2,665	3,119	3,572	4,026
15	879	1,332	1,786	2,240	2,693	3,147	3,600	4,054

*1 lb = 454 gm; 1 kg = 2.2 lb. To convert pounds to grams, multiply by 454.
To convert kilograms to pounds, multiply by 2.2.

Denver II

Name:
Birthdate:
ID No.:

Examiner:
Date:

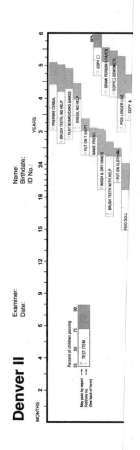

MONTHS   2   4   6   9   12   15   18   24   YEARS   3   4   5   6

Percent of children passing
25 50 75 90
R ↑ ↑ TEST ITEM

May pass by report
Footnote no.
(See back of form)

21. Ask child: What do you do when you are cold?... tired?... hungry? Pass 2 of 3, 3 of 3.
22. Ask child: What do you do with a cup? What is a chair used for? What is a pencil used for?
23. Action words must be included in answers.
    Pass if child correctly places and says how many blocks are on paper. (1, 5).
24. Tell child: Put block on table; under table; in front of me, behind me. Pass 4 of 4.
    (Do not help child by pointing, moving head or eyes.)
25. Ask child: What is a ball?... lake?... desk?... house?... banana?... curtain?... ceiling?... fence? Pass, if defined in terms
    of use, shape, what it is made of, or general category (such as banana is fruit, not just yellow). Pass 5 of 8, 7 of 8.
26. Ask child: If a horse is big, a mouse is ___? If fire is hot, ice is ___? If the sun shines during the day, the moon shines
    during the ___? Pass 2 of 3.
27. Child may use wall or rail only, not person. May not crawl.
28. Child must throw ball overhand 3 feet to within arm's reach of tester.
29. Child must perform standing broad jump over width of test sheet (8 1/2 inches).
30. Tell child to walk forward, ⟶⟵⟶⟵⟶⟵⟶ heel within 1 inch of toe. Tester may demonstrate.
    Child must walk 4 consecutive steps.
31. In the second year, half of normal children are non-compliant.

OBSERVATIONS:

DIRECTIONS FOR ADMINISTRATION

1. Try to get child to smile by smiling, talking or waving. Do not touch him/her.
2. Child must stare at hand several seconds.
3. Parent may help guide toothbrush and put toothpaste on brush.
4. Child does not have to be able to tie shoes or button/zip in the back.
5. Move yarn slowly in an arc from one side to the other, about 8" above child's face.
6. Pass if child grasps rattle when it is touched to the backs or tips of fingers.
7. Pass if child tries to see where yarn went. Yarn should be dropped quickly from sight from tester's hand without arm movement.
8. Child must transfer cube from hand to hand without help of body, mouth, or table.
9. Pass if child picks up raisin with any part of thumb and finger.
10. Line can vary only 30 degrees or less from tester's line.
11. Make a fist with thumb pointing upward and wiggle only the thumb. Pass if child imitates and does not move any fingers other than the thumb.

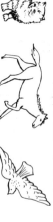

12. Pass any enclosed form. Fail continuous round motions.

13. Which line is longer? (Not bigger.) Turn paper upside down and repeat. (pass 3 of 3 or 5 of 6)

14. Pass any lines crossing near midpoint.

15. Have child copy first. If failed, demonstrate.

When giving items 12, 14, and 15, do not name the forms. Do not demonstrate 12 and 14.

16. When scoring, each pair (2 arms, 2 legs, etc.) counts as one part.
17. Place one cube in cup and shake gently near child's ear, but out of sight. Repeat for other ear.
18. Point to picture and have child name it. (No credit is given for sounds only.)

If less than 4 pictures are named correctly, have child point to picture as each is named by tester.

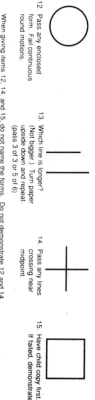

DEVELOPMENT 8

I. **DEFINITIONS:** Since development takes place in an orderly and sequential manner, the phenomena of developmental delay, dissociation, and deviancy are important in the detection of developmental disabilities.

A. **Delay:** Refers to a performance significantly below average in a given area of skill. A developmental quotient below 70 constitutes developmental delay.

B. **Dissociation:** Refers to a substantial difference in the rate of development between two areas of skill. Examples include the cognitive-motor differences in some children with mental retardation or cerebral palsy.

C. **Deviancy:** Refers to nonsequential development within a given area of skill. For example, the development of hand preference at 12 months is a departure from the normal sequence, and may be related to difficulty with the other extremity.

D. **Developmental Quotient (DQ)**
   1. Reflects the child's rate of development:

$$DQ = \frac{\text{developmental age}}{\text{chronological age}} \times 100$$

   2. Two separate developmental assessments are more predictive than a single assessment. Testing must be performed in all areas of development.
   3. Language remains the best predictor of future intellectual endowment. Language development can be divided into two streams, receptive and expressive, each assigned a separate DQ. Language should serve as the common denominator comparing its rate of development with other skills, including gross motor, problem solving, adaptive, and social.

   Ref: Capute AJ, et al Orthop Clin North Am 1981; 12:3–22

II. **MENTAL RETARDATION:** On May 26, 1992, AAMR approved a new definition for mental retardation:

> "Mental retardation refers to substantial limitations in present functioning. It is characterized by significantly subaverage intellectual functioning (IQ below 70–75), existing concurrently with related limitations in two or more of the following adaptive skill areas: communications, self-care, home living, social skills, community use, self direction, health and safety, functional academics, leisure, and work. Mental retardation manifests itself before age 18."

Ref: Mental retardation: Definition, classification, and systems of supports. Special 9th edition. American Association on Mental Retardation, 1992.

Degree of Mental Retardation*	Measured Intelligence Quotient	Expected Mental Age as an Adult (yr)
"Low Normal"	80–90	—
"Borderline"	70–79	—
Mild (Educable)	55–69	9–11
Moderate (Trainable)	40–54	5–8
Severe	25–39	3–5
Profound	Below 25	Below 3

*Based on Wechsler scales.

III. **DEVELOPMENTAL SCREENING**

A. **Denver Developmental Screening Test (Denver II):** (See fold-out following page 130.

B. **CAT/CLAMS**
1. **CLAMS** (Clinical Linguistic and Auditory Milestone Scale): Developed, standardized, and validated for office screening of language development from birth to 36 months of age.
2. **CAT** (Clinical Adaptive Test): Consists of problem-solving items adapted from well-standardized infant psychological tests.
3. **Scoring:** A rate of development can be derived by assigning an age to the child's best performance and dividing it by chronological age (with age adjustments for prematurity). This yields a developmental quotient (DQ). For example a 12 month old performing at a 9 month level has a DQ of 75%. A child with a DQ of less than 80 should have an evaluation to rule out mental retardation or hear-

ing impairment. Dissociation between the CAT/CLAMS components can identify and can help differentiate between cerebral palsy, mental retardation, and communication disorders.

Streams of Development

Disorder	Gross Motor	Language (CLAMS)	Problem Solving (CAT)	Personal/Social
Cerebral palsy	Decreased	Normal	Normal	Normal to decreased
Mental retardation	Normal	Decreased	Decreased	Decreased
Communication disorder	Normal	Decreased	Normal	Normal to decreased

Ref: Capute A et al. Contemp Pediatr 4:(PP), 1987.

Age (mo)	CLAMS	Yes	No	CAT	Yes	No
1	1. Alerts to sound (0.5)*	__	__	1. Visually fixates momentarily upon red ring (0.5)	__	__
	2. Soothes when picked up (0.5)	__	__	2. Chin off table in prone (0.5)	__	__
2	1. Social smile (1.0)*	__	__	1. Visually follows ring horizontally and vertically (0.5)	__	__
				2. Chest off table prone (0.5)	__	__
3	1. Cooing (1.0)	__	__	1. Visually follows ring in circle (0.3)	__	__
				2. Supports on forearms in prone (0.3)	__	__
				3. Visual threat (0.3)	__	__
4	1. Orients to voice (0.5)*	__	__	1. Unfisted (0.3)	__	__
	2. Laughs aloud (0.5)	__	__	2. Manipulates fingers (0.3)	__	__
				3. Supports on wrists in prone (0.3)	__	__
5	1. Orients toward bell laterally (0.3)*	__	__	1. Pulls down rings (0.3)	__	__
	2. Ah-goo (0.3)	__	__	2. Transfers (0.3)	__	__
	3. Razzing (0.3)	__	__	3. Regards pellet (0.3)	__	__
6	1. Babbling (1.0)	__	__	1. Obtains cube (0.3)	__	__
				2. Lifts cup (0.3)	__	__
				3. Radial rake (0.3)	__	__

(Continued.)

Age (mo)	CLAMS	Yes	No	CAT	Yes	No
7	1. Orients toward bell (1.0) *(upwardly/indirectly 90°)	—	—	1. Attempts pellet (0.3)	—	—
				2. Pulls out peg (0.3)	—	—
				3. Inspects ring (0.3)	—	—
8	1. "Dada" inappropriately (0.5)	—	—	1. Pulls out ring by string (0.3)	—	—
	2. "Mama" inappropriately (0.5)	—	—	2. Secures pellet (0.3)	—	—
				3. Inspects bell (0.3)	—	—
9	1. Orients toward bell (upward directly 180°) (0.5)*	—	—	1. Three finger scissor grasp (0.3)	—	—
	2. Gesture language (0.5)	—	—	2. Rings bell (0.3)	—	—
				3. Over the edge for toy (0.3)	—	—
10	1. Understands "no" (0.3)	—	—	1. Combine cube-cup (0.3)	—	—
	2. Uses "dada" appropriately (0.3)	—	—	2. Uncovers bell (0.3)	—	—
	3. Uses "mama" appropriately (0.3)	—	—	3. Fingers pegboard (0.3)	—	—
11	1. One word (other than "mama" and "dada") (1.0)	—	—	1. Mature overhand pincer movement (0.5)	—	—
				2. Solves cube under cup (0.5)	—	—
12	1. One step command with gesture (0.5)	—	—	1. Release one cube in cup (0.5)	—	—
	2. Two word vocabulary (0.5)	—	—	2. Crayon mark (0.5)	—	—
14	1. Three word vocabulary (1.0)	—	—	1. Solves glass frustration (0.6)	—	—
	2. Immature jargoning (1.0)	—	—	2. Out-in with peg (0.6)	—	—
				3. Solves pellet-bottle with demonstration (0.6)	—	—
16	1. Four-six word vocabulary (1.0)	—	—	1. Solves pellet-bottle spontaneously (0.6)	—	—
	2. One step command without gesture (1.0)	—	—	2. Round block on form board (0.6)	—	—
				3. Scribbles in imitation (0.6)	—	—

(Continued.)

Age (mo)	CLAMS	Yes	No	CAT	Yes	No
18	1. Mature jargoning (0.5)	— —		1. Ten cubes in cup (0.5)	— —	
	2. 7–10 word vocabulary (0.5)	— —		2. Solves round hole in form board reversed (0.5)	— —	
	3. Points to one picture (0.5)*	— —		3. Spontaneous scribbling with crayon (0.5)	— —	
	4. Body parts (0.5)	— —		4. Pegboard completed spontaneously (0.5)	— —	
21	1. 20 word vocabulary (1.0)	— —		1. Obtains object with stick (1.0)	— —	
	2. Two word phrases (1.0)	— —		2. Solves square in form board (1.0)	— —	
	3. Points to two pictures (1.0)*	— —		3. Tower of three cubes (1.0)	— —	
24	1. 50 word vocabulary (1.0)	— —		1. Attempts to fold paper (0.7)	— —	
	2. Two-step command (1.0)	— —		2. Horizontal four cube train (0.7)	— —	
	3. Two word sentences (1.0)	— —		3. Imitates stroke with pencil (0.7)	— —	
				4. Completes form board (0.7)	— —	
30	1. Uses pronouns appropriately (1.5)	— —		1. Horizontal-vertical stroke with pencil (1.5)	— —	
	2. Concept of one (1.5)*	— —		2. Form board reversed (1.5)	— —	
	3. Points to seven pictures (1.5)*	— —		3. Folds paper with definite crease (1.5)	— —	
	4. Two digits forward (1.5)*	— —		4. Train with chimney (1.5)	— —	
36	1. 250 word vocabulary (1.5)	— —		1. 3 cube bridge (1.5)	— —	
	2. Three-word sentence (1.5)	— —		2. Draws circle (1.5)	— —	
	3. Three digits forward (1.5)*	— —		3. Names one color (1.5)	— —	
	4. Follows two prepositional commands (1.5)*	— —		4. Draw-a-person with head plus one other part of body (1.5)	— —	

*Note: Items are performed by the examiner.

C. Developmental Milestones

Age	Gross Motor	Visual Motor	Language	Social
1 mo	Raises head slightly from prone, makes crawling movements, lifts chin up	Has tight grasp, follows to midline	Alerts to sound (e.g. by blinking, moving, startling)	Regards face
2 mo	Holds head in midline, lifts chest off table	No-longer clenches fist tightly, follows object past midline	Smiles after being stroked or talked to	Recognizes parent
3 mo	Supports on forearms in prone, holds head up steadily	Holds hands open at rest, follows in circular fashion	Coos (produces long vowel sounds in musical fashion)	Reaches for familiar people or objects, anticipates feeding
4–5 mo	Rolls front to back, back to front, sits well when propped, supports on wrists and shifts weight	Moves arms in unison to grasp, touches cube placed on table	4 mo: orients to voice 5 mo: orients to bell (localizes laterally), says "ah-goo", razzes	Enjoys looking around environment
6 mo	Sits well unsupported, puts feet in mouth in supine position	Reaches with either hand, transfers, uses raking grasp	Babbles 7 mo: orients to bell (localized indirectly) 8 mo: "dada/mama" indiscriminately	Recognizes strangers
9 mo	Creeps, crawls, cruises, pulls to stand, pivots when sitting	Uses pincer grasp, probes with forefinger, holds bottle, fingerfeeds	Understands "no", waves bye-bye 10 mo: "dada/mama" discriminately; orients to bell (directly) 11 mo: 1 word other than "dada/ mama"; follows 1-step command with gesture	Starts to explore environment; plays pat-a-cake

12 mo	Walks alone	Throws objects, lets go of toys, hand release, uses mature pincer grasp	12 mo: uses 2 words other than "dada/mama", immature jargoning (runs several unintelligible words together). 13 mo: uses 3 words 14 mo: Follows 1-step command without gesture	Imitates actions, comes when called, cooperates with dressing
15 mo	Creeps upstairs, walks backwards	Builds tower of 2 blocks in imitation with examiner, scribbles in imitation	15 mo: uses 4–6 words 17 mo: knows 7–20 words, points to 5 body parts, uses mature jargoning (includes intelligible words in jargoning)	
18 mo	Runs, throws toy from standing without falling	Turns 2–3 pages at a time, fills spoon and feeds himself	19 mo: knows 8 body parts	Copies parent in tasks (sweeping, dusting); plays in company of other children
21 mo	Squats in play, goes up steps	Builds tower of 5 blocks, drinks well from cup	21 mo: uses 2-word combinations, uses 50 words, and 2-word sentences	Asks to have food and to go to toilet
24 mo	Walks up and down steps without help	Turns pages one at a time, removes shoes, pants, etc., imitates stroke	24 mo: uses pronouns, (I, you, me) inappropriately, understands 2-step commands	Parallel play

(Continued.)

Developmental Milestones (cont.).

Age	Gross Motor	Visual Motor	Language	Social
30 mo	Jumps with both feet off floor, throws ball overhand	Unbuttons, holds pencil in adult fashion, differentiates horizontal and vertical line	Uses pronouns appropriately, understands concept of "1", repeats 2 digits forward	Tells first and last names when asked; gets self drink without help.
3 yr	Pedals tricycle, can alternate feet when going up steps	Dresses and undresses partially, dries hands if reminded, draws a circle	Uses 3-word sentences, uses plurals, past tense; knows all pronouns; minimum 250 words; understands concept of "2"	Group play, shares toys, takes turns, plays well with others, knows full name, age, sex
4 yr	Hops, skips, alternates feet going downstairs	Buttons clothing fully, catches ball	Knows colors, says song or poem from memory, asks questions	Tells "tall tales", plays cooperatively with a group of children
5 yr	Skips alternating feet, jumps over low obstacles	Ties shoes, spreads with knife	Prints first name, asks what a word means	Plays competitive games, abides by rules, likes to help in household tasks

Ref: Capute AJ, Biehl RF. Pediatr Clin North Am 1973; 20:3–25; Capute AJ, Accardo PJ. Clin Pediatr 1978;17:847–853; Capute AJ, et al. Am J Dis Child 1986; 140:694–8. Capute AJ, et al. Devel Med Child Neurol 1986; 28:762–71. Rounded norms adapted from Capute et al. Devel Med Child Neurol 1986; 28:762–771.

IV. **VISUAL-MOTOR SKILLS:** The Goodenough-Harris draw
   a person test (below) and Gesell figures (see Figure 8.1) are
   two screening tests that focus on visual-motor skills and problem solving abilities. For both it is important to observe *how*
   the pictures are drawn as well as the final product.

A. **Goodenough-Harris Draw-a-Person Test**
   1. **Procedure:** Give the child a pencil (preferably a No. 2
      with eraser) and a sheet of blank paper. Instruct child to
      "Draw a person; draw the best person you can." Supply
      encouragement if needed, i.e., "Draw a whole person";
      however, do not suggest specific supplementation or
      changes.
   2. **Scoring:** Give the child one point for each detail present
      using the following guide:

General
   1. Head present
   2. Legs present
   3. Arms present
Trunk
   4. Present
   5. Length greater than breadth
   6. Shoulders
Arms/legs
   7. Attached to trunk
   8. At correct point
Neck
   9. Present
   10. Outline of neck continuous with head, trunk, or both.
Face
   11. Eyes
   12. Nose
   13. Mouth
   14. 12 and 13 in two dimensions
   15. Nostrils
Hair
   16. Present
   17. On more than circumference; nontransparent
Clothing
   18. Present
   19. Two articles; nontransparent
   20. Entire drawing nontransparent (sleeves and trousers)

(Continued.)

21. Four articles
22. Costume complete

Fingers

23. Present
24. Correct number
25. Two dimension; length, breadth
26. Thumb opposition
27. Hand distinct from fingers and arm

Joints

28. Elbow, shoulder or both
29. Knee, hip, or both

Proportion

30. Head: $^1/_{10}$ to $^1/_2$ of trunk area
31. Arms: Approx. same length as trunk
32. Legs: 1–2 times trunk length; width less than trunk width
33. Feet: $^1/_{10}$ to $^1/_3$ leg length
34. Arms and legs in two dimensions
35. Heel

Motor Coordination

36. Lines firm and well connected
37. Firmly drawn with correct joining
38. Head outline
39. Trunk outline
40. Outline of arms and legs
41. Features

Ears

42. Present
43. Correct position and proportion

Eye Detail

44. Brow or lashes
45. Pupil
46. Proportion
47. Glance directed front in profile drawing

Chin

48. Present; forehead
49. Projection

Profile

50. Not more than one error
51. Correct

3. Goodenough age norms

Age (yr)	3	4	5	6	7	8	9	10	11	12	13
Points	2	6	10	14	18	22	26	30	34	38	42

Ref: Taylor E. Psychological appraisal of children with cerebral defects. Harvard Univ. Press, 1961.

B. Gesell Figures:

15 mos.	Imitates scribble
18 mos.	Scribbles spontaneously
2 yrs.	Imitates stroke
2 1/2 yrs.	Differentiates horizontal and vertical line

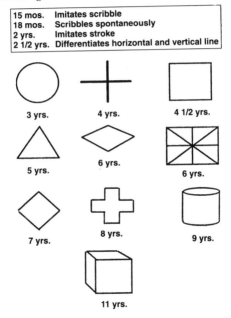

3 yrs.	4 yrs.	4 1/2 yrs.
5 yrs.	6 yrs.	6 yrs.
7 yrs.	8 yrs.	9 yrs.
	11 yrs.	

FIG 8.2.

Gesell figures

Ref: Illingsworth RS: The Development of the Infant and Young Child, Normal and Abnormal, 5th ed., Williams and Wilkins, 1972; p.254; Cattell P: The Measurement of Intelligence of Infants and Young Children. The Psychological Corporation, New York, NY, 1940- revised 1960.

V. **PRIMITIVE REFLEXES:** Intrauterine/birth reflexes appear late in gestation, are present at birth, and are suppressed by 6 months. Late infant reflexes appear following suppression of the birth reflexes. These are the postural reactions which precede voluntary motor function.

Reflex	Age Present (mo)	Age Suppressed (mo)
Intrauterine: birth reflexes		
Palmar grasp	Birth	4
Plantar grasp	Birth	9
Automatic stepping	Birth	2
Crossed extension	Birth	2
Galant	Birth	2
Moro	Birth	3–6
Tonic neck		
Asymmetric	Birth	4
Symmetric	5 mo	8
Lower extremity placing	1 day	—
Upper extremity placing	3 mo	—
Downward thrust	3 mo	—
Late Infant Reflexes		
Landau	3	12–24
(head, trunk and leg extension while prone)		
Derotational righting	4	—
Other Postural Reflexes		
Anterior propping	6	—
Lateral propping	8	—
Posterior propping	10	—

Ref: Adapted in part from: Milani-Comparetti A, Gidoni EA. Dev Med Child Neurol 1967; 9:631; Capute AJ. Pediatr Ann 1986; 15:217.

ENDOCRINOLOGY 9

I. **NORMAL VALUES:** Normal values may differ among laboratories because of variation in technique and in type of radioimmunoassay used. Unless otherwise noted (*), values that follow come from laboratory standards at the Johns Hopkins Hospital. Ranges include 2 SD above and below the mean.

A. **Gonadotropins***

	FSH (mIU/ml)	LH (mIU/ml)
Adult males	1.0–10.3	1.0–10.0
Adult females (not mid-cycle)	1.9–10.2	2.1–15.3
Prepubertal children	0.0–2.0	0.0–1.9

*Normal infants have transient rise in FSH and LH to pubertal levels or higher during the first 3 mo. There is no rise with central gonadotropin deficiency.

Ref: Winter, J. J Clin Endocrinol Metab 1975; 40:545.

B. **Steroid Hormones**
   1. Plasma
      a. Total Testosterone, ng/dl

Adult male	275–875
Adult female	23–75
Pregnancy	35–195*
Prepubertal	10–20
Male, Tanner stage	
2	25–85*
3	52–328*
4	134–532*

   b. Free Testosterone, ng/dl

Adult male	1.4–5.79
Adult female	0.2–0.73
Prepubertal	0.06–0.38

c. Estradiol, pg/ml

Adult male	6–44
Adult female	
Luteal phase	15–260
Follicular	10–200
Mid-cycle	120–375
Prepubertal	<25

d. Androstenedione, ng/dl (increased in most forms of congenital adrenal hyperplasia)

Adult male	69–149
Adult female	74–230
Pregnancy	85–413*
Prepubertal	0–50

e. Dehydroepiandrosterone (DHEA), ng/dl (increased in most forms of CAH and adrenal tumors)

Adult male	195–915
Adult female	215–855
Prepubertal	0–100

f. Dehydroepiandrosterone sulfate (DHEAS), μg/dl (increased in most forms of CAH and adrenal tumors)

Adult male	200–335
Adult female	82–338
Prepubertal	10–60

g. 17,OH-progesterone, ng/dl (increased in most forms of CAH)

Adult male	36–154
Adult female	
(non-pregnant)	
Follicular	15–102
Luteal	150–386
Prepubertal	
Male	0–81
Female	0–92
CAH (well-controlled)	0–430

h. Cortisol, mcg/dl

Any age/sex, 8 A.M.	6–18

2. Urine
   a. 17-ketosteroids, mg/24h (increased in most forms of CAH and adrenal tumors)

Adult male	6–18
Adult female	4–13
Prepubertal	
<1 mo	<2.0
1 mo–5 yr	<0.5
6–8 yr	1.0–2.0
>8 yr	Gradually increases to adult levels

b. DHEA, mg/24h (increased in adrenal tumors)

<15% of total 17-ketosteroids

c. 17, OH-corticosteroids (increased in Cushing's syndrome; decreased in adrenal insufficiency)

Adult male	3–9 mg/24h
Adult female	2–8 mg/24h
Prepubertal	1–5 mg/m^2/24h

d. Free cortisol, mcg/d: 25–125

Ref: Migeon CJ. In Rudolf AM (ed). Pediatrics. Norwalk, Appleton-Lange, 1987; 1474–5; Penny R. Pediatr Clin North Am 1979; 26:113.

C. **Catecholamines:** Urinary catecholamines are elevated with neuroblastoma, ganglioneuroma, ganglioblastoma, and pheochromocytoma. Any urinary catecholamine (total catecholamines, Homovanillic acid (HVA), vanillylmandelic acid (VMA), metanephrines (and dopamine) may be elevated with neuroblastoma, ganglioneuroma, or ganglioblastoma; HVA and dopamine usually are not elevated with neuroblastoma.

24-hour Urine	
Dopamine	100–440 mcg/24 hr
Epinephrine	<15 mcg/24 hr
Norepinephrine	11–86 mcg/24 hr
Metanephrines	<0.9 mg/24 hr
HVA	1–10 mg/24 hr
VMA	2–10 mg/24 hr

Ref: Smith Klein Beecham Clinical Laboratories

D. **Miscellaneous**
   1. Insulin-like growth factor 1, IGF-1, ng/ml (<25 in most growth hormone deficient subjects; elevated with growth hormone excess)

Age	Males	Females
2 mo–6 yr	17–248	17–248
6 yr–9 yr	88–474	88–474
9 yr–12 yr	110–565	117–771
12 yr–16 yr	202–957	261–1096
16 yr–26 yr	182–780	182–780
>26 yr	123–463	123–463

   2. Insulin (fasting), 0–20 microU/ml
   3. Glycosylated Hgb, 5.3–7.9%
   4. Prolactin <18 ng/ml (may be increased with pituitary and hypothalamic tumors and hypothyroidism)

E. Thyroid Function Tests

1. Routine studies

Test	Age	Normal	Comments
T_4RIA (μg/dL)	Cord	6.6–17.5	Measures total T_4 by radioimmunoassay. Values for premature infants below.
	1–3 d	11.0–21.5	
	1–4 wk	8.2–16.6	
	1–12 mo	7.2–15.6	
	1–5 yr	7.3–15.0	
	6–10 yr	6.4–13.3	
	11–15 yr	5.6–11.7	
	16–20 yr	4.2–11.8	
	21–50 yr	4.3–12.5	
T_3RU		25–35%	Measures thyroid hormone binding, not T_3.
T index		1.25–4.20	T_4RIA $\times$ T_3RU
Free T_4 (ng/dl)	1–10 d	0.6–2.0*	Metabolically active form.
	>10 d	0.7–1.7*	
T_3RIA (ng/dL)	Cord	14–86	Measures triiodothyronine by radioimmunoassay.
	1–3 d	100–380	
	1–4 wk	99–310	
	1–12 mo	102–264	
	1–5 yr	105–269	
	6–10 yr	94–241	
	11–15 yr	83–213	
	16–20 yr	80–210	
	21–50 yr	70–204	
TSH-RIA (MIU/ml)	Cord	<2.5–17.4	Best sensitivity for primary hypothyroidism. TSH surge peaks at 80–90 MIU/ml in term newborn by 30 min after birth.*
	1–3 d	<2.5–13.3	
	1–4 wk	0.6–10.0	
	1–12 mo	0.6–6.3	
	1–5 yr	0.6–6.3	
	6–10 yr	0.6–6.3	
	11–15 yr	0.6–6.3	
	16–20 yr	0.2–7.6	
	21–50 yr	0.2–7.6	
TBG (mg/dL)	Cord	0.7–4.7	
	1–3 d	—	
	1–4 wk	0.5–4.5	
	1–12 mo	1.6–3.6	
	1–5 yr	1.3–2.8	
	6–10 yr	1.4–2.6	
	11–15 yr	1.4–2.6	
	16–20 yr	1.4–2.6	
	21–50 yr	1.2–2.4	

2. **Thyroid Antibodies:** High titers are consistent with Hashimoto's thyroiditis.

Interpretation	Antithyroglobulin	Antimicrosomal
Insignificant	<1:40	<1:400
Borderline	1:80	1:400
Significant	1:160–1:640	1:1600–1:6400
Very Significant	>1:640	>1:6400

F. Thyroid Function: Premature Infants

1. Serum T_4(mcg/dl)*

	Estimated Gestational Age (wk)				
Age	30–31	32–33	34–35	36–37	Term
Cord	4.5–8.5	3.3–11.7	4.3–9.1	1.9–13.1	4.6–11.8
12–72 hr	7.3–15.7	5.9–18.7.	6.2–18.6	10.3–20.7	14.8–23.2
3–10 day	4.1–11.3	4.7–12.3	5.2–14.8	7.7–17.7	9.9–21.9
11–20 day	3.9–11.1	5.1–11.5	6.9–14.1	5.4–17.0	8.2–16.2
21–45 day	4.8–10.8	4.6–11.4	6.7–11.9	3.0–19.8	9.1–15.1
46–90 day	6.2–13.0	6.2–13.0	6.2–13.0	6.2–13.0	6.4–14.0

2. Free T_4 (ng/dl)*

GA (wk)[a]	27–28	29–30	31–32	33–34	35–36	37–38
Free T_4	0.03–1.3	0.3–1.2	0.2–1.6	0.5–1.4	0.5–1.7	0.6–1.9

[a]GA = Estimated gestational age (wk)

Ref: LaFranchi SH. Ped Clin North Am 1979; 26:46. Travert G, et al. Clin Chem 1985; 31:1830. Migeon CJ. In Rudolf AM (ed). Pediatrics. Norwalk, Appleton-Lange 1987:1510. Cuestas RA. J Pediatr 1978; 92:963.

II. Sexual Development

A. Penile Length:
Measured from pubic ramus to tip of glans while traction is applied along length of phallus to point of increased resistance. Penile length >2.5 SD below mean is considered abnormal.

1. Newborn: 0 to 5 months (mean ± SD) = 3.9 ± 0.8 cm
2. Premature: Ranges published in Feldman and Smith.
3. Child: Data published in Lee et al.

Ref: Feldman KW, and Smith DW. J Pediatr 1975; 86:395–398. Lee PA, et al. Johns Hopkins Medical Journal 1980; 146:156–163.

B. Testicular Volume (TV) (mean ± SD)

| | \multicolumn{5}{c}{Tanner Stage (Genital)} |
	I	II	III	IV	V
Age (yr)	8.5 ± 3.4	13.0 ± 1.0	14.4 ± 1.2	15.5 ± 1.3	16.6 ± 1.3
TV (ml)	2.3 ± 0.8	5.2 ± 3.0	14.6 ± 3.8	18.6 ± 4.1	22.7 ± 3.3

Ref: Lee VWK, Burger HG. Monogr Endocrinol 1983; 25:44.

C. Clitoris

1. Width: Measured with the labia majora spread and redundant prepuce skin retracted (mean ± SEM).

| 0–6 mo | 3.72 ± 0.25 mm |
| 6–12 mo | 3.94 ± 0 .25 mm |

Ref: Riley RJ, Rosenbloom AL. J Pediatr 1980; 96:918.

2. Anogenital ratio: Distance between anus and posterior fourchette divided by distance between anus and base of clitoris. Ratio >0.5 suggests virilization with labioscrotal fusion.
Ref: Callegari C. J Pediatr 1987; 111:240.
3. Length: Newborn (mean ± SD) = 4.3 ± 1.1 mm.
Ref: Yoyaka S. Horumon To Rinsho 1983; 31:69.
4. Premature infants: Clitoris normally is more prominent because clitoral size is fully developed by 27 weeks gestation and there is less fat in labia majora.

D. Secondary Sex Characteristics

1. Tanner Stages (mean age ± SD)

a. Breast development

Stage I	Preadolescent; elevation of papilla only.
Stage II	Breast bud; elevation of breast and papilla as small mound; enlargement of areolar diameter (11.15 ± 1.10).
Stage III	Further enlargement and elevation of breast and areola; no separation of their contours (12.15 ± 1.09).
Stage IV	Projection of areola and papilla to form secondary mound above level of breast (13.11 ± 1.15).
Stage V	Mature stage; projection of papilla only due to recession of areola to general contour of breast (15.33 ± 1.74).

Note: Stages IV and V may not be distinct in some patients.

b. Genital development (male)

Stage I	Preadolescent; testes, scrotum, and penis about same size and proportion as in early childhood.
Stage II	Enlargement of scrotum and testes; skin of scrotum reddens and changes in texture; little or no enlargement of penis (11.64 ± 1.07).
Stage III	Enlargement of penis, first mainly in length; further growth of testes and scrotum (12.85 ± 1.04).
Stage IV	Increased size of penis with growth in breadth and development of glans; further enlargement of testes and scrotum and increased darkening of scrotal skin (13.77 ± 1.02).
Stage V	Genitalia adult in size and shape (14.92 ± 1.10).

c. Pubic hair (male and female)

Stage I	Preadolescent; vellus over pubes no further developed than that over abdominal wall, i.e. no pubic hair.
Stage II	Sparse growth of long, slightly pigmented downy hair, straight or only slightly curled, chiefly at base of penis or along labia. (Male: 13.44 ± 1.09. Female: 11.69 ± 1.21)
Stage III	Considerably darker, coarser and more curled; hair spreads sparsely over junction of pubes. (Male: 13.9 ± 1.04. Female: 12.36 ± 1.10)
Stage IV	Hair resembles adult in type; distribution still considerably smaller than in adult. No spread to medial surface of thighs. (Male: 14.36 ± 1.08. Female: 12.95 ± 1.06)
Stage V	Adult in quantity and type with inversion of the horizontal pattern. (Male: 15.18 ± 1.07. Female: 14.41 ± 1.12)
Stage VI	Spread up linea alba: "male escutcheon".

Ref: Kaye R, Oski FA, Barness LA. Core Textbook of Pediatrics. Philadelphia: J.B. Lippincott 1988; 188, as adapted from Marshall WA, Tanner JM. Archives Dis Childhood 1969; 44:291 and Marshall WA, Tanner JM. Archives Dis Childhood 1970; 45:13.

2. Pubertal events
   (Mean ages [years ± SD] in American adolescents.)

Male		Female	
Gynecomastia	13.2 ± 0.8	Peak height velocity	12.5 ± 1.5
Voice break	13.5 ± 1.0	Peak weight gain	12.4 ± 1.4
Peak height velocity	13.8 ± 1.1	Axillary hair	13.1 ± 0.8
Peak weight velocity	13.9 ± 0.9	Acne	13.2 ± 0.5
Axillary hair	14.0 ± 1.1	Menarche	13.3 ± 1.3
Acne	14.3 ± 0.8	Regular menses	13.9 ± 1.0

Ref Lee, PA Adolesc. Health Care, 1980; 1:26.

III. TESTS AND PROCEDURES
A. Sexual development
1. **Karyotype:** Purpose: to determine chromosomal sex in patients with ambiguous genitalia. Mosaicism and structural abnormalities (e.g., partial deletions and translocations) may be missed on buccal smear. May take two weeks; if result is needed more quickly, Y-fluorescence can be done within 3 days.
2. **Vaginal Smear**
   a. Purpose: To test for estrogenization of vaginal mucosa; useful in evaluating precocious puberty.
   b. Method: Moisten sterile cotton swab with normal saline and express excess fluid. Carefully insert swab into introitus, scrape vaginal wall and withdraw; avoid contaminating with cells from introitus or perineum. Spread vaginal secretions on glass slide. Add a few drops of saline to make a wet mount. Methylene blue may be used to stain nuclei, but an unstained preparation can also be read. To make a permanent slide for cytopathology, place in 95% ethanol fixative.
   c. Interpretation: Low estrogen states: predominance of round or oval parabasal cells with thick cytoplasm and vesicular nuclei displaying chromatin detail. High estrogen states: predominance of polygonal squamous cells with small pyknotic nuclei and thin cytoplasm. Intermediate cells with squame-like cytoplasm and nuclei with a reticular chromatin pattern may be vari-

ably present, but will predominate in high cortisol or progestin states.

Ref: Frost JK, in Novak ER, Woodruff JD (eds). Novak's Gynecologic and Obstetric Pathology 8th ed. Philadelphia: WB Saunders 1979:689.

3. **Dexamethasone suppression test (DST)**
   a. Purpose: To evaluate premature adrenarche or precocious puberty.
   b. Interpretation: Increased urinary 17-KS (see Section III.C.8.) confirm the diagnosis of CAH. Incomplete suppression of 17-KS suggests that patient has entered puberty. Markedly increased, nonsuppressible 17-KS suggests the presence of an androgen-producing tumor, most likely adrenal in origin.

   Ref: Kelch RP. In Rudolf AM (ed). Pediatrics. Norwalk, Appleton and Lange 1987;1550.

4. **Gonadotropin releasing hormone (LHRH) stimulation test**
   a. Purpose: Measures pituitary LH and FSH reserve. Helpful in the differential diagnosis of precocious or delayed sexual development.
   b. Interpretation: Normal prepubertal children should show no or minimal response to an LHRH injection. Central precocious puberty will have a rise of LH into the adult range.

   Ref: Kelch RP. In Rudolf AM (ed). Pediatrics. Norwalk, Appleton and Lange 1987;1549; Reiter EO et al. Pediatr Res 1975; 9:111.

5. **Human Chorionic Gonadotropin (HCG) stimulation test:** Used to differentiate cryptorchidism (undescended testes) from anorchia (absent testes). In cryptorchidism, following IM HCG testosterone rises to adult levels; in anorchia there is no rise. A 6 week course of HCG may be used to induce descent of cryptorchid testes; the timing and value of this procedure is controversial.

   Ref: Penny, R. In Kaplan SA (ed). Clinical Pediatric and Adolescent Endocrinology. Philadelphia, W.B. Saunders Co. 1982; 312. Lee PA, et al. Johns Hopkins Medical Journal, 1980; 146:159; Garagorri, et al. J Pediatr 1982; 101:923.

B. **Growth**
1. **Adult Height Prediction**
   a. Bayley-Pinneau Method: Uses Greulich and Pyle bone age.
   b. RWT Method: Uses Greulich and Pyle bone age and midparental heights.
   c. Genetic potential formula:
      Boys: Pat + Mat + 5 in/2
      Girls: Pat + Mat − 5 in/2

   Ref: Roche A, et al. Monogr Paediatr 1975; 3:1; Himes JH, et al. Monogr Paediatr 1981;13:1; Roche A, Pediatrics 1975; 56:1026; Tanner JM, et al. Assessment of Skeletal Maturity and Prediction of Adult Height (TW-2 Method). New York: Academic Press, 1975.

2. **Growth Hormone (GH) Detection:** Because GH secretion is pulsatile, a random GH may be low in normal individuals. Diagnosis of GH deficiency requires two abnormal stimulation tests (not screening tests). A single value of >10 ng/ml on a screening or stimulation test will rule out GH deficiency. Patients must be euthyroid for these tests to be valid.
   a. Screening tests
      1) Sleep specimen: Draw GH samples from an indwelling catheter 30 and 60 minutes after onset of sleep. Most subjects will have a rise in GH 45–60 minutes after the onset of nocturnal sleep.
      2) Exercise test: Fast the patient for at least 4h. Get baseline GH level. Exercise the patient for 20 minutes (steady jogging) and obtain a GH sample immediately; 80% or more of normal persons will release significant amounts of GH after vigorous exercise.
      3) IGF-1 (Somatomedin C): May be drawn at any time during the day. May be useful in detecting patients with quantitative or qualitative deficiencies in growth hormone not picked up by standard provocative tests. A clearly normal SM-C level argues against GH deficiency, athough in young children there is considerable overlap between normals and those with GH deficiency. (For normal values see Section I.D.1.)

      Ref: Eisenstein E, et al. Pediatrics 1978; 62:526; Reiter E. Compr Ther 1983; 9(2):45.

b. Stimulation tests: Growth hormone secretion may be stimulated by arginine, insulin-induced hypoglycemia, L-dopa, glucagon, and clonidine. A growth hormone level >10 ng/ml effectively rules out GH deficiency. (Note that some labs use 7 ng/ml as the cutoff for normal/abnormal.) Values between 5–10 ng/ml are equivocal and may indicate partial deficiency. Results less than 5 ng/ml are definitely abnormal.

Ref: Bacon GE, et al. Pediatric Endocrinology, 2nd Edition. Chicago: Year Book Medical Publishers 1982; 85. Weldon VV, et al. J Pediatr 1975; 87:540. Vanderschueren-Lodeweyckx M, et al. J Pediatr 1974; 85:182. Gil-Ad J, et al. Lancet 1979; 2:278. Lanes R, et al. Am J Dis Child 1985; 139:87.

C. **Adrenal and Pituitary Function** (for normal values, see section I.B.)

1. Urinary 17-hydroxycorticosteroids (17-OHCSs)
   a. Measures approximately ⅓ of the end products of cortisol metabolism.
   b. Method: Collect a 24 hour urine specimen. Refrigerate during collection and process immediately (17-OHCSs are destroyed at room temperature).
   c. Interpretation
      1) Decreased in inanition states (anorexia nervosa); pituitary disorders involving ACTH; Addison's disease; administration of synthetic, potent corticosteroids (prednisone, dexamethasone, triamcinolone); 21-hydroxylase deficiency; liver disease; hypothyroidism; newborn period (due to decreased glucuronidation).
      2) Increased in Cushing's syndrome; ACTH, cortisone, or cortisol therapy; medical or surgical stress; obesity (occasionally); hyperthyroidism; 11-hydroxylase deficiency.

2. **Urinary 17-ketosteroids (17-KS)**
   a. Measures some end products of androgen metabolism.
   b. Method: Collect and refrigerate 24 hour urine specimen.
   c. Interpretation
      1) Increased in adrenal hyperplasia (in congenital adrenal hyperplasia it may take 1–2 weeks for 17-KS

to rise above the normally high newborn levels; other signs of CAH would be hyponatremia, hyperkalemia, high 17-OH progesterone, and high androstenedione). Also increased in virilizing adrenal tumors; Cushing's syndrome; exogenous ACTH, cortisone, or androgen administration (except methyltestosterone); stressful illness (burns, radiation illness, etc.); and androgen-producing gonadal tumors.

2) Decreased in Addison's disease, anorexia nervosa, panhypopituitarism.

3. **Plasma corticosteroids**
   a. Method: Collect heparinized blood and separate plasma immediately. Measure cortisol (corticosterone and 11-deoxycortisol sometimes may be needed). Because of the diurnal variation in cortisol concentration, 8 a.m. (the time of peak cortisol level) is the best time to draw plasma cortisol level.
   b. Interpretation: Same as for 17-OHCSs (see above); except usually normal in anorexia nervosa, liver disease, hypo- and hyperthyroidism, and obesity. Elevated levels by protein binding assay occur during pregnancy and during estrogen administration.

4. **Plasma 17-OH progesterone (17-OHP):** Collect heparinized blood and separate plasma immediately. Measures precursor which is elevated with 21- and 11-hydroxylase deficiency forms of CAH.

5. **Adrenal Capacity Test (ACTH Stimulation Test):** Used to evaluate adrenal insufficiency, either primary (Addison's disease), secondary (ACTH deficiency), or due to adrenal suppression after long term steroid treatment. With a normal pituitary-adrenal axis there will be a rise in serum cortisol after IV ACTH. With ACTH deficiency or prolonged adrenal suppression, there will not be a rise in cortisol after a single IV dose, as this will not produce adrenal reactivation. After 3 days of IM ACTH, however, there will be adrenal reactivation with a rise in urinary 17-OHCSs. A lack of response to the IM ACTH stimulation is seen in Addison's disease; a sub-

normal response may be seen with adrenal hyperplasia; a normal response is seen with ACTH deficiency.

Ref: Migeon CJ. In Rudolf AM (ed). Pediatrics. Norwalk, Appleton-Lange 1987; 1474. Styne DM. Pediatric Endocrinology for the House Officer. Baltimore, Williams & Wilkins 1988; 171.

6. **Pituitary ACTH Capacity (Metyrapone) Test:** Metyrapone inhibits 11-hydroxylase in the adrenal and blocks cortisol production. This causes a rise in ACTH, which increases production of cortisol precursors, which accumulate (the measured precursor is 17-deoxycortisol) and are excreted as 17-OHCSs. A failure of 17-deoxycortisol and 17-OHCSs to rise occurs with pituitary ACTH deficiency, hypothalamic tumors, and with pharmacologic doses of steroids.

   Warning: test can precipitate adrenal crisis.

   Ref: Migeon CJ. In Rudolf AM (ed). Pediatrics. Norwalk, Appleton-Lange; 1987:1474.

7. **Insulin-Induced Hypoglycemia:** With insulin-induced (or spontaneous) hypoglycemia, plasma cortisol will normally rise by >10 mcg/dl or to a level of >20 mcg/dl.

8. **Dexamethasone Suppression Test (DST)**

   a. Dexamethasone suppresses secretion of ACTH by the normal pituitary, decreasing endogenous production of cortisol and, hence, also the excretion of 17-OHCSs. Dexamethasone is not excreted as 17-OHCSs.

   b. Standard low-dose and high-dose DST

      1) Method: Give dexamethasone PO for 3 days (low dose: 1.25 mg/m²/day; high dose: 3.75 mg/m²/day divided q6h) and collect 24 hour urine for 17-OHCS. (If using DST to evaluate premature adrenarche, also measure urinary 17-KS and pregnanetriol.)

      2) Interpretation: Normally, and in obesity, low dose DST will cause 17-OHCS to fall to >1 mg/m²/24h. In Cushing's syndrome secondary to adrenal hyperplasia, 17-OHCSs are not suppressed by the low dose DST, but fall with the high dose DST, unless the hyperplasia is due to ectopic ACTH production (lung, mediastinal tumor, etc.). With

Cushing's syndrome due to adrenocortical carcinoma, and with some hypothalamic tumors, 17-OHCSs are not suppressed even with the high dose DST.

c. Overnight screening DST

Give 1 mg dexamethasone at 11 P.M. At 8–9 A.M. the following day, draw a fasting serum cortisol level. In normal or in obese patients, the serum cortisol should fall below 5 μg/dl.

Ref: Migeon CJ. In Rudolf AM (ed). Pediatrics. Norwalk, Appleton-Lange 1987; 1474; Bongiovanni AM. In Kaplan SA (ed). Clinical Pediatric and Adolescent Endocrinology. Philadelphia, W.B. Saunders Co. 1982; 180.

9. **Water Deprivation Test**

a. Used to diagnose diabetes insipidus. Requires careful supervision since dehydration and hypernatremia may occur.

b. Method: Begin the test in the morning after a 24 hour period of adequate hydration and stable weight. Have the patient empty his bladder and obtain a baseline weight. Restrict fluids for 7 hours. Measure body weight, and urinary specific gravity and volume hourly. Check serum sodium and urine and serum osmolality every 2 hours. Hematocrit and BUN also may be obtained at these times but are not critical. Monitor carefully to assure that fluids are not ingested during the test. Terminate the test if weight loss approaches 5%.

c. Interpretation: Normal individuals who are water deprived will concentrate their urine between 500 and 1400 mOsm/L and plasma osmolality will range between 288 and 291 mOsm/L. In normal children and those with psychogenic DI, urinary specific gravity rises to at least 1.010 and usually greater. The urinary-to-plasma osmolality ratio exceeds 2. Urine volume decreases significantly, and there should be no appreciable weight loss. Specific gravity remains below 1.005 in patients with ADH-deficient or nephrogenic DI. Urine osmolality remains below 150 mOsm/L, with no significant reduction of urine volume. A weight loss up to 5% usually occurs. At the end of the test, a serum osmolality >290 mOsm/L, Na >150 mEq/L and a rise of BUN and hematocrit provide evidence that the patient did not receive water.

10. **Vasopressin Test**

a. To test for nephrogenic versus ADH-deficient diabetes insipidus, vasopressin is given subcutaneously and urine output, urine concentration, and water intake are monitored. Intranasal vasopressin is not recommended for this test.

b. Interpretation: Patients with ADH-deficient DI concentrate their urine (to 1.010 and usually greater) and also demonstrate a reduction of urine volume and decreased fluid intake. Patients with nephrogenic DI have no significant change in intake, urine volume, or specific gravity. Constant intake associated with decreased output and increased specific gravity suggests psychogenic DI.

Ref: (For sections 7–10 above): Bacon GE, et al. Pediatric Endocrinology, 2nd Edition. Chicago, Year Book 1982; 258.

D. Thyroid Function

1. Thyroid Function Tests: Interpretation

	T_4RIA	T_3RU	T index	Free T_4	TSH
1st-degree hypothyroidism	L	L	L	L	H
2nd-degree hypothyroidism	L	L	L	L	nl or L
TBG deficiency	L	H	nl	nl	nl
Hyperthyroidism	H	H	H	H	L
L = low; H = high; nl = normal.					

2. **Thyroid Scan:** Used to assess thyroidal clearance, localize ectopic thyroid tissue, and study structure-function of the thyroid. Localizes hyper- and non-functioning thyroid nodules. Chronic lymphocytic (Hashimoto's) thyroiditis frequently will be seen as an abnormal distribution of isotope with irregular thyroidal iodine kinetics (though a scan is generally not necessary to make this diagnosis). Uptake is increased in most types of dyshormonogene-

sis. ^{99m} Technetium-pertechnetate and ^{123}I isotopes are preferred because of their markedly decreased radiation dose compared with ^{131}I.

Ref: Heyman S, et al. J Pediatr 1982; 101:571, Bauman RA, et al. J Pediatr 1976; 89:268; Fisher DA. J Pediatr 1973; 82:1.

3. **Technetium Uptake:** Measures uptake of technetium by thyroid gland during the first 20 minutes after administration. Normal: 0.24–3.4%. Increased in hyperthyroidism. Decreased in TBG deficiency and in hypothyroidism (except dyshormonogenesis, when it may be increased).

4. **Pituitary TSH Reserve Test:** Synthetic TRH can be given IV, which will normally cause a rise in TSH. No rise in TSH in the face of a high T_4 is confirmatory of hyperthyroidism. No rise in TSH in the face of a low T_4 and low TSH suggests pituitary dysfunction. An exaggerated delayed peak TSH response is suggestive of hypothalamic hypothyroidism, but the distinction from normal is not always clear.

Ref: Lee WP. In Kaplan SA (ed). Clinical Pediatric and Adolescent Endocrinology. Philadelphia, W.B. Saunders Co. 1982; 80.

E. Pancreatic Endocrine Function

1. A **random plasma glucose** of >200 mg/dl in the presence of classic symptoms of diabetes (polyuria, polydipsia, ketonuria, and weight loss) is diagnostic of diabetes mellitus.

2. **Oral Glucose Tolerance Test (OGTT)**
   a. Pretest preparation: Calorically adequate diet required for 3 days prior to the test, with 50% of total calories as carbohydrate.
   b. Delay test 2 weeks after period of illness. Discontinue all hyper- or hypoglycemic agents (salicylates, diuretics, oral contraceptives, phenytoin, etc.).
   c. Method: Give 1.75 gm/kg (**max.** 100 gm) of glucose orally after a 12 hour fast allowing up to 5 minutes for ingestion. Mix glucose with water and lemon juice as a 20% dilution. Quiet activity is permissible during the OGTT. Draw blood samples at 0, 30, 60, 120, 180 and 240 minutes.

d. Interpretation: (Venous plasma using autoanalyzer ferricyanide method.) In asymptomatic individuals, diabetes mellitus is diagnosed if the fasting venous plasma glucose is >140 mg/dl and two OGTTs are abnormal. The OGTT is abnormal if the 2 hour sample and one other sample show plasma venous glucose >200 mg/dl.

Ref: American Diabetes Association, 1989.

Note: For management of diabetic ketoacidosis and adrenal crisis, see the Emergency Management chapter.

FLUIDS AND ELECTROLYTES

10

I. MAINTENANCE REQUIREMENTS

A. Caloric Expenditure Method: This method is based on the understanding that water and electrolyte requirements parallel caloric expenditure but not body weight. It is effective for all ages, shapes, and clinical states.

1. Determine the child's standard basal caloric expenditure (SBC):

Age	Weight (kg)	Caloric Expenditure (cal/kg/24 hr)
Newborn	2.5–4	50
1 wk–6 mo	3–8	65–70
6–12 mo	8–12	50–60
1–2 yr	10–15	45–50
2–5 yr	15–20	45
5–10 yr	20–35	40–45
10–16 yr	35–60	25–40
Adult	70	15–20

2. Add 12% of SBC for each degree that patient's rectal temperature is above 37.8°C.
3. Add 0–30% of SBC to account for activity level; e.g., coma (add nothing) or thrashing/tachypnea (add 30%).

4. For each 100 calories metabolized in 24 h, the average patient will need 100–120 cc H_2O*, 2–4 mEq Na^+, and 2–3 mEq K^+, as derived from the table below:
Average water (cc) and electrolyte (mEq) requirements for different clinical states per 100 calories per 24 h

Clinical State	H_2O	Na	K
Average patient receiving parenteral fluids*	110–120	2–4	2–3
Anuria	45	0	0
Acute CNS infections and inflammation	80–90	2–4	2–3
Chronic renal disease with fixed specific gravity	14	Var†	Var
Diabetes insipidus	Up to 400	Var	Var
Hyperventilation	120–210	2–4	2–3
Heat stress	120–240	Var	Var
High humidity environment	80–100	2–4	2–3

*Adequate maintenance solution: dextrose 5%–10% (as needed) in 0.2% NaCl + 20 mEq/L of KCl (= 30 mEq Na and 50 mEq of Cl/L).
†Var = variable requirement.

5. Average water (cc) and electrolyte (mEq) expenditures per 100 calories metabolized over 24 h

Route	Usual			Range*		
	H_2O	Na	K	H_2O	Na	K
Lungs	15	0	0	10–60	0	0
Skin	40	0.1	0.2	20–100	0.1–3.0	0.2–1.5
Stool	5	0.1	0.2	0–50	0.1–4.0	0.2–3.0
Urine	65	3.0	2.0	0–400	0.2–30	0.4–30
Total	125†	3.2	2.4	30–610	0.4–37	0.8–34.5

*High values represent abnormal losses due to environmental variation or pathological states.
†Maintenance H_2O requirements are less than estimated total expenditure, because 5–15 cc of H_2O is produced endogenously during oxidation of carbohydrate, fat, and protein.

B. Holliday-Segar Method: This is a quick, simple formula which estimates caloric expenditure from weight alone; it assumes that for each 100 calories metabolized, 100 cc of H_2O will be required. This method is not suitable for neonates

<14 days old, or for conditions associated with abnormal losses.

	Water (cc/kg)	Electrolytes (per 100 cc H_2O)	
1st 10 kg body weight	100	Na	3 mEq
2nd 10 kg body weight	50	Cl	2 mEq
Each additional kg	20	K	2 mEq

C. **Body Surface Area Method:** This method is based on the assumption that caloric expenditure is proportional to surface area. It should not be used for children <10 kg. It provides no convenient method of taking into account changes in metabolic rate.

H_2O	1500 cc/M^2/24 h
Na	30–50 mEq/M^2/24 h
K	20–40 mEq/M^2/24 h

Ref: Finberg L, et al. Water and Electrolytes in Pediatrics. Philadelphia: WB Saunders, 1982. Behrman R, et al. Nelson Textbook of Pediatrics. 13th ed. Philadelphia: WB Saunders, 1987.

II. DEFICIT THERAPY
A. Clinical Assessment
  1. Clinical observation

% Dehydration	Clinical Observation
5%–6%	HR (10%–15% above baseline)
	Slightly dry mucous membranes
	Concentration of the urine
	Poor tear production*
7%–8%	Increased severity of above
	Decreased skin turgor
	Oliguria
	Sunken eyeballs*
	Sunken anterior fontanelle*
>9%	Marked severity of above signs
	Decreased blood pressure
	Delayed capillary refill
	Acidosis (large base deficit)

*These signs may be less sensitive indicators of dehydration.

2. In hypotonic dehydration (Na^+ <130) all manifestations appear with less fluid deficit, while in hypertonic dehydration (Na^+ >150), the circulating volume is relatively preserved at the expense of cellular water, so that circulatory disturbance is seen later.

B. Deficit Calculation

1. **Intracellular and extracellular fluid composition**

	Intracellular	Extracellular
Na^+	20 mEq/L	145 mEq/L
K^+	150 mEq/L	3–5 mEq/L
Cl^-	—	110 mEq/L
HCO_3^-	10 mEq/L	20–25 mEq/L
PO_4^-	110–115 mEq/L	5 mEq/L
Protein	75 mEq/L	10 mEq/L

Note: Dehydration for <3 days: 80% ECF and 20% ICF losses. Dehydration for ≥3 days: 60% ECF and 40% ICF losses.

2. **Correction of symptomatic electrolyte disturbances**

   a. Formula:

   mEq required = (CD − CA) × fD × weight (kg)
   CD = concentration desired (mEq/L)
   CA = concentration present (mEq/L)
   fD = distribution factor as fraction of body weight
   Wt = baseline weight prior to illness.

   b. Apparent distribution factor (fD):

Electrolyte	fD
HCO_3^-	0.4–0.5
Cl^-	0.2–0.3
Na^+	0.6–0.7

3. **Correction of free H_2O deficit in hypernatremic dehydration:** Free H_2O Deficit = 4 cc/kg for every mEq that the serum Na exceeds 145 mEq/L.

C. Oral Rehydration

1. **Indications:** This method of rehydration has been shown to be effective for treating patients with mild to moderate dehydration. It may be contraindicated in patients with shock, severe dehydration, intractable vomiting, >10 cc/kg/hr losses, coma, or severe gastric distention.

2. **Hemodynamic instability:** In patients with severe dehydration, intravenous therapy should be used initially until pulse, blood pressure, and level of consciousness return to normal. At that time, oral hydration can be safely instituted.

3. **Technique**

   a. Give 5–10 cc of fluid every 5–10 minutes, and increase amount gradually as tolerated. See table of oral rehydration solutions (ORS) in Section II.C.5. Monitor this phase of rehydration in the office, clinic, or emergency room.

   b. Consider administering this fluid with a spoon or small syringe to limit the rate of fluid consumption by the child. Instruct parents to give 1 teaspoon every minute, or every 5 minutes if the child is vomiting. Increase the rate of fluid administration as tolerated.

   c. **STOP** if severe vomiting occurs; small amounts of vomiting should not warrant abandoning this mode of rehydration.

4. **Deficit replacement**

   a. Mild dehydration: 60 cc/kg over 2 h.

   b. Moderate dehydration: 80 cc/kg over 2 h.

   c. Regardless of the degree of dehydration, give 10 cc/kg of rehydration solution for each diarrheal stool seen in the E.R.

5. **Oral rehydration solutions (ORS)**

	Glucose (g/dl)	Na (mEq/L)	K (mEq/L)	Cl (mEq/L)	Base (mEq/L)
WHO Solution*	2.0	90	20	80	30 bicarbonate
Rehydralyte†	2.5	75	20	65	30 citrate
Pedialyte†‡	2.5	45	20	35	30 citrate
Lytren†	2.0	50	25	45	30 citrate
Ricelyte†	3.0	50	25	45	34 citrate
Naturalyte	2.5	45	20	35	48 citrate

*Must be reconstituted with water. Available in the USA from Jianas Bros. Packaging Co., Kansas City, MO.
†Ready to use.
‡Note that there are now many generic products available with compositions identical to Pedialyte.

Ref: MMWR 16 Oct, 1992;41:7.

6. **Maintenance replacement**
   a. For breast-fed infants, give 100 cc/kg of rehydration solution in addition to breast milk ad lib.
   b. For formula-fed infants, give lactose-free formula, or half-strength lactose-containing formula at 100–150 cc/kg/24 hours, alternating with an equal volume of rehydration solution.
   c. For children on a regular diet, give 100 cc/kg of rehydration solution and continue the regular diet. However, avoid products such as carbonated drinks and Kool-Aid, which have a high carbohydrate content. Good food to suggest includes:

Category	Example Foods
Parents should try	
Starchy foods	Rice, potatoes, noodles, crackers, toast, bananas
Cereals	Rice, cream of wheat, shredded wheat, oatmeal, rice or "bran"-based cereals
Soups	Soups with rice or noodles, meat and vegetables
Yogurt	
Vegetables	All kinds, but without butter
Fresh fruits	All kinds, but not packed in syrup
Parents should avoid	
Primarily sugar	Ice cream, sherbet, Popsicles, gelatin, pudding, sweetened cereals
Fatty foods	
Plain water	
Fruit juices	Apple, orange, grape juice, colas, ginger ale, Gatorade

7. Ongoing loss replacement: Instruct parents to give 4–8 ounces of rehydration solution for every diarrheal stool.
   Ref: Santosham M, et al. Ped Rev 1987; 8:273.

D. **Parenteral Rehydration**
   1. Phase 1: For symptomatic dehydration, rapidly expand the extracellular volume in order to preserve the circulation and renal function.
      a. Give Ringer's lactate or 0.9% (normal) NaCl 20-40 ml/kg in the first hour.
      b. Consider blood or plasma 10 ml/kg, if patient not responding to above solutions, or if the patient has had acute blood loss.
      c. For shock, give above fluids at a maximal rate until hemodynamic stability is achieved.

2. Phase 2
    a. Calculate fluid and electrolyte requirements for the next 24 h.
        1) Deficits: Use table, section II.A. above to approximate magnitude of deficits. In hypernatremic dehydration, calculate the free water deficit as described in Section II.B.3. In hyponatremic dehydration, calculate the sodium deficit as described in section II.B.2.
        2) Maintenance: Use methods described in Section I to determine maintenance requirements.
    b. Replace phase 2 fluid and electrolytes as follows:
        1) For isotonic or hyponatremic dehydration, add all of phase 2 requirements and replace 50% over 8 h, 50% over next 16 h.
        2) For hypernatremic dehydration, add all of phase 2 requirements and replace over 48 h; avoid dropping serum sodium >15 mEq/L over 24 h.
3. Continued abnormal losses
    a. Use the following table to estimate ongoing electrolyte losses.

Fluid	Na (mEq/L)	K (mEq/L)	Cl (mEq/L)	Protein (g/dl)
Gastric	20–80	5–20	100–150	—
Pancreatic	120–140	5–15	40–80	—
Small bowel	100–140	5–15	90–130	—
Bile	120–140	5–15	80–120	—
Ileostomy	45–135	3–15	20–115	—
Diarrhea	10–90	10–80	10–110	—
Burns	140	5	110	3–5

    b. Losses should be determined and replaced Q6h–Q8h. Because of the wide range of normal values, specific analyses are suggested in individual cases.

III. SERUM ELECTROLYTE DISTURBANCES
A. Hyponatremia
1. Factitious
    a. Hyperlipidemia: Na ↓ by 0.002 × lipid (mg/dl).
    b. Hyperproteinemia: Na ↓ by 0.25 × [protein (g/dl) − 8].

c. Hyperglycemia: Na ↓ 1.6 mEq/L for each 100 mg/dl rise in glucose.
2. Etiology and management

| | Decreased Weight | | Increased or Normal Weight |
	Renal Losses	Extrarenal Losses	
Cause	Na-losing nephropathy Diuretics Adrenal Insufficiency Hyperglycemia	G.I. loss Third space Skin losses Other losses	Nephrotic syndrome Congestive heart failure S.I.A.D.H
Laboratory data	↑ Urine Na ↑ Urine volume ↓ Specific gravity ↓ Urine osmolality	↓ Urine Na ↓ Urine volume ↑ Specific gravity ↑ Urine osmolality	↓ Urine Na* ↓ Urine volume ↑ Specific gravity ↑ Urine osmolality
Management	Replace losses Treat cause	Replace losses Treat cause	Restrict fluids Treat cause

*Urine Na may be appropriate for level of Na intake in patients with S.I.A.D.H.

B. Hypernatremia

| | Decreased Weight | | Increased Weight |
	Renal Losses	Extrarenal Losses	
Cause	Nephropathy Diuretic use Adrenal insufficiency Diabetes insipidus	G.I. losses Respiratory* Skin/other sites	Exogenous Na Mineralocorticoid excess
Laboratory data	↑ Urine volume ↑ Urine Na ↓ Specific gravity	↓ Urine volume ↓ Urine Na ↑ Specific gravity	Relative ↓ urine volume Relative ↓ urine Na Relative ↑ specific gravity
Management	Replace losses Treat cause	Replace losses Treat cause	Give low Na fluid Consider natriuretic agent Treat cause

*These causes of hypernatremia are usually secondary to free water loss so that fractional excretion of sodium may be decreased or normal.

C. Hypokalemia: Diagnosis

	Decreased Stores			Normal Stores
			Normal BP	
	Hypertension	Renal	Extrarenal	
Causes	Renovascular disease	R.T.A.	Skin losses	Alkalosis
	Excess renin	Fanconi syndrome	GI losses	↑ Insulin
	Congenital adrenal hyperplasia	Bartter syndrome	High CHO diet	Leukemia
	Excess mineralocorticoid	Antibiotics	Enema abuse	
	Cushing's syndrome	Diuretics	Laxative abuse	
			Anorexia nervosa	
Laboratory data	↑ Urine potassium	↑ Urine potassium	↓ Urine potassium	↑ Urine potassium
Management	Replace potassium in all cases. Treat cause.			

D. Hyperkalemia
1. Etiology

Increased Stores		Normal Stores
Increased Urine Potassium	Decreased Urine Potassium	
Cell breakdown	Renal failure	Leukocytosis
Transfusion with aged blood	Hypoaldosteronism	Thrombocytosis >750K /mm^3
NaCl substitutes	Aldosterone insensitivity	Metabolic acidosis*
Spitzer syndrome	↓ Insulin	Blood drawing
	K-sparing diuretics	

*For every 0.1 unit reduction in arterial pH there is an approximately 0.2–0.4 mEq/L increase in plasma potassium.

2. Treatment: See Emergency Management, Chapter 2.

E. Abnormal Serum Potassium: Symptoms

Serum K⁺	ECG Changes	Other Symptoms
2.5	AV conduction defect, prominent U wave, ventricular arrhythmia, S-T segment depression	Apathy, weakness, paresthesias
~7.5	T-wave elevation	Weakness, paresthesias
~8	Loss of P wave, widening of QRS	
~9	S-T depression, further widening of QRS	Tetany
~10	Bradycardia, sine-wave QRS-T, primary AV block, ventricular arrhythmia, cardiac arrest	

Ref: Feld, et al. Adv Pediatr 1988; 35:497.

IV. ANION GAP

A. **Definition:** The anion gap represents the difference between unmeasured cations (UC) and unmeasured anions (UA). Clinically it is measured by:

$$AG = UC - UA = Na + K - (Cl + HCO_3)$$
Normal: 12 mEq/L ± 2 mEq/L

B. **Increased Anion Gap: Causes**
   1. Decreased unmeasured cation: Hypokalemia, hypocalcemia, hypomagnesemia.
   2. Increased unmeasured anion
      a. Organic anions: lactate, ketones.
      b. Inorganic anions: phosphate, sulfate.
      c. Proteins: hyperalbuminemia (transient).
      d. Exogenous anions: salicylate, formate, nitrate, penicillin, carbenicillin, etc.
      e. Incompletely identified anions: anions accumulating with paraldehyde, ethylene glycol, methanol and salicylate poisoning, uremia, hyperosmolar hyperglycemic nonketotic coma.

    3. Laboratory error
      a. Falsely increased serum sodium.
      b. Falsely decreased serum chloride or bicarbonate.

C. **Decreased Anion Gap: Causes**
    1. Increased unmeasured cation.
    2. Increased normally present cation: Hyperkalemia, hyper-
       calcemia, hypermagnesemia.
    3. Retention of abnormal cation: IgG globulin, tromethamine
       (TRIS buffer), lithium.
    4. Decreased unmeasured anion: Hypoalbuminemia.
    5. Laboratory error
      a. Systematic error: Hyponatremia due to viscous serum,
        hyperchloremia in bromide intoxication.
      b. Random error: Falsely decreased serum sodium, falsely
        increased serum chloride or bicarbonate.

Ref: Emmett M, Narins R. Medicine 1977; 56:38. Oh MS, Carroll HJ. N Engl J Med 1977; 297:814.

V. **MISCELLANEOUS**
A. **Atomic Weights**

Aluminum (Al)	26.97	Lead (Pb)	207.21
Calcium (Ca)	40.08	Magnesium (Mg)	24.32
Carbon (C)	12.01	Manganese (Mn)	54.93
Chlorine (Cl)	35.46	Nitrogen (N)	14.01
Copper (Cu)	63.57	Oxygen (O)	16.00
Fluorine (F)	19.00	Phosphorus (P)	30.98
Gold (Au)	197.20	Potassium (K)	39.10
Hydrogen (H)	1.01	Sodium (Na)	23.00
Iodine (I)	126.92	Sulfur (S)	32.06
Iron (Fe)	55.85		

B. **Serum Osmolality**
    1. Defined as the number of particles per liter. May be ap-
      proximated by:

$$2 \, (Na) + \frac{glucose \ (mg/dl)}{18} + \frac{BUN \ (mg/dl)}{2.8}$$

    2. Normal range: 285–295 mOsm/L.

VI. PARENTERAL FLUID COMPOSITION

Composition of Frequently Used Parenteral Fluids

Liquid	CHO	Protein	Cal/L	Na	K	Cl	HCO₃†	Ca	P‡
	(gm/100 ml)			(mEq/L)				(mg/dl)	
D₅W	5	—	170	—	—	—	—	—	—
D₁₀W	10	—	340	—	—	—	—	—	—
Normal saline (0.9% NaCl)	—	—	—	154	—	154	—	—	—
½ Normal saline (0.45% NaCl)	—	—	—	77	—	77	—	—	—
D₅ (0.2% NaCl)	5	—	170	34	—	34	—	—	—
3% Saline	—	—	—	513	—	513	—	—	—
8.4% Sodium bicarbonate (I mEq/ml)	—	—	—	1000	—	—	1000	—	—
Ringer's	0–10	—	0–340	147	4	155.5	—	4.5	—
Ringer's lactate	0–10	—	0–340	130	4	109	28	3	—
Amino acid 8.5% (Travasol)	—	8.5	340	3	—	34	52	—	—
Plasmanate	—	5	200	110	2	50	29	—	—
Albumin 25% (salt poor)	—	25	1000	100–16	—	<120	—	—	—
Intralipid (Cutter)§	2.25	—	1100	2.5	0.5	4.0	—	—	0.8

*Protein or amino acid equivalent.
†Bicarbonate or equivalent (citrate, acetate, lactate).
‡Approximate values: actual values may vary somewhat in various localities depending on electrolyte composition of water supply used to reconstitute solution.
§Values are approximate—may vary from lot to lot.

GASTRO- ENTEROLOGY

11

I. STOOL EXAMINATION

A. Occult Blood (Guaiac Method)

1. **Purpose:** To screen for the presence of heme in stool.
2. **Method**
   a. Reagents: Glacial acetic acid, guaiac, hydrogen peroxide (fresh).
   b. Directions: Make thin stool smear on filter paper. Serially apply 2 drops of each in this order: acetic acid, guaiac, hydrogen peroxide.
3. **Interpretation:** A royal blue color is 4+; a green color is negative. Other gradations of blue are 1 to 3+. Medicinal iron does not give a positive guaiac.
   Note: This method has almost entirely been replaced by the use of Gastrocult and Hemoccult cards.

B. Fetal Hemoglobin (Apt Test)

1. **Purpose:** To differentiate fetal blood from swallowed maternal blood.
2. **Method:** Mix specimen (stool, vomitus, etc.) with an equal quantity of tapwater. Centrifuge or filter. Supernatant must have pink color to proceed. To 5 parts of supernatant, add 1 part of 0.25 N (1%) NaOH.
3. **Interpretation:** A pink color persisting over 2 minutes indicates fetal hemoglobin. Adult hemoglobin gives a pink color that becomes yellow in 2 minutes or less, indicating denaturation of hemoglobin.

   Ref: Apt L, Downey WS. J Pediatr 1955; 47:6.

C. Fecal Leukocyte Examination

1. **Purpose:** To aid in the early diagnosis of diarrhea by noting the presence or absence of leukocytes.
2. **Method:** Place a small fleck of stool or mucus (ideally from a rectal swab) on a clean glass slide. Mix thoroughly with 2 drops of 0.5% methylene blue stain. Wait 2–3 min-

utes for good nuclear staining, cover with coverslip and examine under low power.

3. **Interpretation:** PMNs are seen with any inflammatory enterocolitis, most commonly shigellosis, salmonellosis, *Yersinia, Campylobacter,* invasive *E. coli* infections, and ulcerative or granulomatous colitis. A predominance of mononuclear cells is seen in typhoid fever.

Ref: Harris, JC, et. al. Ann Intern Med 1972; 76:697-703.

D. Fecal pH

1. **Purpose:** To screen for carbohydrate malabsorption.
2. **Method:** Dip a portion of nitrazine pH paper into the liquid portion of the stool specimen and compare the color with the color chart provided.
   (normal ≥ 5.5)
3. **Interpretation:** A pH of <5.5 suggests carbohydrate malabsorption.

E. Sugar (Reducing Substances)

1. **Purpose:** Detection of carbohydrate malabsorption by measuring reducing substances in stool.
2. **Method:** Place a small amount of fresh liquid stool in a test tube and dilute with twice its volume of water. To look for sucrose malabsorption (sucrose is not a reducing substance) use 1 N HCl instead of water and boil briefly. Place 15 drops of this suspension in second test tube containing a Clinitest tablet. Compare the resulting color with the chart provided for urine testing.
3. **Interpretation**
   a. Values $<0.25\%$ are normal.
   b. Values of 0.25% to 0.5% are questionable.
   c. Values $>0.5\%$ are abnormal and suggest carbohydrate malabsorption.

F. Fecal Fat

1. **Neutral fat** (fat which has not been degraded by pancreatic enzymes): Obtain stool specimen (avoid oil or petroleum jelly if obtaining specimen via a rectal exam). Place a small amount of stool on a microscope slide and add two drops of 95% ethanol and two drops of Sudan III stain. Mix the suspension. Neutral fat will appear as orange globules. Steatorrhea is suspected if there are >60 globules per high-power field.

2. **Fatty acids:** Obtain specimen as above. Add two drops of 36% acetic acid and two drops of Sudan III stain. Fatty acids will stain orange. Malabsorption (mucosal defect) is suggested when 100 globules are noted per high-power field.

   Ref. Kleinman, Ronald, Malabsorption: Screening tests, Pediatric Gastroenterology and Nutrition News, vol. 1, no. 4, 1987.

G. Parasites

1. **Direct smear:** Add a small amount of feces to a drop of saline mix and remove feces with applicator stick. Cover. Examine under low power to locate the parasite and high dry for identification. Species identification of protozoan cysts can be made by adding iodine stain (KI 1% saturated with crystalline iodine) to smear, or by making an additional prep in a drop of stain.

2. **Preservatives:** Specimens should be delivered to the laboratory immediately. If delays are expected, place in either polyvinyl alcohol fixatives or formalin.

3. *Giardia lamblia:* The use of string test collection system (Entero/Test) can be helpful. The Entero/Test is available in sizes for both children and adults.

4. **Pinworms (cellophane tape method):** Obtain smear in the morning before the child has had a bath. Cover one end of a tongue depressor with clear cellophane tape, sticky side out. Apply to perianal area with mild pressure. Put 1 drop of xylol on a glass slide, then apply tape to slide. Look for ova under the microscope.

II. MALABSORPTION (SPECIFIC EXAMS AND TESTS)
A. Carbohydrates

1. **Breath Hydrogen Test**

   a. **Principle:** Hydrogen gas is produced by bacterial fermentation of undigested carbohydrate that reaches the colon. Hydrogen is absorbed into the blood and diffuses into the expired air. A rise in expired hydrogen concentration after oral loading with a particular carbohydrate indicates its malabsorption.

   b. **Method:** Fast infants for 4–6 h; fast older children for 12 h. Give 2 gm/kg (max: 50 gm) of desired carbohydrate as a 20% solution (10% in infants less than 6 months). Collect end-expired air by aspirating 5 ml of air after each breath to a total of 20–30 ml via nasal prong attached to a gas-tight syringe or via gas balloon attached to a face mask. H_2 is measured by gas chromatography on baseline sample (before carbohydrate load) and on q30 min samples for 3 h.

c. **Interpretation:** Elevation in H_2 concentration >20 ppm above baseline is considered significant. Bacterial overgrowth is suggested by:

   1) An early rise in H_2.
   2) An elevated basal value after a fast in the first 30 min after the substrate load.

   Ref. Perman, JA, et. al., J Pediatrics, 1978; 93: 17. Montez, R, Perman, JA, Seminars in Pediatric Gastroenterology and Nutrition, vol. 2, no. 3, Fall, 1991: p. 2. Barr, Rg, et. al., Pediatrics 1981; 68: 526.

2. **Monosaccharide and Disaccharide Absorption**

   a. **Purpose:** To diagnose malabsorption of a specific carbohydrate by measuring the change in blood glucose following an oral dose of the carbohydrate in question.

   b. **Method**

      1) Have patient fast 4–6 h prior to test. Give test carbohydrate (lactose, sucrose, maltose, glucose, galactose) orally or by gastric tube in a dose of 2.0 gm/kg as a 10% solution (maximum dose of 50 gm). For maltose, the dose is 1.0 gm/kg.

      2) Measure serum glucose prior to carbohydrate dose and 30, 60, 90, and 120 minutes following the dose. Note the number and character of stools. Perform a Clinitest determination for reducing substances on all stools passed during the test and for 8 h after the test is completed.

   c. **Interpretation**

      1) A rise in blood glucose 25 mg/dl over the fasting level within the test period is considered normal. An increase of <20 mg/dl is abnormal and suggests malabsorption of the test carbohydrate.

2) Malabsorption also is suggested if during or within 8h of test the patient develops diarrhea, stool pH <5.5, >0.5% stool reducing substances.

Ref. Silverman A, Roy CC, Pediatric Clinical Gastroenterology, CV Mosby, 1983: 895.

3. **D-Xylose Test**

   a. **Purpose:** To estimate the functional surface area of the duodenojejunal intestinal mucosa by measuring the absorption of an oral dose of D-xylose. Either the elevation in serum concentration or the urinary excretion of D-xylose may be used to quantitate D-xylose absorption. Absorption is independent of bile salts, pancreatic exocrine secretions, and intestinal mucosal disaccharidases. Unreliable in patients with edema, renal disease, delayed gastric emptying, severe diarrhea, rapid transit time, or small bowel bacterial overgrowth.

   b. **Method:** Have older children fast for 8 h prior to the test; younger infants need fast for only 4–6 h. Give D-xylose 14.5 gm/m^2 BSA (max: 25 gm) as a 10% water solution orally or via nasogastric tube. Collect all urine for 5 h. Ensure adequate urine flow using supplementary oral or IV fluid.

   c. **Interpretation (urine):** The quantity of xylose is measured colorimetrically; 5 h urinary excretion ≥25% of the administered dose is normal for children over 6 months. Values between 15 and 23% are questionable. Urinary excretion of <15% is abnormal. In infants < 6 months, values <10% are abnormal.

   d. **Interpretation (serum) (infants):** Determine serum D-xylose concentration in fasting state and at 30, 60, 90, and 120 minutes following the D-xylose dose. Normal response: serum level exceeding 25 mg/dl in any of the post-absorptive specimens.

   Ref. Santiago-Borrero P, et al., Pediatrics, 1971; 48: 55. Anderson CM, Burke A, Pediatric Gastroenterology, CV Mosby, 1975: 623–70. Silverman A, Roy CC, Pediatric Clinical Gastroenterology, CV Mosby, 1983: 894.

B. Fat

1. **Quantitative Fecal Fat**

   a. **Purpose:** Quantitative determination of fecal fat excretion to aid in diagnosis or management of fat malabsorption syndromes.

b. **Method**
1) Patient should be on a normal diet with adequate fat content (35% of diet) and caloric intake for 2 days before beginning the test. No meals should be omitted and no medications given during the test period. Exclude medium chain triglyceride oil from the diet.
2) Adjust amount of fat administered to the child according to age. Attempt to deliver:
    a) >25 gm/day in infants
    b) >50 gm/day in toddlers
    c) 100 gm/day in school-aged children. Record all foods given to estimate fat intake.
3) Collect and freeze all stools passed within 72 h. Determine total fecal fatty acid content. For children with diarrhea or constipation, give carmine red marker (0.6 to 0.9 gm) at beginning of test and again 72 h later. Collect all stools appearing between the marker regardless of time interval.

c. **Interpretation**
1) Normal: Total fecal fatty acid (FA) excretion of <5.0 gm fat/24h for children >2 years old.
2) Coefficient of absorption (CA):
    a) Fat absorption can be more accurately expressed as the coefficient of absorption, which should not vary with dietary fat intake. Its determination requires a strict record of dietary fat intake and output and is therefore best reserved for patients whose fecal fat excretion is borderline abnormal.

$$CA = \frac{gm\ fat\ ingested\ -\ gm\ fat\ excreted}{gm\ fat\ ingested} \times 100$$

    b) Normal:

Premature infants	60–75%
Newborn infants	80–85%
10 mo–3 yr	85–95%
>3 yr	95%

Ref: Silverman A, Roy CC. Pediatric Clinical Gastroenterology. CV Mosby, 1983:901. Shmerling DH, et al. Pediatrics 1970; 46:690.

III. GASTROINTESTINAL HEMORRHAGE
A. **Etiology (by Age)**
   1. **Neonate**
      a. Swallowed maternal blood (at birth or breast nipple)
      b. Hemorrhagic disease of the newborn
      c. Hemorrhagic gastritis
      d. Protein induced enterocolitis
      e. Necrotizing enterocolitis
      f. Hirschsprung's enterocolitis
      g. Midgut volvulus
   2. **0 to 6 months**
      a. Protein-induced enterocolitis
      b. Intussusception
      c. Lymphonodular hyperplasia
      d. Hirschsprung's enterocolitis
   3. **6 months to 5 years**
      a. Epistaxis
      b. Esophageal varices
      c. *C. difficile* colitis
      d. Lymphonodular hyperplasia
      e. Intussusception
      f. Meckel's diverticulum
      g. Hemolytic uremic syndrome
      h. Henoch-Schonlein purpura
      i. Neutropenic typhlitis
      j. Polyps
      k. Inflammatory bowel disease
      l. Hemorrhoids
   4. **Any age**
      a. Anal fissure, gastritis *(H. pylori),* stress ulcers, infective enterocolitis, duplication cysts, vascular malformation, esophagitis
   5. **False-positive Guaiac test**
      a. Meat in the diet within 96 h, inorganic iron ingestion.
B. **Suggested Evaluation and Management of Gastrointestinal Bleeding**

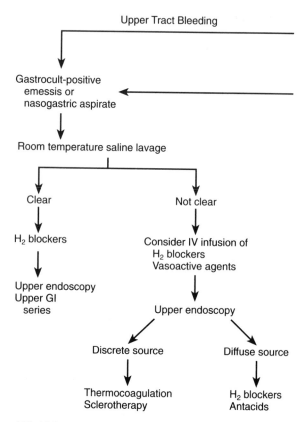

FIG 11.1.

Algorithm for evaluation and management of GI tract bleeding.
*Chemistries should include complete blood cell count, chemistry
panel including BUN, liver enzymes, PT, PTT, type and cross-
match of blood products. **Nasogastric intubation with gastric lavage should be performed in all patients with hematemesis, hema-
tochezia, melena, and hypotension to evaluate for upper GI tract
bleeding. A negative aspirate does not rule out bleeding just distal

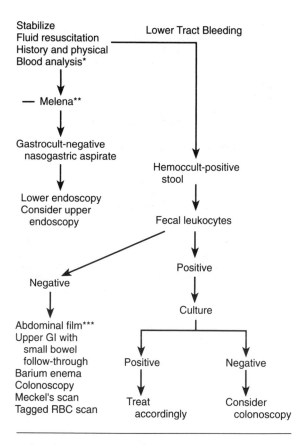

to the pylorus. ***Evaluation will be highly dependent on history and physical. Arteriography may be indicated when active bleeding continues or bleeding occurs repeatedly and cannot be localized by other tests.

Stockman, James A., et. al, The Pediatric Book of Lists, Mosty-Year Book, Inc., St. Louis, 1991. Oski, Frank A., Principles and Practice of Pediatrics, J.B. Lippincott Co., Philadelphia, 1990.

IV. DIARRHEA

A. **Definition:** Diarrhea is the passage of frequent, loose, or watery stools caused by a derangement in intestinal water and electrolyte transport due to an increased osmolar load or active secretion of water into the lumen.

B. **Etiologies**

  1. **Acute** (course self-limited, lasting <14 days).

    a. Infectious (bacterial, viral, parasitic):

      rotavirus, Norwalk agent, adenovirus, *Yersinia, Salmonella, Shigella,* enterotoxic *E. coli, C. difficile, Campylobacter jejuni, Klebsiella*

  2. **Chronic** (course lasting >14 days)

    a. Infectious (bacterial, viral, parasitic):

      Enteroadherent *E. coli, Giardia,* amebiasis, cryptosporidium, *C. difficile.*

    b. Inflammatory: Ulcerative colitis, Crohn's disease

    c. Malabsorption

      1) Impaired intraluminal digestion: Cystic fibrosis, Shwachman syndrome, interrupted enterohepatic circulation (Crohn's disease, ileal resection), Johanson-Blizzard syndrome, biliary atresia, impaired bile acid synthesis, bacterial overgrowth.

      2) Mucosal malabsorption: Celiac disease, combined immune deficiency, hypogammaglobulinemia, IgA deficiency, A-betalipoproteinemia, food protein sensitivity, intestinal lymphangiectasia, short bowel syndrome, congenital sucrose-isomaltase deficiency, lactase deficiency.

    d. Allergic

    e. Malignancy: Neuroblastoma, ganglioneuroma

    f. Intestinal obstruction: Hirschprung's disease, malrotation

    g. Malnutrition

    h. Radiation

    i. HIV

C. **Stool Screening Procedures (Refer to Section I.)**

  1. Fecal Leukocytes: The presence of white cells suggests bacterial infection.

  2. pH and Reducing Substances: To screen for carbohydrate malabsorption and colonic fermentation; stool will be

acidic and reducing substances will be present if malabsorption is occurring.

3. Occult Blood (Gastrocult/Hemocult): Blood present in stool may indicate bacterial infection, inflammation, or protein allergy intolerance.

4. Sudan III: To screen for fecal fat malabsorption.

5. Stool Electrolytes and Osmotic Gap: Stool osmotic gap may be calculated with the formula:

$$290* - 2 \times ([Na] \times [K])$$

Secretory diarrheas tend to have elevated stool [Na] and a resultant lower osmotic gap (<100 mOsm/L). In malabsorption or viral illness, the stool tends to have decreased [Na] and increased stool osmotic gap (>100 mOsm/L).

*Plasma osmolality of 290 is used because stool osmolarity will increase after stool excretion due to bacterial fermentation which continues in the sample.

D. Additional investigational studies: The results of the history and physical exam and the above stool screening procedures should help to direct further studies including: complete white blood cell count, erythrocyte sedimentation rate, electrolytes, radiographic studies, cultures for bacteria, viruses, and parasites, fecal fat collection, breath hydrogen test, sweat chloride tests, endoscopy with intestinal biopsy.

E. Management: Treatment of diarrhea will depend on the ultimate diagnosis. Initial management should focus on correction of fluid and electrolyte abnormalities and on preventing or correcting resultant malnutrition and nutrient deficiencies.

Ref. Walker, Alan, Pediatric Gastrointestinal Disease, B.C. Decker Inc., Vol. I, 1991: p.62–78.

V. CONSTIPATION

A. Definition: A decreased frequency of stooling associated with painful or difficult passage of hard stool.

B. Etiology

1. "Functional": idiopathic.
2. Dietary: low dietary fiber, starvation
3. Psychosocial: Emotional disturbance, mental retardation
4. Anatomic/obstructive: Hirschsprung's disease, imperforate/stenotic anus, stenotic/atretic intestine, anterior placement of anus, meconium ileus (cystic fibrosis)

5. Endocrine: hypothyroidism
6. Electolyte abnormalities: hypokalemia, hypocalcemia
7. Drugs: antacids, anticonvulsants, diuretics, lead, opiates, phenothiazines
8. Spinal abnormalities: meningomyelocele, spinal cord injury, spinal tumors
9. Distal ileal obstructive syndrome (cystic fibrosis)

C. **Presentation:** Accompanying symptoms will depend on the underlying etiology. "Functional" constipation tends to present with encopresis, recurrent periumbilical pain (60% of patients), enuresis (30% of those with encopresis), large, bulky dry stool, abdominal distention, poor appetite, poor growth.

D. **Investigational Studies**
1. Abdominal radiograph: looking for evidence of bowel obstruction.
2. Barium enema (without bowel prep): this test is most useful when an anatomic abnormality or Hirschsprung's disease is suspected.
3. Motility/manometry: functional abnormalities have been noted in almost all cases of chronic constipation on motility testing, although at this time testing parameters and methodologies vary. Anorectal manometry is useful in identifying those patients with Hirschsprung's disease. In normal individuals, there is relaxation of the internal anal sphincter upon distention of the rectal ampulla. This rectal inhibitory reflex is absent in patients with Hirschsprung's disease.
4. Rectal suction biopsy: may reveal additional pathologic causes of chronic constipation including intestinal neuronal dysplasia and aganglionosis.

E. **Treatment:** Therapy for constipation will be directed by the history, physical exam, and underlying diagnosis. This section will focus on one suggested approach to the management of "functional" or idiopathic constipation, DIOS, and spinal abnormalities.
1. Neonates: nonabsorbable carbohydrate (Maltsupex)
2. Older infants and children
   a. Intial management involves an effective emptying of the rectal vault to permit rectal/colonic size and function to normalize.

1) Mineral oil enema: softener and lubricant
2) Phosphosoda enema: Fleets enema
3) In patients with long-standing "functional" constipation and limited response to enemas, nasogastric tube placement and administration of Colyte or Golitely (hyperosmotic electrolyte solutions) may be required. These should be given at a rate of 15–20 cc/kg/hr until the bowel is clear. Monitor patient for vomiting and abdominal distention.

b. Laxation: Titrate to a stool pattern of approximately 2–3 stools qd.
   1) Mineral oil
   2) Milk of magnesia
   3) Lactulose
   4) Bulking agents: Perdiem, Metamucil

c. Follow-up: Patients should be followed at 1–2 month intervals. May begin to taper therapy once normal rectal function has resumed and stooling pattern is established.

Ref. Oski, FA, Principles and Practice of Pediatrics, J.B. Lippincott Co., 1990; p. 1682–1694. Walker, Alan, Pediatric Gastrointestinal Disease, B.C. Decker Inc., 1991, vol. I; p. 90–110.

VI. NEONATAL DIRECT HYPERBILIRUBINEMIA

A. Definition: The presence of conjugated (direct-acting) bilirubin fraction 2 mg/dl or 20% of the total bilirubin.

B. Goals of the Evaluation

1. To differentiate intrahepatic (parenchymal vs. intrahepatic bile duct disease) from extrahepatic (biliary tract) disorders.

2. To identify diseases for which therapy is available (anatomic, i.e., biliary atresia which will require surgical intervention, infectious, metabolic, and endocrinologic).

3. To recognize and stabilize the clinical sequelae of cholestasis (fat malabsorption, coagulopathy).

C. Staged Evaluation

Evaluation	Test/Study
Clinical evaluation	History, physical exam (liver size, consistency, spleen size, presence of abnormalities), stool color
Biochemical/serological evaluation	Serum bilirubin fractionation, hepatic synthetic function (albumin, coagulation profile), viral and bacterial cultures (blood, urine, spinal fluid), viral serology (HBsAg, TORCH), and VDRL titers, alpha-$_1$-antitrypsin pheno, thyroxine and thyroid stimulating hormone, metabolic screen (urine/serum amino acids, urine-reducing substances), ferritin, serum bile acid determination, sweat chloride test
Special studies	Ultrasonography, hepatobiliary scintigraphy, liver biopsy

Ref: Balistreri, William, M.D., Foreward Neonatal Cholestasis: Lessons from the Past, Issues for the Future, Seminars in Liver Disease, vol. 7, no. 2, 1987.

GENETICS *12*

I. GENETIC CONSULTATION
A. Indications for Referral to a Genetics Center
1. Known or suspected hereditary disorder.
2. Major physical anomalies, unusual body proportions, short stature.
3. Major organ malformation.
4. Developmental delay, mental retardation, or learning disability in females who have brothers with mental retardation.
5. Complete or partial blindness or hearing loss.
6. Loss or deterioration of motor or speech abilities in a child who was previously thriving.
7. Evidence of maternal exposure to drugs, alcohol, or radiologic agents during pregnancy.

B. Indications for Prenatal Counseling
1. Genetic disorder or birth defect in 1 partner.
2. Previous child with a known or suspected genetic disorder.
3. Maternal age of ≥35 yr.
4. Family history of known or suspected chromosome error(s).
5. Multiple early miscarriages or stillbirths.
6. Membership in an ethnic group known to have a higher incidence of a specific genetic disorder than the general population.
7. Known carrier of a gene for a genetic disorder.

C. Indications for Karyotype: Draw 3 cc of blood in a green-topped tube that contains sodium heparin. Keep tube at room temperature.
1. Two or more major malformations (small for gestational age and mental retardation are considered major malformations for this purpose.
2. Features of specific chromosomal syndrome.
3. At risk for a familial chromosomal aberration.

    4. Ambiguous genitalia.

    5. Malignancies.

    6. Recurrent spontaneous abortions (>2) or history of infertility (karyotype both father and mother).

D. DNA Testing (partial list)

    1. Direct DNA analysis

       a. Sickle cell disease (Hb SS, Hb SC)

       b. Thalassemias

       c. Cystic fibrosis

       d. Fragile X mental retardation

       e. Medium-chain acyl-coenzyme A dehydrogenase (MCAD) deficiency

       f. Myotonic dystrophy

       g. Muscular dystrophy (Duchenne/Becker)

    2. Linkage analysis (requires family members)

       a. Hemophilia A, B

       b. Muscular dystrophy (Duchenne/Becker)

       c. Neurofibromatosis, type 1, 2

       d. Von Hippel-Lindau

       e. PKU (phenylketonuria)

       f. Polycystic kidney disease

       g. Spinal muscular atrophy (Werdnig Hoffman)

       h. Hypertrophic cardiomyopathy

II. NORMAL MORPHOLOGY: Unless otherwise stated, illustrations in this section have been reproduced with permission from Hall JG, et al., Handbook of Normal Physical Measurements. 1989; Oxford Medical Publications.

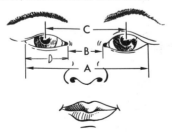

FIG 12.1. Diagram of Face

A. Outer canthal distances

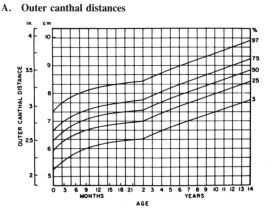

FIG 12.2. Outer Canthal Distance. Ref: Feingold M, Bossert WH. Birth Defects: Original Article Series, 1974; 10(13):8–9. (With permission.)

B. Inner canthal distances

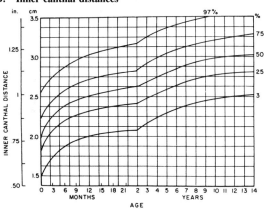

FIG 12.3. Inner Canthal Distance

C.   **Interpupillary distance**

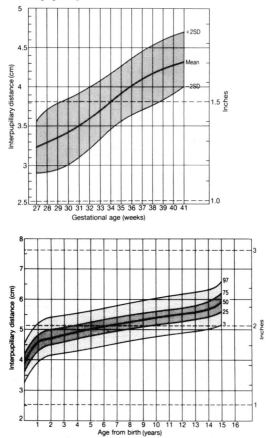

FIG 12.4. Interpupillary Distances

D. Palpebral fissure length

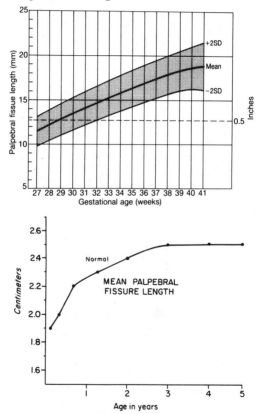

FIG 12.5.
Palpebral Fissure Length. Ref: Thomas IT, Gaintantzis Ya, Frias
JL. J Pediatr 1987;111:268 (With permission).

E. Total ear length

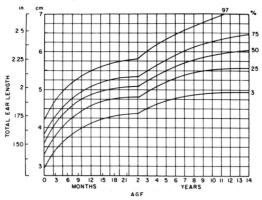

FIG 12.6. Total Ear Length

F. Total hand length

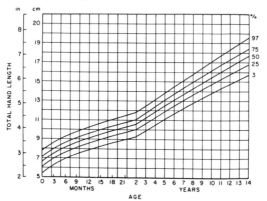

FIG 12.7. Total Hand Length

G. Upper-lower segment ratio

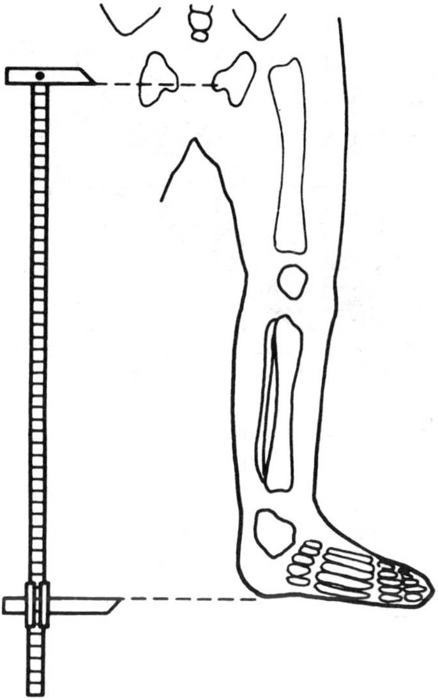

FIG 12.8.
To calculate upper:lower segment ratio:

$$\frac{\text{upper segment}}{\text{lower segment}} = \frac{\text{height} - \text{lower segment}}{\text{lower segment}}$$

H.   Internipple distance

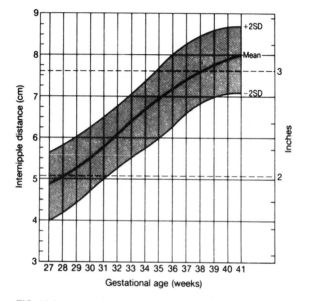

FIG 12.9.   Internipple Distance, Both Sexes, at Birth

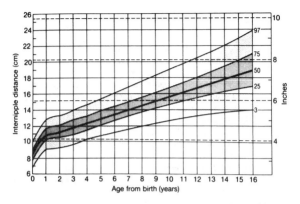

FIG 12.10.
Internipple Distance, Both Sexes, Birth to 16 Years

III. INBORN ERRORS OF METABOLISM (IEM)
A. Initial Laboratory Tests
1. **Blood**
    a. CBC (neutropenia, thrombocytopenia seen in organic acidemias).
    b. Serum electrolytes, glucose, anion gap.
    c. Arterial blood gas.
    d. Plasma ammonium.
2. **Urine:**
    Check **odor, pH, ketones, reducing substances.**
B. Advanced Studies: If any of the initial studies are abnormal, consider the following advanced studies:
1. **Blood:** Plasma amino acids, plasma carnitine.
2. **Urine**
    a. Metabolic screen: The JHH urine metabolic screen includes pH, specific gravity, protein, glucose, ketones, reducing substances (Clinitest), ferric chloride, DNPH (dinitrophenylhydralizine for alpha-ketoacids), nitrosonapthal (for tyrosine metabolites), nitroprusside (for sulfhydryl groups), and a mucopolysaccharide spot test.
    b. Organic acids, amino acids.

C. Sample Collection

1. Plasma amino acids and plasma carnitine each require 3 cc of blood in a green-topped (sodium heparin) tube. Samples should be drawn after an overnight fast (or at least a 4 hour fast in an infant). Deliver on ice or separate and freeze plasma for later analysis.
2. Urine amino and organic acid assays each require 5–10 ml of urine. If fresh urine cannot be delivered immediately to the lab, freeze samples.
3. Plasma ammonium values increase rapidly on standing. Collect on ice and deliver immediately to lab.
4. Skin biopsy for fibroblasts studies: Specimen should be stored in tissue culture medium at 4°C. When this is unavailable, store specimen in the patient's serum. Refrigerate, but do not freeze specimen. Keep the tissue immersed in the culture media.

D. Unusual Urine Odor

	Odor
Acute disease	
Maple syrup urine	Maple syrup, burned sugar
Isovaleric acidemia	Cheesy, or sweaty feet
Multiple carboxylase deficiency	Cat's urine.
3-OH, 3-methyl glutaryl-CoA, lyase deficiency	Cat's urine.
Nonacute disease	
Phenylketonuria	Musty
Hypermethioninemia	Rancid butter, rotten cabbage

E. Ferric Chloride Reaction

1. Ferric iron forms colored derivatives when combined with many organic compounds. Results depend on methodology.
2. Place 2 drops of 10% ferric $FeCl_3$ in 1 ml of fresh urine; mix and observe color immediately and upon standing.
3. The test is relatively insensitive and usually requires high concentrations of the reacting metabolite. Salicylate is an exception. Phosphate ions yield cloudy precipitates, which may mask positive results. A negative test does not rule out the disease.

4. Interpretation

Color	Interpretation
Green	PKU, tyrosinemia, direct hyperbilirubinemia, L-dopa.
Blue-green	Histidinemia, pheochromocytoma.
Gray-green	MSUD, formiminotransferase deficiency.
Purple	Salicylates, methionine malabsorption.
Blue-purple	Phenothiazines.

Ref: Buist NRM. Brit Med J 1968; 2:745; Thomas GH, Howell RR. Selected screening tests for genetic metabolic disease. Chicago: Year Book, 1973.

F. Urine Reducing Substance: For method see Nephrology, Section I.C.3.b. Metabolic disorders associated with a positive test include:
   1. Galactose: Galactosemia, galactokinase deficiency, severe liver disease.
   2. Fructose: Hereditary fructose intolerance, essential fructosuria.
   3. Glucose: Diabetes mellitus, renal glycosuria, Fanconi's type RTA.
   4. p-Hydroxyphenyl pyruvic acid: Tyrosinemia.
   5. Xylulose: Pentosuria

   Ref: Burton BK, Nadler HL. Pediatrics 1978; 61:398; Aleck KA, Shapiro LJ, Pediatr Clin North Am 1978; 25:431.

G. Neonatal Hyperammonemia
   1. Respiratory alkalosis is present early.
   2. Detected by gas chromatography—mass spectroscopy. Includes propionic, methylmalonic, and isovaleric acidemias, type II glutaric acidemia, and others. Hyperglycinemia is characteristic of proprionic and methylmalonic acidemia.

	Index
CPS	Carbamyl phosphate synthetase deficiency
OTC	Ornithine transcarbamylase deficiency
AL	Argininosuccinase deficiency
AS	Argininosuccinic acid synthetase deficiency

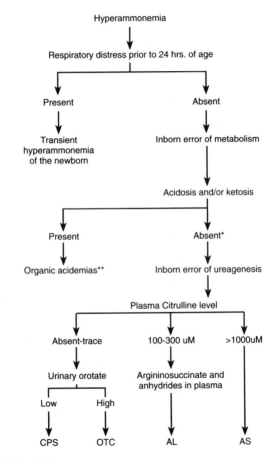

FIG 12.11.
The workup of neonatal hyperammonemia.
Ref: Arn PH, Valle DL, Brusilow SW. Contemp OB/Gyn, April, 1989.

IV. **NEWBORN METABOLIC SCREEN:** See table, next page. For interpretation of hemoglobin patterns, **see Chapter 14, Hematology.**

V. **GENETIC SUPPORT GROUPS:** A network for families and individuals affected by genetic disorders is available through the Alliance of Genetic Support Groups (35 Wisconsin Circle, Suite 440, Chevy Chase, MD 20815; 800/336-GENE). This group is dedicated to patients and professionals, and provides information, awareness, genetic services, and referrals.

Disease	Newborn Screening Level	Diagnostic Test	Immediate Clinical Response
Phenylketonuria	Phe (4–6 mg/dl) Phe (6–12 mg/dl) Phe (>12 mg/dl)	Plasma amino acids (Phe, Tyr); urine phenyl acids; genotyping	1. For mild elevation: Evaluate nutritional developmental, neurological status, hepatic, and renal function. Repeat screening test. 2. For moderate elevation: Consult referral center and send frozen urine and plasma. 3. For high levels: Arrange for hospitalization and diagnostic evaluation.
Maple syrup urine disease	Leu (4 mg/dl) Leu (4–8 mg/dl) Leu (>8 mg/dl)	Plasma amino acids (Val, Leu, Ileu)	
Homocystinuria	Meth (2–6 mg/dl) Meth (>6 mg/dl)	Plasma amino acids (homocystine, Met)	
Tyrosinemia	Tyr (6–12 mg/dl) Tyr (12–20 mg/dl) Tyr (>20 mg/dl)	Plasma amino acids (Tyr, Phe); blood spot for succinylacetone	
Galactosemia	Beutler test, positive; *E. coli* phage test negative. Beutler test, positive; *E. coli* phage test positive.	Galactose-1-P uridyl transferase; galactokinase; UPD-gal-4-epimerase galactose; galactose-1-P	Evaluate for jaundice, sepsis, cataracts, urine reducing substances. Send blood for enzyme analysis. Remove lactose from diet.
Hypothyroidism	RIA (T_4 = 5–7.6 µg/dl) (TSH <25 µIU/ml) RIA (T_4 <5 µg/dl) (TSH >25 µIU/ml)	T_4, T_3, TSH, TBG, thyroid antibodies, bone age	Evaluate for hypothermia, hypoactivity, poor feeding, jaundice, constipation.

Ref: Maryland State Department of Health and Hygiene Laboratories Administration

GROWTH CHARTS *13*

Note: "Normal" growth curves are available for children with specific disease syndromes, for example:

Down Syndrome: Developmental Evaluation Clinic of the Children's Hospital, Boston; the Child Development Center of Rhode Island Hospital; and Clinical Genetics Service of Children's Hospital of Philadelphia.

Turner Syndrome: Lyon AH, et al. Am J Dis Child 1985;60:932.

Cystic Fibrosis: Cystic Fibrosis Foundation, 1985.

Sickle Cell Anemia: Platt OS, New Eng J Med 1984; 311:7.

I. GIRLS: BIRTH TO 36 MONTHS
A. Length and Weight.

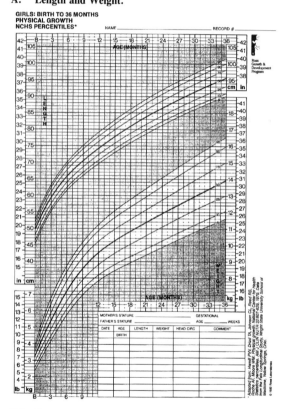

FIG 13.1. Length and weight for girls, birth to 36 months. Ref: Adapted from Hamill PV, et al. Physical Growth: National Center for Health Statistics percentiles, Am J Clin Nutr 1979; 32:607. Data from the Fels Longitudinal Study, Wright State Univ School of Medicine, Yellow Springs, Ohio. Copyright Ross Laboratories 1982. Reproduced with permission.

B. Head Circumference and Length-Weight Ratio.

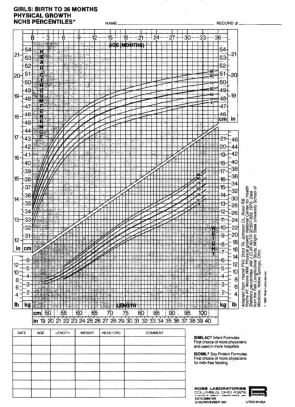

FIG 13.2. Head circumference and length-weight ratio for girls, birth to 36 months. Ref: Adapted from Hamill PV, et al. Physical Growth: National Center for Health Statistics percentiles, Am J Clin Nutr 1979; 32:607. Data from the Fels Longitudinal Study, Wright State Univ School of Medicine, Yellow Springs, Ohio. Copyright Ross Laboratories 1982. Reproduced with permission.

II. BOYS: BIRTH TO 36 MONTHS
A. Length and Weight.

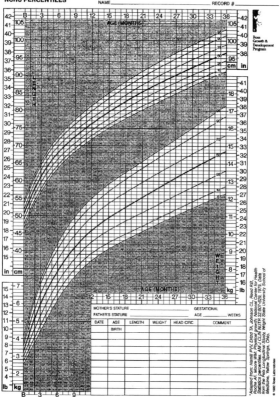

FIG 13.3. Length and weight for boys, birth to 36 months. Ref: Adapted from Hamill PV, et al. Physical Growth: National Center for Health Statistics percentiles, Am J Clin Nutr 1979; 32:607. Data from the Fels Longitudinal Study, Wright State Univ School of Medicine, Yellow Springs, Ohio. Copyright Ross Laboratories 1982. Reproduced with permission.

B. Head Circumference and Length-Weight Ratio.

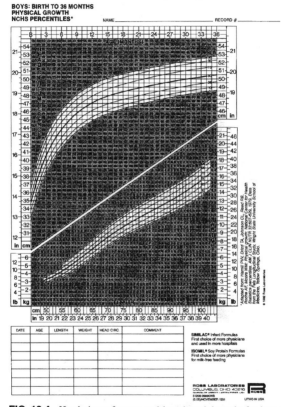

FIG 13.4. Head circumference and length-weight ratio for boys, birth to 36 months. Ref: Adapted from Hamill PV, et al. Physical Growth: National Center for Health Statistics percentiles, Am J Clin Nutr 1979; 32:607. Data from the Fels Longitudinal Study, Wright State Univ School of Medicine, Yellow Springs, Ohio. Copyright Ross Laboratories 1982. Reproduced with permission.

III. GIRLS: 2 TO 18 YEARS
A. Stature and Weight.

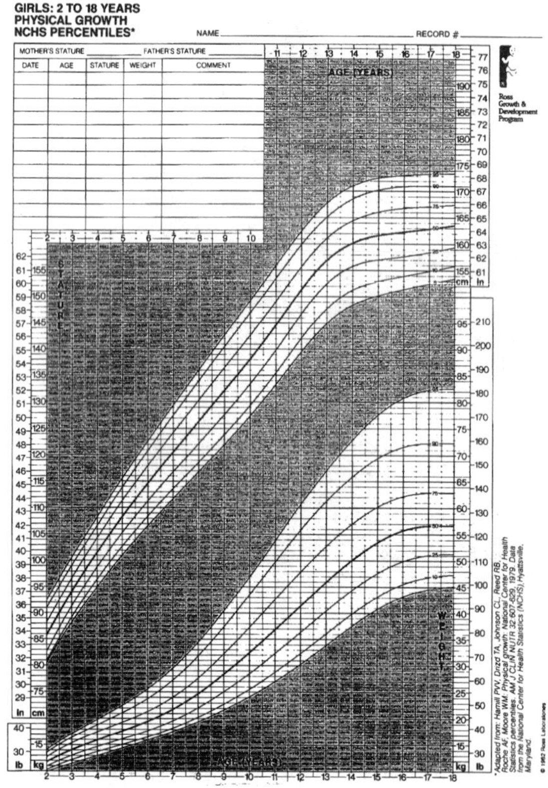

FIG 13.5. Stature and weight for girls, 2 to 18 years.

B. Stature-Weight Ratio.

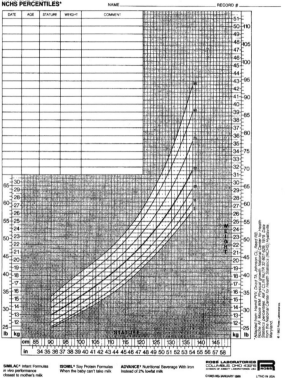

FIG 13.6. Stature-weight ratio for girls, 2 to 18 years.

C. Height Velocity.

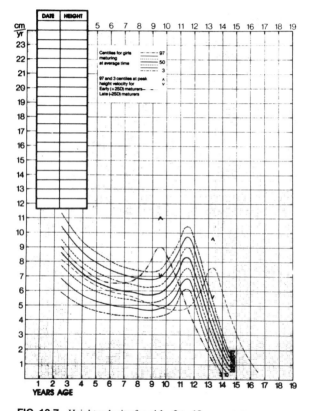

FIG 13.7. Height velocity for girls, 2 to 18 years. Ref: Adapted from Tanner JM, Davis PSW. J Pediatrics 1985; 107:317. Copyright Castlemead Publications, 1985. Distributed by Sereno Laboratories.

IV. BOYS: 2 TO 18 YEARS
A. Stature and Weight.

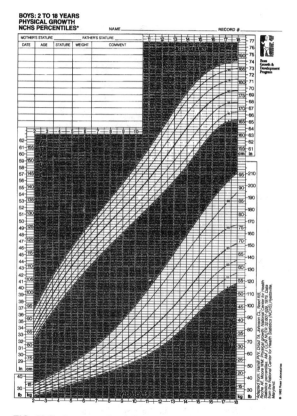

FIG 13.8. Stature and weight for boys, 2 to 18 years.

B.   Stature-Weight Ratio.

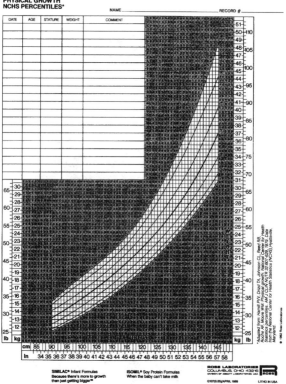

FIG 13.9. Stature-weight ratio for boys, 2 to 18 years.

C. Height Velocity.

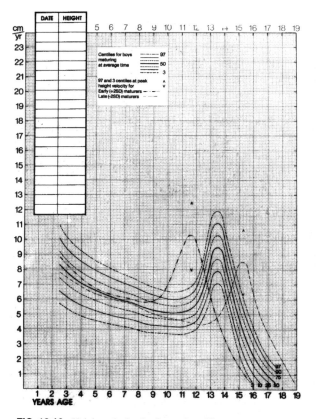

FIG 13.10. Height velocity for boys, 2 to 18 years. Ref: Adapted from Tanner JM, Davis PSW. J Pediatrics 1985; 107:317. Copyright Castlemead Publications, 1985. Distributed by Sereno Laboratories.

V. HEAD CIRCUMFERENCE: GIRLS AND BOYS 2 TO 18 YEARS

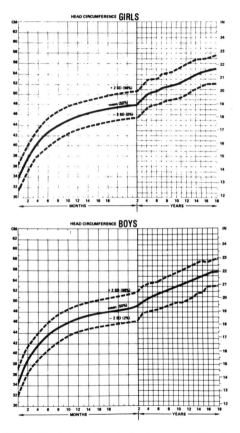

FIG 13.11. Head circumference for boys and girls, 2 to 18 years. Ref: Nelhaus G. Pediatrics 1968; 41:106. Reproduced with permission.

VI. BODY SURFACE AREA NOMOGRAM

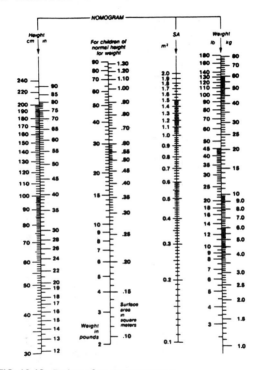

FIG 13.12. Body surface area nomogram.

VII. DENTAL DEVELOPMENT

| | Deciduous Teeth | | | | Permanent Teeth | |
| | Eruption | | Shedding | | Eruption | |
	Maxillary	Mandibular	Maxillary	Mandibular	Maxillary	Mandibular
Central incisors	6–8 mo	5–7 mo	7–8 yr	6–7 yr	7–8 yr	6–7 yr
Lateral incisors	8–11 mo	7–10 mo	8–9 yr	7–8 yr	8–9 yr	7–8 yr
Cuspids	16–20 mo	16–20 mo	11–12 yr	9–11 yr	11–12 yr	9–11 yr
1st premolar	—	—	—	—	10–11 yr	10–12 yr
2nd premolar	—	—	—	—	10–12 yr	11–13 yr
1st molars	10–16 mo	10–16 mo	10–11 yr	10–12 yr	6–7 yr	6–7 yr
2nd molars	20–30 mo	20–30 mo	10–12 yr	11–13 yr	12–13 yr	12–13 yr
3rd molars	—	—	—	—	17–22 yr	17–22 yr

Note: Sexes are combined, although girls tend to be slightly more advanced (at least with respect to tooth eruption), than boys. Averages are approximate values derived from various studies.

Ref: Vaugh VC, et al (eds): Nelson's Textbook of Pediatrics. Philadelphia: W. B. Saunders 1987:30.

HEMATOLOGY   *14*

I.   **ROUTINE HEMATOLOGY:** Methods adapted from Williams WJ, et al., eds. Hematology. New York: McGraw-Hill, 1983. For normal values, see section VIII.

A.   **Microhematocrit**

    1. Fill standard microhematocrit tube with blood and seal one end with clay. Centrifuge (12,000 g) for 5 minutes.

    2. Falsely high hematocrits caused by increased plasma trapping occur with short centrifugation time and in disorders with decreased red cell deformability.

B.   **Wright's Staining Technique**

    1. Place air-dried blood smears, film side up, on staining rack.

    2. Cover smear with undiluted Wright's stain and leave for 2 to 3 minutes.

    3. Add equal volume of distilled water and blow gently on the surface until a greenish metallic sheen appears. Leave diluted stain on smear for 2 to 6 minutes.

    4. Without disturbing the slide, flood with water and wash until stained smear is pinkish-red. Blot dry.

C.   **Hematologic Indices**

    1. **Mean Corpuscular Volume (MCV):** Average RBC volume. Usually measured directly by electronic counters. Expressed in femtoliters (fl, 10^{-15} L).

$$MCV = \frac{Hct~(\%) \times 10}{RBC~count~(millions/mm^3)}$$

    2. **Mean Corpuscular Hemoglobin (MCH):** Average quantity of Hb per red cell expressed in picograms (pg, 10^{-12} g).

$$MCH = \frac{Hb~(gm~\%) \times 10}{RBC~count~(millions/mm^3)}$$

3. **Mean Corpuscular Hemoglobin Concentration (MCHC):** Grams of Hb per 100 cc packed cells. High in congenital spherocytic hemolytic anemia and hemoglobin SC disease; may be low in iron deficiency.

$$\text{MCHC} = \frac{\text{Hb (gm \%)} \times 100}{\text{Hct (\%)}}$$

4. **Red Cell Distribution Width (RDW):** Statistical description of heterogeneity of red cell size. Increases with anisocytosis, reticulocytosis, iron deficiency. Increased in newborns. Normal in thalassemia minor.

$$\text{RDW} = \frac{\text{Standard deviation of MCV} \times 100}{\text{MCV}}$$

D. **Reticulocyte Count**
   1. Mix equal amounts of new methylene blue or brilliant cresyl blue with whole blood. After 10–20 minutes, prepare thin smears.
   2. Count the number of reticulocytes (cells containing reticulum or blue granules) per 1000 red cells and report as % of RBCs.

E. **Platelet Estimation:** Use Wright's stained blood smear to approximate platelet count. Always examine periphery of smear or coverslip as platelet clumps may be deposited there. For rough approximation, 1 platelet/oil immersion field corresponds to 10,000–15,000 platelets/mm³. Platelet clumps usually indicate >100,000 platelets/mm³.

II. **HEMATOLOGIC INDICATORS OF SYSTEMIC DISEASE**

A. **Erythrocyte Sedimentation Rate (ESR):** Should be determined within 1 hour after obtaining blood.
   1. Collect venous blood in EDTA or oxalate-containing tube.
   2. Place 1 ml in a Wintrobe tube, using a long Pasteur pipette. Fill carefully from the bottom of the tube; do not shake tube or allow air bubbles to form in the column of blood. Place the tube vertically.

3. Read depth of fall of RBC column at the end of 60 minutes.

4. Anemia, tilting of column, warming, shaking may artificially increase the ESR. Hypo or afibrinogenemia, old or cold blood, excessive anticoagulant, sickle cell anemia, congestive heart failure, polycythemia, trichinosis, and pertussis may decrease the ESR. Elevated in newborns with infections, or with ABO hemolysis.

   Ref: Cartwright, GE. Diagnostic Laboratory Hematology 4th ed. New York: Grune & Stratton, 1968.

B. **Cold Agglutinins: Rapid Screening Test**

1. Collect 4–5 drops of blood in 60×7 mm Wasserman tube containing about 0.2 ml of 3.8 NaEDTA.

2. Cap tube and place in ice water bath for 30–60 seconds.

3. Tilt tube and observe blood as it runs down wall of tube.

4. Definite floccular agglutination (seen with unaided eye) which disappears upon warming to 37° C is considered a positive (3–4+) test. A control sample is useful for interpretation.

5. Positive test frequently correlates with cold agglutinin titer of >1:64. 75–85% of patients with atypical pneumonia and a positive test will develop serologic evidence of mycoplasma pneumonia infection.

   Ref: Griffin JP. Ann Intern Med 1969; 70:701; Coradero L, et al. J Pediatr 1967; 71:1.

III. **ANEMIA: EVALUATION**

A. **General Studies:** Anemia is defined by age-specific norms. Common screening studies include:

1. Complete blood count (CBC) with differential and reticulocyte count

2. Blood smear to examine morphology of cells

3. Urinalysis for bilirubin, blood, protein, glucose. Also perform microscopic exam.

4. Stool for occult blood

5. Serum bilirubin, blood urea nitrogen, creatinine

6. Coombs test

B. **Specific Tests**

1. Tests to diagnose sickle hemoglobin: Any substance that reduces O_2 tension will cause red cells containing

Hb S to sickle. A positive "sickle prep" is found in the sickle hemoglobinopathies (SS, SC, S thal, and others), as well as in sickle trait; 8% of black children will have a positive sickle prep. All positive tests should be confirmed with cellulose acetate electrophoresis.

   a. Sulfite solution—"sickle prep": Mix one or two drops of 2% sodium metabisulfite or sodium hyposulfite on a slide with one drop of blood; apply coverslip. Read preparation at 30 minutes and again at 3 hours. Positive test: presence of sickled cells.

   b. "Sickledex": A solubility test using dithionate reduction of Hb S. Used in many commercial and hospital diagnostic laboratories.

2. Hemoglobin electrophoresis: Cellulose acetate electrophoresis: separation of hemoglobin variants based on molecular charge. Hemoglobins found are reported in order of relative abundances in the sample; e.g., sickle cell trait is ASA_2, sickle cell disease is SFA_2.

3. Bone marrow aspiration

4. G6PD, pyruvate kinase

5. Iron trial: Adequate iron therapy should result in reticulocytosis peaking 7–10 days into therapy. A significant increase in Hb concentration should be evident after 3–4 weeks of therapy.

6. Ferritin: Serum ferritin is an accurate reflection of total body iron stores after 6 months of age. Ferritin may be falsely elevated with infection or inflammation.

   Ref: Siimes MA, et al. Blood 1974; 43:581.

7. Indicators of Hemolysis

   a. Haptoglobin: binds free hemoglobin. Decreased with intravascular and extravascular hemolysis, and hepatocellular disease. Falsely normal or increased levels may occur in association with inflammation, infection, or malignancy.

   b. Hemopexin: binds free heme groups. Decreased with intravascular hemolysis, renal disease, and hepatocellular disease. Hemopexin usually not increased with inflammation, infection, or malignancy.

8. Free erythrocyte protoporphyrin (FEP): Accumulates when the conversion of protoporphyrin to heme is blocked. Elevated in iron deficiency, plumbism, and erythropoietic protoporphyria. Levels >300 mcg/dl PRBC generally found only with lead intoxication.

IV. ANEMIA: DIAGNOSIS
A. **Diagnostic Categories:** Please refer to age-related normal values of MCV in hematology, Section A.

Reticulocyte Count	Microcytic Anemia*	Normocytic Anemia	Macrocytic Anemia

Low	Iron deficiency†
	 Lead poisoning
	 Chronic disease
	 Aluminum toxicity
		Chronic disease
		 Red cell aplasia
		 (TEC, infection,
		   drug-induced)
		 Splenomegaly
		 Malignancy
		 Endocrinopathies
		 Renal failure
			Folate deficiency
			 Vitamin B^{12}
			   deficiency
			 Diamond-Blackfan
			 anemia
			 Aplastic anemia

Normal	Thalassemia trait Sideroblastic anemia	Acute bleeding Dyserythropoietic anemia II	Drug-induced

High	Thalassemia
	 syndromes
	 Hb C disorders
	 (↑ MCV)
		Antibody-mediated
		 hemolysis
		 Fragmentation
		 (HUS, TTP, DIC,
		   Kassaback-Merritt)
		 Membrane
		   abnormalities
		   (spherocytosis,
		   elliptocytosis),
		 Enzyme disorders
		 (G6PD, pyruvate
		   kinase,
		   hemoglobinopathies)
			Dyserythropoetic
			 anemia I, III
			 Active hemolysis

*As a rule of thumb, the lowest limit of normal for MCV is age + 70.
†An easy way to differentiate iron deficiency from thalassemia minor is to calculate the discriminate index: MCV/RBC >13.5 suggests iron deficiency; <11.5 is suggestive of thal minor.

Ref: (F. Oski, Personal communication.)

B.   Distinguishing Common Causes of Anemia

	Iron Deficiency	β-Thalassemia Trait	Chronic Inflammation	Lead Poisoning
Reticulocyte count	Low	Low	Normal	Low
RDW	↑	↓	Normal	↓
Ferritin	↓	Normal to ↑	Normal	↓ to normal
FEP	↑	Normal	↑	↑
Iron	↓	Normal	↓	↓ to normal
TIBC	↑	Normal	↓	
Electrophoresis	Normal	↑ HbA$_2$ or F	Normal	Normal
ESR	Normal	Normal	↑	Normal
Smear	Hypochromic, target cells	Normochromic, microcytic	Varies	Basophilic stippling

C.   Interpretation of Hemoglobin Patterns

FA   Designation for adult normal hemoglobin with fetal hemoglobin, which is the normal hemoglobin pattern for a newborn.

FAV   Indicates the presence of both hemoglobin A and F as would be expected in the newborn. However, an anomalous band (V) is present which does not appear to be any of the common hemoglobin variants.

FAS   Indicates the presence of adult normal hemoglobin and hemoglobin S. This preliminary finding is consistent with the benign Sickle Cell *trait*.

FS   Designates the presence of sickle hemoglobin without detectable adult normal hemoglobin A. This is consistent with homozygous sickle hemoglobin genotype (S/S) and could lead to manifestations of Sickle Cell Anemia during infancy.

FC[1]   Designates the presence of hemoglobin C without adult normal hemoglobin A. This finding is consistent with the clinically significant monozygous hemoglobin genotype (C/C) and could result in a hematologic disorder during childhood.

FSC   Indicates the presence of both hemoglobins S and C. This heterozygous condition could lead to manifestations of sickle cell disease during childhood.

FAC   Indicates the presence of hemoglobin C and adult normal hemoglobin A. This finding is consistent with the benign hemoglobin C *trait*.

FSAA$_2$ Designates heterozygous S Beta Thalassemia which is a clinically significant sickling disorder.

FAA₂   Designates heterozygous hemoglobin A Thalassemia which is a clinically significant hematologic disorder.

F[1]   Designates the presence of fetal hemoglobin F without adult normal hemoglobin A. Although this may indicate a delayed appearance of hemoglobin A, it may also represent a potential hereditary persistence of fetal hemoglobin. It is not possible to interpret this finding without further laboratory studies.

FV[1]   Indicates the presence of fetal hemoglobin F and an anomalous hemoglobin variant (V). The potential clinical significance can only be ascertained after laboratory studies.

AF   If this is the case, another filter paper blood specimen must be submitted when the infant is about 4 months of age at which time the transfused blood cells should have been cleared.

---

[1]Repeat blood specimen should be submitted to confirm the original interpretation.

V.   **COAGULATION:** Normal clotting depends on adequate platelet number and function as well as intact coagulation cascade (see Figure 14.1).

A.   **Platelet Function:** Adequacy of platelet function and number can be measured by bleeding time, for example by Ivy technique:

1. Place blood pressure cuff on upper arm and inflate to 40 mm Hg. Clean forearm with alcohol and allow to dry.

2. Make a standardized incision with a nonheparinized long point disposable lancet (3 mm deep) or with a commercially available template. Avoid lancing a superficial vein.

3. Gently absorb the blood onto filter paper every 30 seconds, without disturbing the wound. Bleeding time = time required for bleeding to cease. A prolonged bleeding time in a nonhemophiliac patient with normal platelet count indicates von Willebrand's disease, platelet dysfunction, or aspirin ingestion within the past week.

B.   **Activated Partial Thromboplastin Time (APTT):** Measures intrinsic system; requires factors XII, XI, IX, VIII, V, II, I. May be prolonged with polycythemia, inadequate sample volume, blood drawn from heparin-containing catheter. Useful for monitoring heparin therapy.

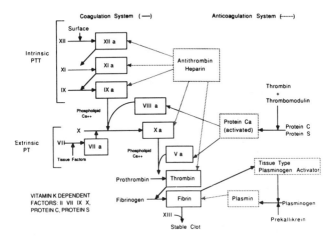

FIG 14.1.
Coagulation Cascade
Modified from Rosenberg RD, Bauer KA. Hospital Practice 1986; March (with permission)

C. **Prothrombin Time (PT):** Measures extrinsic pathway; requires factors VII, X, V, II, I. May be prolonged with decreased liver synthetic capacity, decreased vitamin K absorption, warfarin therapy, inadequate sample volume and drawing from heparin containing catheter. Useful for monitoring warfarin therapy; systemic heparin has little effect at usual therapeutic doses.

D. **Disseminated Intravascular Coagulation:** Usually associated with fragmented RBCs, low or decreasing platelet count, hemoglobinemia (pink plasma), prolonged PT and APTT, and low or decreasing fibrinogen. Confirm by measuring fibrin split products (present), and factors V and VIII (decreased).

VI. BLOOD COMPONENT REPLACEMENT
A. Approximate Blood Volume

Age	Total Blood Volume
Premature infants	90–105 ml/kg
Term newborns	78–86 ml/kg
>1 mo	78 ml/kg
>1 yr	74–82 ml/kg
Adult	68–88 ml/kg

Ref: Oski FA. In Nathan DG, Oski FA: Hematology of Infancy and Childhood. Philadelphia: WB Saunders, 1993; 29, 1916.

B. Required Packed Cell Volume: Infuse no faster than 2–3 ml/kg/hr or in 10 ml/kg aliquots over several hours.

$$\text{Vol of cells (ml)} = \frac{\text{Est blood vol (ml)} \times \text{desired Hct change}}{\text{Hct of PRBC}}$$

Note: The usual Hct of PRBC is 65%.

C. Partial Exchange Transfusion
(See Procedures, Chapter 4, for technique in newborns.)

Diagnosis		Vol of Exchange (ml)
Symptomatic polycythemia	Use fresh frozen plasma or 5% albumin solution	$\dfrac{\text{Est blood vol (ml)} \times \text{desired Hct change}}{\text{Starting Hct}}$
Severe anemia: rapid correction	Use PRBC (about 22 g/dl)	$\dfrac{\text{Blood vol (ml)} \times \text{desired Hb rise}}{22\ \text{gm/dl} - \text{HbR}}$
		$\text{HbR} = \dfrac{\text{Hb (initial)} + \text{Hb (desired)}}{2}$
Sickle cell crisis: double red blood cell volume exchange	Usually reduces sickle cells to <40%; follow Hct during transfusion; use Sickledex negative PRBC.	$\dfrac{\text{Est blood vol (ml)} \times \text{patient's Hct (\%)} \times 2}{\text{Hct of PRBC (\%)}}$

Ref: Nieburg PI, et al. Am J Dis Child 1977; 131:60. Zinkham WH, Personal Communication, 1989.

D.   Platelet Transfusions: Usually give 4 units/m^2. Hemorrhagic complications rare with platelet counts $>20,000/mm^3$. Platelet counts $>50,000/mm^3$ advisable for lumbar puncture. One unit of platelets/m^2 raises platelet count $10,000/mm^3$ in the absence of platelet destruction or antiplatelet antibodies.

$$\text{Platelet increment/mm}^3 = \frac{30,000 \times \text{(number of units)}}{\text{Est blood vol (L)}}$$

E.   Coagulation Factor Replacement
   1.   Background
     a.   1 unit Factor activity = activity in 1 ml normal plasma.
     b.   1 unit Factor VIII/kg raises VIII levels 2%.
     c.   1 unit Factor IX/kg raises IX levels 1%.
   2.   Desired factor level

Bleeding Site	Desired Level
Joint or simple hematoma	20–40%
Simple dental extraction*	50%
Major soft tissue bleed	80–100%
Serious oral bleeding*	80–100%
Head injury	100+%
Major surgery (dental, orthopedic, other)	100+%

*Aminocaproic acid, 100 mg/kg IV or PO q6h (up to 24 gm/d); may be useful for treatment of oral bleeds and prophylaxis for dental extractions.

F.   Blood Products
   1.   **Whole blood:** Use emergently for hypovolemia due to blood loss.
   2.   **PRBC:** Contains WBC but few platelets. Usual choice for RBC transfusion.
   3.   **Leukocyte-poor PRBC:** Use if history of nonhemolytic transfusion reaction, or in immunocompromised patients or neonates.
     a.   Washed: $>90\%$ of WBCs and $>99\%$ plasma removed.

      b. Leukofiltered or frozen deglycerolized: >95% WBCs removed.

  4. **Platelets**

      a. Pooled-concentrates: From multiple donors.

      b. Single donor product: From hemapheresis. Use in patients with antibodies from multiple transfusions.

      c. Leukocyte-poor: Use if history of significant platelet transfusion reactions.

  5. **Granulocytes:** Use only in selected patients with very low WBC count and documented severe infection.

  6. **Fresh Frozen Plasma:** Contains all clotting factors.

  7. **Cryoprecipitate:** Contains factor VIII (5-10 U/cc), VWF, fibrinogen. Do not use in factor IX deficiency.

  8. **Monoclonal Factor VIII:** Relatively purified factor VIII. Use in factor VIII deficiency.

  9. **Prothrombin Complex Concentrates (Konyne, Proplex):** Contains factors II, IX, X, protein C, and some VII and XI. Used in patients with inhibitors and factor IX or VIII deficiency.

  10. **Activated Prothrombin Complex Concentrates (FEIBA, Autoplex):** Contain above factors with some activated IX and X (and VII in some). Consider in factor VIII deficiency with high titer inhibitors.

G.   **Irradiated Blood Products**

  1. Principle: Many blood products (PRBC, platelet preparations, leukocytes, FFP, and others) contain viable lymphocytes capable of sustained survival in recipient. Irradiation with 1500 rad prior to transfusion may prevent graft vs. host disease in immunocompromised patients.

  2. Indications: Intensive chemotherapy, leukemia, lymphoma, bone marrow transplantation, known or suspected T-cell deficiencies, intrauterine transfusions for erythroblastosis fetalis, and possibly transfusions in neonates.

Ref: Von Fliedner V, et al. Am J Med 1982; 72:951.

H.   **CMV Negative Blood:** Desirable in neonates who are CMV-antibody negative.

Ref: Yeager A, et al. J Pediatr 1981; 98:281.

VII. SCREENING FOR LEAD TOXICITY

A. **Sources of Lead:** Lead-based paint, leaded gasoline, soil, and dust; drinking water from lead-soldered pipes, food stored in leaded cans or pottery.

B. **Effect of Lead:** Inhibits enzyme heme synthetase, which prevents incorporation of iron into protoporphyrin III to produce heme, resulting in anemia.

C. **Minimal Screening:**
(Age 6 mos-36 mos)

Risk Groups	Blood Pb Level (μg/dL)	Treatment Plan
Low risk: Initial test at 12 months.	<10	Retest at 24 mo
	10–14	Retest every 3–4 mo; once 2 consecutive tests are <10 μg/dL, or 3 are <15 μg/dL, test once a year.
	≥15	See next section, below.
High risk: Initial test at 6 months	<10	Retest every 6 mo; once two consecutive tests are <10 μg/dL, or 3 <15 μg/dL, test once a year.
	10–14	Retest every 3–4 mo; once two consecutive tests are <10 μg/dL, or 3 are <15 μg/dL, test once a year.
	≥15	See below.

1. Follow-up of children with Pb >15 μg/dL:
    a. >15–19 μg/dL: Screen every 3–4 months; family education and nutrition counseling; identify source of exposure. When Pb is 15–19 in 2 consecutive tests, 3–4 months apart, investigate environment and consider abatement.
    b. ≥20 μg/dL: Confirm with venous blood. If still > 20 μg/dL, refer for medical evaluation.
    c. >45 μg/dL: Confirm with venous blood. If still >45 μg/dL, urgent medical and environmental intervention is needed.
    d. >70 μg/dL: Immediate inpatient chelation therapy.
    Ref: Centers for Disease Control. Preventing lead poisoning in young children. U.S. Department of Health and Human Services Public Health Service, Oct. 1991.

VIII. **NORMAL VALUES:** The following normal values are compiled from published literature and The Johns Hopkins Hospital Department of Laboratory Medicine. Values may vary depending upon analytic technique used. International System (SI) values are in parentheses.

A. **Blood Levels**

Bilirubin	See Blood Chemistries	
Bleeding Time	<9 min	
D-Dimer	Any positive test is significant	
Erythrocyte Sedimentation Rate		
Newborn (0–48 h)	0–4 mm/hr	
Child	4–20 mm/hr	
Adult male	0–10 mm/hr	[Mean, 4]
Adult female	0–20 mm/hr	[Mean, 4]
Ferritin		
Child	7–144 mcg/L	(Same)
Adult male	30–265 mcg/L	(Same)
Adult female	10–110 mcg/L	(Same)
Fibrin Degradation Products		
Titer of 1:25	Borderline positive	
Titer of 1:50	Positive	
Fibrinogen	200–400 mg/dl	(2–4 g/L)
Folate (RBCs)	150–450 mcg/ml	(340–1020 nmol/PRBC)
Free Erythrocyte Protoporphyrin	<3 mcg/g Hb	
	<50 mcg/dl whole blood	
	<130 mcg/dl PRBC	
Haptoglobin	40–180 mg/dl	(0.4–1.8 g/L)
Hemoglobin A$_1$C	3.9%–7.7% of total Hb	(Same)
Hemopexin		
Premature	2–26 mg/dl	
Newborn	8–42 mg/dl	
1–12 yr	40–70 mg/dl	
>12 yr	50–100 mg/dl	
Iron		
Newborn	110–270 mcg/dl	20–48 mmol/L
4–10 mo	30–70 mcg/dl	5.4–12.5 mmol/L
3–10 yr	53–119 mcg/dl	9.5–27.0 mmol/L
Adult	72–186 mcg/dl	13–33 mmol/L

(Continued.)

Blood Levels (cont.).

Lead	See Section VII	
Partial Thromboplastin Time Activated (APTT)		
Preterm	70 sec	
Full-term	45–65 sec	
Child/adult	30–45 sec	
Prothrombin Time (PT)		
Preterm	17 (range, 12–21) sec	
Full-term	16 (range, 13–20) sec	
Child/adult	13 (range, 12–14) sec	
Red Cell Distribution Width (RDW)		
Adults	11.5–14.5%	
Transferrin		
Newborn	130–275 mg/dl	(1.3–2.75 g/L)
Adult	220–400 mg/dl	(2.2–4.0 g/L)
Vitamin B_{12}	30–785 pg/ml	(96–579 pmol/L)

B. Age-Specific Indices

Age	Hgb (gm%), Mean (−2 SD)	Hct (%), Mean (−2 SD)	MCV (fl), Mean (−2 SD)	MCHC (gm/% RBC), Mean (−2 SD)	Retic (%)	WBC/mm³ × 1000, Mean (+2 SD)	Platelets (10³/mm³), Mean (+2 SD)
26–30 wk gestation*	13.4 (11)	41.5 (34.9)	118.2 (106.7)	37.9 (30.6)	—	4.4 (2.7)	254 (180–327)
28 wk	14.5	45	120	31.0	(5–10)	—	275
32 wk	15.0	47	118	32.0	(3–10)	—	290
Term† (cord)	16.5 (13.5)	51 (42)	108 (98)	33.0 (30.0)	(3–7)	18.1 (9–30)‡	290
1–3 days	18.5 (14.5)	56 (45)	108 (95)	33.0 (29.0)	(1.8–4.6)	18.9 (9.4–34)	192
2 wk	16.6 (13.4)	53 (41)	105 (88)	31.4 (28.1)		11.4 (5–20)	252
1 mo	13.9 (10.7)	44 (33)	101 (91)	31.8 (28.1)	(0.1–1.7)	10.8 (4–19.5)	
2 mo	11.2 (9.4)	35 (28)	95 (84)	31.8 (28.3)			
6 mo	12.6 (11.1)	36 (31)	76 (68)	35.0 (32.7)	(0.7–2.3)	11.9 (6–17.5)	(150–350)
6 mo–2 yr	12.0 (10.5)	36 (33)	78 (70)	33.0 (30.0)		10.6 (6–17)	"
2–6 yr	12.5 (11.5)	37 (34)	81 (75)	34.0 (31.0)	(0.5–1.0)	8.5 (5–15.5)	"
6–12 yr	13.5 (11.5)	40 (35)	86 (77)	34.0 (31.0)	(0.5–1.0)	8.1 (4.5–13.5)	"
12–18 yr							
Male	14.5 (13)	43 (36)	88 (78)	34.0 (31.0)	(0.5–1.0)	7.8 (4.5–13.5)	"
Female	14.0 (12)	41 (37)	90 (78)	34.0 (31.0)	(0.5–1.0)	7.8 (4.5–13.5)	"
Adult							
Male	15.5 (13.5)	47 (41)	90 (80)	34.0 (31.0)	(0.8–2.5)	7.4 (4.5–11)	"
Female	14.0 (12)	41 (36)	90 (80)	34.0 (31.0)	(0.8–4.1)	7.4 (4.5–11)	"

*Values are from fetal samplings.

†Under 1 m/o, capillary Hgb exceeds venous: 1 hr-3.6 gm difference; 5 days-2.2 gm difference; 3 wks-1.1 gm difference.

‡Mean (95% confidence limits.)

Ref: Adapted from: Forestier F. et al. Pediatr Res 1986; 20:342; Oski FA, Naiman JL. Hematological Problems in the Newborn Infant. WB Saunders 1982; Nathan D, Oski FA. Hematology of Infancy and Childhood. WB Saunders, 1981; Metoth Y, et al. Acta Paed Scand 1971; 60:317; Wintrobe. Clinical Hematology. Lea & Febiger, 1981.

C.   **Hemoglobin and MCV Percentiles**

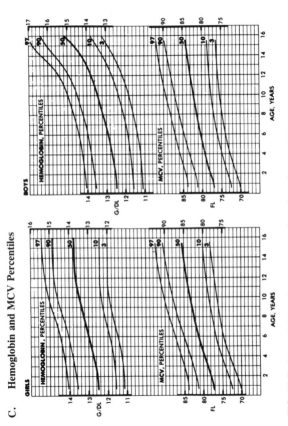

FIG 14.2.   Hemoglobin and mean corpuscular volume by age. Ref:
Dallman PR and Siimes MA: J Pediatr 1979; 94:26 (with permission).

D. Age-Specific White Cell Differential: Number of leukocytes are in thousands per mm^3; ranges are estimates of 95% confidence limits, and percentages refer to differential counts

Age	Total Leukocytes		Neutrophils*			Lymphocytes			Monocytes		Eosinophils	
	Mean	Range	Mean	Range	%	Mean	Range	%	Mean	%	Mean	%
Birth	—†	—	4.0	2.0–6.0	—	4.2	2.0–7.3	—	0.6	—	0.1	—
12 hr	—	—	11.0	7.8–14.5	—	4.2	2.0–7.3	—	0.6	—	0.1	—
24 hr	—	—	9.0	7.0–12.0	—	4.2	2.0–7.3	—	0.6	—	0.1	—
1–4 wk	—	—	3.6	1.8–5.4	—	5.6	2.9–9.1	—	0.7	—	0.2	—
6 mo	11.9	6.0–17.5	3.8	1.0–8.5	32	7.3	4.0–13.5	61	0.6	5	0.3	3
1 yr	11.4	6.0–17.5	3.5	1.5–8.5	31	7.0	4.0–10.5	61	0.6	5	0.3	3
2 yr	10.6	6.0–17.0	3.5	1.5–8.5	33	6.3	3.0–9.5	59	0.5	5	0.3	3
4 yr	9.1	5.5–15.5	3.8	1.5–8.5	42	4.5	2.0–8.0	50	0.5	5	0.3	3
6 yr	8.5	5.0–14.5	4.3	1.5–8.0	51	3.5	1.5–7.0	42	0.4	5	0.2	3
8 yr	8.3	4.5–13.5	4.4	1.5–8.0	53	3.3	1.5–6.8	39	0.4	4	0.2	2
10 yr	8.1	4.5–13.5	4.4	1.8–8.0	54	3.1	1.5–6.5	38	0.4	4	0.2	2
16 yr	7.8	4.5–13.0	4.4	1.8–8.0	57	2.8	1.2–5.2	35	0.4	5	0.2	3
21 yr	7.4	4.5–11.0	4.4	1.8–7.7	59	2.5	1.0–4.8	34	0.3	4	0.2	3

*Neutrophils include band cells at all ages and a small number of metamyelocytes and myelocytes in the first few days of life.

†Insufficient data for a reliable estimate.

Ref: Dallmann PR. "Developmental Changes in Number," in Pediatrics, Rudolph AM (ed), 18th ed. Norwalk: Appleton and Lange, 1987, 1061, (with permission). (Data on infants under the age of 1 month are derived from Monroe, et al. J Pediatr 1979: 95:89, and Ewinberg, et al: J Pediatr 1985; 106:462. Other values are from Albritton EC (ed). Standard Value in Blood. W. B. Saunders, 1952.)

IMMUNOLOGY

15

I. LABORATORY EVALUATION OF SUSPECTED IM-MUNODEFICIENCY

Suspected Abnormality	Screening Tests	Advanced Tests
B-cell (antibody) deficiency	Antibody levels (IgG, IgM, IgA)	IgG antibody subclass levels
	Antibody titers to protein vaccines (tetanus, diptheria)	B-cell enumeration
	Antibody titers to polysaccharide vaccines (Pneumovax)	
T-cell (cell-mediated immunity) deficiency	Total lymphocyte count	T-cell (CD2 or CD3) enumeration
	Delayed hypersensitivity skin tests (Candida, tetanus toxoid, mumps, trichophyton)	T-cell subset (CD4, CD8) enumeration
		In vitro T-cell proliferation to mitogens, antigens, or allogeneic cells
	HIV test	
Phagocytic/splenic deficiency	WBC count and morphology	Nitroblue tetrazolium (NBT) dye test
	Peripheral blood smear for Howell-Jolly bodies	Chemotactic assay
		Phagocytic and bactericidal assay
		Spleen scan
Complement deficiency	Total hemolytic complement CH_{50}	Classic and alternative pathway assays
		Individual component assays

Ref: Modified from Stiehm RE. Pediatr Rev, 1985;7:53.

II. INTRAVENOUS IMMUNE GLOBULIN (IVIG)

A. **Purpose:** Provides immediate antibody levels with a half-life of 3–4 weeks.

B. **Indications**
1. Humoral immune deficiency
   a. IVIG replaces IgG, but contains only trace amounts of IgA and IgM.
   b. IVIG and all other blood products containing IgA are relatively contraindicated in patients with selective IgA deficiency.
   c. Dose: 300–400/mg/kg IV per month. Determine optimal frequency and dose of IVIG by monitoring clinical response.
2. Idiopathic thrombocytopenic purpura
   a. Initial therapy: 1–2 g/kg IV over 1–4 days.
   b. Maintenance therapy: 0.5–1 g/kg IV per month as needed.
3. Kawasaki disease
   Dosage: 2 g/kg IV as a single dose, or 1 g/kg/day IV × 2 days.
   Ref: 1991 Report of the Committee of Infectious Disease. (Red Book)

III. INTRAMUSCULAR IMMUNE GLOBULIN

A. **IVIG is the drug of choice for the above indications. Recommended doses cannot be given using IM immune globulin, which is supplied as a 16.5% solution (165 mg/ml).**

B. **Intramuscular immune globulin preparations contain IgG aggregates; IMIG *never* should be given intravenously.**

C. **Indications for intramuscular immunoglobulin.**
1. Hepatitis A exposure
2. Travel prophylaxis
3. Measles exposure
   a. Nonvaccinated normal individuals: dose, 0.25 ml/kg IM.
   b. Immunocompromised individuals: dose, 0.5 ml/kg IM; maximum dose, 15 ml.
   Ref: Red Book, 1991.

IV. REFERENCE VALUES
A. Serum Immunoglobulin Levels

Age	IgG (mg/dl)	IgM (mg/dl)	IgA (mg/dl)
Newborn	1031 ± 200	11 ± 5	2 ± 3
1–3 mo	430 ± 119	30 ± 11	21 ± 13
4–6 mo	427 ± 186	43 ± 17	28 ± 18
7–12 mo	661 ± 219	54 ± 23	37 ± 18
13–24 mo	762 ± 209	58 ± 23	50 ± 24
25–36 mo	892 ± 183	61 ± 19	71 ± 37
3–5 yr	929 ± 228	56 ± 18	93 ± 27
6–8 yr	923 ± 256	65 ± 25	124 ± 45
9–11 yr	1124 ± 235	79 ± 33	131 ± 60
12–16 yr	946 ± 124	59 ± 20	148 ± 63
Adults	1158 ± 305	99 ± 27	200 ± 61

Ref: Modified from Pediatrics 1966; 37:715.

B. Serum IgG Subclass Levels: Mean (95th% Confidence Interval)

Age (yr)	IgG1 (mg/dl)	IgG2 (mg/dl)	IgG3 (mg/dl)	IgG4 (mg/dl)*
0–1	340 (190–620)	59 (30–140)	39 (9–62)	19 (6–63)
1–2	410 (230–710)	68 (30–170)	34 (11–98)	13 (4–43)
2–3	480 (280–830)	98 (40–240)	28 (6–130)	18 (3–120)
3–4	530 (350–790)	120 (50–260)	30 (9–98)	32 (5–180)
4–6	540 (360–810)	140 (60–310)	39 (9–160)	39 (9–160)
6–8	560 (280–1120)	150 (30–630)	48 (40–250)	81 (11–620)
8–10	690 (280–1740)	210 (80–550)	85 (22–320)	42 (10–170)
10–13	590 (270–1290)	240 (110–550)	58 (13–250)	60 (7–530)
13–Adult	540 (280–1020)	210 (60–790)	58 (14–240)	60 (11–330)

* 10% of individuals appear to have absent IgG4 levels.

Ref: Modified from Schur PH. Ann Allergy 1987; 58:89.

C. Lymphocyte Enumeration

1. T cells: Normal values (5th-95th percentile) for T-Lymphocytes in peripheral blood.

Age	CD3 (Total T-Cells)	CD4 (T-Helper/Inducer)	CD8 (T-Suppressor/ Cytotoxic)	CD4/CD8 Ratio
2-3 mo	60-87% (2.07-6.54)*	41-64% (1.46-5.11)*	16-35% (0.65-2.45)*	1.32-3.47
4-8 mo	57-84% (2.28-6.45)*	36-61% (1.69-4.60)*	16-34% (0.72-2.49)*	1.20-3.48
12-23 mo	53-81% (1.46-5.44)*	31-54% (1.02-3.60)*	16-38% (0.57-2.23)*	0.95-2.95
2-6 yr	62-80% (1.61-4.23)*	35-51% (0.90-2.86)*	22-38% (0.63-1.91)*	1.05-2.07
Adult	59-81% (558-1948)†	31-55% (350-1334)†	17-38% (147-812)†	0.84-3.05

*Absolute number of T-cells $\times 10^9$/liter
†Absolute number of T-cells per milliliter

2. B Cells: Total B cells comprise about 5-20% of total lymphocytes.

Ref: (1) Denny, T. et al. JAMA 267:1484; 1992. (2) The Johns Hopkins Hospital Laboratory Medicine Department. (3) Manual of Clinical Laboratory Immunology, 3rd ed.; American Society of Microbiology: Washington DC,1986.

D. Serum Complement Levels

C1 esterase inhibitor	17.4-24 mg/dl
C3	
1-6 mo	53-175 mg/dl
7-12 mo	75-180 mg/dl
1-5 yr	77-166 mg/dl
6-10 yr	88-199 mg/dl
Adult	83-177 mg/dl
C4	
1-6 mo	7-42 mg/dl
7-12 mo	9.5-39 mg/dl
1-5 yr	9-40 mg/dl
6-10 yr	12-40 mg/dl
Adult	15-45 mg/dl
CH$_{50}$	75-160 U/ml

E. Complement Cascade

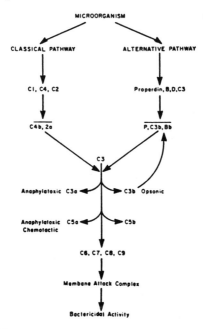

FIG 15.1.
Complement Cascade

Ref: Oski, FA et al. Principles and Practice of Pediatrics; JB Lippincott Company; Philadelphia 1990; p. 172.

IMMUNO-PROPHYLAXIS

16

Note: For more detailed and updated information on immunizations, please refer to the current issues of Morbidity and Mortality Weekly Report, the package inserts of individual vaccines, or the current edition of the Report of the Committee on Infectious Diseases of the American Academy of Pediatrics (the "Red Book").

I.   IMMUNIZATION SCHEDULES

Ref: MMWR 1991; 40:No. RR-1, RR-10, RR-13. MMWR 1992; 41:No. RR-1. Red Book, 1991.

A.   Routine Immunizations

Birth						Birth	HBV[1]	
2 mo	DTP	Polio	Hib[1]	Hib[2]		1-2 mo	HBV[1]	HBV[2]
4 mo	DTP	Polio	Hib[1]	Hib[2]		4 mo		HBV[2]
6 mo	DTP	Polio[+]	Hib[1]					
12 mo				Hib[2]				
15 mo	DTP/ DTaP	Polio	Hib[1]		MMR	6-18 mo	HBV[1]	HBV[2]
18 mo								
4–6 yr	DTP/ DTaP	Polio						
11–12 yr					MMR[3]			
14–16 yr	Td (repeat every 10 yr)							

HIB[1] and HIB[2]: Alternate schedules for vaccine produced by different manufacturers.

HBV[1] and HBV[2]: Alternate schedules for the recombinant hepatitis vaccine for routine primary immunization for infants of HBsAg negative mothers.

MMR[3]: Local regulations may differ. 2nd dose may be required upon entry into primary school.

+: Third dose in endemic area.

B. Alternative Schedule: Unimmunized Children (See Schedule C for Hib Alternative Schedule)

Interval after 1st visit	Age < 7 yr at 1st visit			Age ≥ 7 yr at 1st visit		
1st Visit	DTP	Polio	MMR if age ≥ 15 mo	Td	Polio	MMR
2 mo	DTP	Polio		Td	Polio	
4 mo	DTP	Polio*		Td [2]	Polio [2]	
10–16 mo	DTP/DTaP	Polio+				
4–6 yr	DTP or DTaP	Polio++	MMR[3]			
11–12 yr						MMR

++Not given if 3rd dose is after 4th birthday
+Not given if 3rd dose is given earlier
*Give only in endemic areas.
[3]Local regulations may differ; 2nd dose may be required upon entry into primary school.
[2]8-14 months after 1st visit

C. *Haemophilus influenzae:* Primary Series and Booster Schedule

Conjugate Vaccine	Age (mo) at 1st Dose	Series Interval	Age (mo) at Booster*
HbOC	2–6	3 doses, 2 mo-interval	15
	7–11	2 doses, 2 mo-interval	15
	12–14	1 dose	15
	15–59	1 dose	—
PRP-OMP	2–6	2 doses, 2 mo-interval	12
	7–11	2 doses, 2 mo-interval	15
	12–14	1 dose	15
	15–59	1 dose	—
PRP-D	15–59	1 dose	—

*Booster doses should be given at least 2 months after previous dose.

II. GENERAL INFORMATION: IMMUNIZATION GUIDELINES

A. Immunocompromised Hosts and Their Contacts

1. **Contraindiciations for live viral vaccines**
   a. Children with decreased immune function (see below for exception in children with HIV disease).
   b. Immunosuppressive therapy
      Give live viral vaccines three or more months after immunosuppressive treatment has been discontinued.
   c. Household contacts of persons with an immunologic deficiency should not receive oral polio virus vaccine (OPV). Give IPV, MMR following the routine schedule.

2. **Immunization of children with known or suspected HIV disease**
   a. DTP, IPV, Hib, MMR according to routine schedule.
   b. Pneumococcal vaccine at 2 years of age.
   c. Yearly influenza vaccine beginning at 6 months of age.
   d. **With the exception of MMR, do not give BCG or live viral vaccines to symptomatic children.**
   e. Passive immunization with specific immune globulin when exposed to measles, varicella, or tetanus (see specific disease guidelines in this chapter).

3. **Immunization of children with Hodgkin's disease**
   a. Pneumococcal vaccine if 24 months of age or older.
   b. *Haemophilus influenzae* vaccine, using the routine schedule.
      Note: Immunize at least two weeks before or three months after chemotherapy.

B. Asplenic Children:
Children with functional or anatomic asplenia are at high risk for fulminant bacteremia. Pneumococcal and meningococcal vaccines are recommended for asplenic children 2 years and older. Follow routine schedule for Hib vaccine.

C. Premature Infants

1. Premature infants should be immunized based on chronological age.
2. If the child remains hospitalized, IPV should be used, or OPV may be given upon discharge if the timing is correct to prevent transmission of live virus in the nursery.
3. Full dose (0.5 ml IM) of DTP should be given.

D. **Pregnant Women and Adolescents:** All live virus vaccines are contraindicated in pregnancy unless the woman is at high risk of exposure to the disease and a threat is posed to the mother and fetus if infected.

E. **Patients Treated With Immune Globulin:** Individuals who have received immune globulin (Ig) or blood products should not receive MMR until 3–12 months later, because the Ig may interfere with the desired immune response. See current Red Book for specific recommendation.

F. **Febrile Illness:** Immunizations should be deferred in the presence of significant febrile illness (see specific vaccine guidelines for further recommendations).

III. IMMUNIZATION GUIDELINES FOR SPECIFIC DISEASES: Please refer to Section I for recommended vaccination schedules.

A. **Diphtheria/Tetanus/Pertussis Vaccine**
  1. Vaccine Types
    a. DTP: adsorbed triple vaccine; dose, 0.5ml IM.
    b. DTaP: contains an acellular pertussis component.
      1) Recommended only for the the fourth and fifth doses of the series.
      2) DTaP currently is not licensed for use in children less than 15 months of age.
  2. Side Effects and Contraindications
    a. **Common side effects of pertussis component,** occurring within several hours of vaccination (not contraindications for further immunization):
      1) Redness
      2) Swelling or pain at the injection site
      3) Slight to moderate fever
      4) Drowsiness
      5) Anorexia
    b. **Contraindications to pertussis immunization**—indications for the use of DT vaccine:
      1) Evolving neurologic disorders
      2) Poorly controlled seizures
      3) A history of severe reactions to DTP:
        a) Unexplained fever >40.5° C within 48 hours
        b) Unconsolable screaming for > 3 hours within 48 hours

    c) Somnolence or shock within 48 hours

    d) Convulsions within 72 hours

    e) Encephalopathy within 7 days

    f) Immediate anaphylactic reaction

    Note: DTaP is not a substitute for DTP in children in whom there is a contraindication for the use of pertussis vaccine.

  c. **Children with febrile seizures or seizure disorders:** There are few specific guidelines for immunizations in children with a history of febrile seizures or other seizure disorders. The value of immunization must be weighed against the possibility of adverse reactions. Children with neurologic disorders identified in the first year of life may require temporary deferment of DTP and DT (see Red Book 1991, pp 322–324 for details). Prophylactic antipyretics may be considered for children deemed to be at high risk for convulsions.

    Ref: MMWR, 1992: 41. RR-1

  d. The following are not contraindications to DTP vaccinations:

    1) Temperature <40.5° C

    2) Redness, swelling at site of previous DTP vaccination

    3) Mild acute illness with low grade fever in an otherwise healthy child

    4) Recent exposure to infectious disease

    5) Prematurity

    6) Family history of SIDS, convulsions or adverse reactions to DTP vaccination

    Ref: MMWR 1991,40: RR-10

3. **Pertussis outbreak:** During pertussis outbreak, monovalent pertussis vaccine, 0.25cc IM, may be given to previously immunized children and adults. A child with culture proven pertussis need not receive further pertussis vaccination; use DT for boosters if child is less than 7 years, and dT if older than 7 years.

B. *Haemophilus influenzae* **Type B Vaccine**
1. **Vaccine Types:** Each polysaccharide conjugate vaccine has a different immunization schedule. Use the same type of vaccine throughout the primary series. See Section I for details.

Vaccine Abbreviation*	Trade Name	Dose	Comments
HbOC	HibTITER	0.5 ml IM ⎫	Approved for infants of all
PRP-OMP	PedvaxHIB	0.5 ml IM ⎬	ages
PRP-D	ProHIBit	0.5 ml IM	Available only for children ≥ 15 mo

*A third conjugate vaccine, PRP-T, may be licensed soon.

2. **Side Effects of Hib Vaccines:** To date, no vaccine-related side effects have been reported.
3. **Special Circumstances**
   a. Any child less than 24 months old who has had invasive *Haemophilus influenzae* B disease may not have developed an adequate immunity. They should continue to receive the vaccine series beginning 1 to 2 months after the acute illness.
   b. Unimmunized children ≥ 5 years of age, who are at increased risk for *Haemophilus influenzae* B invasive disease (including children with functional or anatomic asplenia), should receive a single dose of any conjugate vaccine.
   c. Vaccinate children with Hodgkin's disease 2 or more weeks before chemotherapy or 3 months after chemotherapy has ended.

C. Hepatitis A Prophylaxis
1. **Indications**
   a. Anyone inoculated with a contaminated needle.
   b. Anyone who has had open lesions directly in contact with material (blood, serum, saliva or other body fluids) from a person known to have hepatitis A.
   c. All household contacts and sexual partners of individuals infected with hepatitis A.
   d. Schoolmates in classes where more than one case has been documented.

    e. All employees and children at daycare centers where one case has been documented.

    f. Consider in infants born to mothers with hepatitis A infection if mother is jaundiced at time of delivery.

    g. Travelers to developing countries may require prophylaxis.

2. **Treatment**

    a. Give 0.02 ml/kg of immune globulin (Ig), IM.

    b. For continuous exposure >3 months, give 0.06 ml/kg of Ig every 5 months.

D. Hepatitis B Vaccine and Immunoprophylaxis

  1. **Vaccine types**

Vaccine Name	Age (Range)	Dose (IM)	Comments
Energerix-B	< 11 yr	10 µg (0.5 ml)	May be given in a four dose schedule (see MMWR).
	≥ 11 yr	20 µg (1.0 ml)	
Recombivax HB	< 11 yr	2.5 µg (0.25 ml)	
	11–19 yr	5 µg (0.5 ml)	
	> 19 yr	10 µg (1.0 ml)	
	Infants of HIV+ mothers	5 µg (0.5 ml)	
Hepatovax			Only available in the United States for hemodialysis patients, immunocompromised hosts, or patients with yeast allergy (see Red Book for details).

2. **Side effects and contraindications:** Most frequent side effects are pain at the injection site, and a low grade fever.

3. **Specific Guidelines**

    a. Routine immunization for:

       1) Infants born to hepatitis B surface antigen (HBsAg)-negative mothers

       2) All adolescents, resources permitting

3) Patients at high risk of developing hepatitis B infection:
   a) Chronically institutionalized children and their caretakers
   b) Health professionals
   c) Hemodialysis patients
   d) Intravenous drug abusers
   e) Sexually active homosexual males
   f) Patients with multiple sex partners (>1 partner/6 months)
   g) Chronic blood product recipients (e.g., hemophiliac patients receiving clotting factors)
   h) Household and sexual contacts of HBV carriers
   i) Infants of (HBsAg)-positive mothers
   j) Travelers or adopted children living >6 months in areas of high hepatitis B endemicity
   Ref: Pediatrics, 1992; 89:795.

b. Recommendation for treament of individuals exposed to the hepatitis B virus.
   (Ref: Red Book, 1991;250.).

Exposure	Treatment
Perinatal*	0.5 ml HBIg within 12 hours of birth; first dose of vaccine within 7 days; preferably simultaneous with HBIg
Sexual	0.06 ml/kg HBIg (max, 5 ml); first dose of vaccine with HBIg; repeat at 1 and 6 mo
Acute hepatitis B in household contact	Infants <12 mo; give HBIg and initiate 3-dose vaccine schedule as soon as possible; infants >12 mo; follow serologies of index case; if HBsAg carrier-all household contacts receive vaccine
Percutaneous or permucosal exposure to blood or body fluids	Single dose HBIg 0.06 ml/kg within 24 hours; initiate vaccine series within 7 days (0, 1, and 6 mo)

*Children born to mothers who are HBsAg-positive at delivery, have unknown serologies, or have known third-trimester HBV infection should receive hepatitis immune globulin (HBIg) at birth and the first in the primary series of recombinant vaccine. Test at 9 mo of age for HBsAg and anti-HBsAg. If negative, a fourth dose of vaccine should be given. If HBsAg-positive, serologies should be monitored for evidence of a chronic carrier state. Breast-feeding is not contraindicated if infant has received appropriate immunoprophylaxis.

E. Influenza Vaccine
1. **Vaccine information**
   a. Preparations
      1) Subvirion (split) vaccine.
      2) Whole inactivated virus vaccine. Not used in children >12 years.
   b. Doses: Antigenic makeup varies from year to year. Administer during autumn in preparation for winter influenza season.
      1) Age 6 to 35 months: 2 doses (0.25 ml IM) of split virus vaccine at 0 and 1 months for 1st year of immunization; thereafter, single dose yearly, amount based on age.
      2) Age 3–8 years: 2 doses (0.5 ml IM) of split virus vaccine at 0 and 1 months for the 1st year of immunization; thereafter, single 0.5 ml IM dose yearly.
      3) Age 9–12 years: one dose (0.5 ml IM) of split virus vaccine.
      4) Age ≥12 years: one dose (0.5 ml IM) of either split or whole virus vaccine.
   c. May be given simultaneously (separate sites) with MMR, Hib conjugate, pneumococcal or polio vaccines, but should not be given within 3 days of DTP.
2. **Contraindications**
   a. Not routinely recommended for
      1) Children <6 months old.
      2) Normal children not in close contact with someone who would be placed at high risk with influenza disease.
3. **Indications**
   a. Indicated for children >6 months of age with:
      1) Chronic pulmonary disease
      2) Hemodynamically significicant cardiac disease
      3) HIV
      4) Hemoglobinopathies
      5) Immunosuppression

    b. Consider vaccinating other high-risk children over 6 months of age:
      1) Chronic renal or metabolic diseases
      2) Diabetes
      3) Children on long-term aspirin therapy who would be at risk for developing Reye's syndrome with influenza.

      Ref: MMWR, 1991;40:No.RR-6

F. Measles/Mumps/Rubella

1. **Vaccine types**

    a. A combined vaccine composed of live, attenuated viruses. Measles and mumps vaccines prepared in chick embryo cell culture; rubella vaccine prepared in human diploid cell culture. Dose, 0.5 ml SC. Each is available in monovalent form

2. **Side effects and contraindications**

    a. Contraindications include:
      1) Pregnancy or pregnancy expected within 3 months
      2) Transfusion of immune globulin, plasma, or whole blood within 3 months
      3) Altered immunity (except HIV infection)
      4) Egg or neomycin anaphylactic allergy.

3. **Special Guidelines**

    a. Measles epidemic: During an epidemic, MMR vaccine may be given to children at age 12 months, or monovalent vaccine to infants 6 months or older.

    b. Treatment of patients exposed to measles
      1) Live measles vaccine given within 72 hours of exposure can effectively prevent disease. Monovalent vaccine may be given to infants as young as six months.
      2) Give immune globulin (Ig), 0.25 ml/kg (max, 15 ml) IM for normal unvaccinated children or asymptomatic HIV-infected children within 6 days of exposure. Immunization should be given no sooner than 5 months after Ig administration.
      3) Give 0.5 ml/kg (max, 15 ml) Ig to children with symptomatic HIV infection with or without previous vaccination, or unvaccinated children with ma-

lignancies, immunodeficiencies, or receiving immunosuppressive therapy. Not required if IVIG received within 2 weeks.

  c. Rubella passive immunization

    1) Ig may modify rubella disease. Not generally recommended for children. Dose is 0.55 ml/kg IM of immune globulin.

    2) Routine use of Ig following rubella exposure in early pregnancy is not recommended. Post-exposure prophylaxis may be considered for pregnant women exposed during the first trimester if termination of the pregnancy is not an option.

G. Pneumococcal Vaccine

1. Vaccine: Purified capsular polysaccharide antigen from 23 serotypes. Dose is 0.5 ml SC or IM.
2. Indications and Contraindications

  a. Indicated for children > 2 years of age with:

    1) Sickle cell disease

    2) Functional or anatomic asplenia*

    3) Chronic renal failure

    4) Nephrotic syndrome

    5) HIV infection

    6) Immunosuppressive therapy or chemotherapy*

  b. Consider revaccination in 3–5 years in children <10 years, or in older children at high risk of developing fatal pneumococcal disease (e.g., asplenic or sickle cell patients).

  c. Recommendations are not to vaccinate during pregnancy but must balance unknown risk to fetus with that of pneumococcal sepsis in the mother.

H. Poliomyelitis Vaccine

1. Oral polio virus vaccine

  a. Live trivalent vaccine produced in monkey kidney cell cultures. Dose varies by manufacturer.

  b. Contraindicated in children with altered immunity (from primary disease or therapy) and household contacts of immunodeficient individuals. Avoid in pregnancy unless immediate protection is needed.

*Give vaccine 2 weeks before elective splenectomy, chemotherapy, or immunosuppressive therapy.

2. Inactivated Polio Virus Vaccine: Polio vaccine of choice for immunodeficient children and children with immuno-compromised households contacts. Schedule is the same as for OPV. Dose, 0.5 ml IM.

I. Rabies

1. Vaccines
   a. Two vaccines available
      1) Human diploid cell vaccine (HDCV)
      2) Rabies vaccine adsorbed (RVA)
   b. Usual dose is 1.0 ml IM given on days 0, 3, 7, 14, and 28 if unimmunized. Give 1.0 ml on days 0 and 3 to previously immunized individuals.

2. Immune globulin: Human rabies immune globulin (HRIG) is given in postexposure prophylaxis with the vaccine as soon as possible after exposure, but no later than the seventh day of vaccine schedule. For persons not previously immunized, give HRIG 20 IU/kg, infiltrate one-half dose at site of bite/wound, if possible. Give remainder IM. If HRIG unavailable, give equine serum RIG-40 IU/kg IM after a SC test dose. People previously immunized do not receive HRIG.

3. Post-exposure Treatment: Possible rabies exposure should be evaluated by type of exposure, animal species, vaccination status of animal, prevalence of rabies in locale, and nature of the attack. Decision to immunize should be made in conjunction with local health officials.
   a. All wound care should begin with an immediate and thorough cleansing with soap and water. Consider tetanus prophylaxis and antibacterial management as indicated.

Postexposure Antirabies Treatment

Species of Animal	Condition of Animal at Time of Attack	Treatment of Exposed Patient
Wild*	Regard as rabid	HRIG + vaccine
Domestic†	Known healthy	None
	Unknown (escaped) rabid; or suspected rabid	

*Skunk, fox, coyote, raccoon, bat, other carnivores
†Dog, cat. If livestock, rodents, rabbits, etc., consider individually.

J. Tetanus Immunoprophylaxis
1. Passive immunization
   a. Give tetanus immune globulin (TIG) 3,000 to 6,000 units IM (with some placed into wound).
   b. If TIG not available, give equine antitoxin after testing for hypersensitivity. Give 3,000 to 5,000 units for those with susceptible wounds and 50,000 to 100,000 units (20,000 given IV, and the rest given IM) for clinical illness.
   c. Parenteral penicillin G or tetracycline may be considered for 10-14 days duration.
2. Tetanus prophylaxis in wound management

Previous Tetanus Immunization	Clean Minor Wound	Tetanus-Prone Wound
Uncertain or < 3 doses	Td only*	Td and TIG within 3 days
3 doses	Td (4th dose)*	Td (4th dose)*
> 3 doses	Td if last dose > 10 years ago	Td if last dose > 5 years ago

*In child ≥ 7 years, use Td for vaccination. If < 7 yrs use DPT (or DT if pertussis is contraindicated.)

3. **Any child with AIDS should receive TIG for tetanus-prone wounds, regardless of vaccination status!**

K. Varicella Zoster Immunoprophylaxis
   Note: Exposed children who receive monthly infusions of IVIg (100-400 mg/kg) should not require VZIG if last dose IVIg within 3 weeks.
1. Indications for varicella zoster immunoglobulin (VZIG): Significant exposure in:
   a. Susceptible, immunocompromised children
   b. Normal, nonimmune adolescents and adults
   c. Infants born to mothers who have had the onset of chicken pox within 5 days before or 2 days after delivery.
   d. Hospitalized premature infants (>28 weeks gestation) with a nonimmune mother.
   e. Any hospitalized premature infant <28 weeks gestation or ≤ 1000 grams.

2. Dose of VZIG
   a. Give 1 vial (125 units) for each 10 kg IM (min, 125 units, max, 625 units).
   b. Optimal if given within 48 hours, effective if given within 96 hours.

INFECTIOUS DISEASES

17

I. **HUMAN IMMUNODEFICIENCY VIRUS (HIV) AND THE ACQUIRED IMMUNODEFICIENCY SYNDROME (AIDS):** HIV infection causes a disorder of immune function that may affect multiple organ systems. Latent period may extend from months to years. (For the most recent information in the diagnosis and management of children with HIV infection, contact the National Pediatric HIV Resource Center, 1–800–362–0071.)

A. **Counseling and Testing:** Legal requirements vary by state. Counseling should include informed consent for testing, implications of positive test results and prevention of transmission.

B. **Diagnosis of HIV Infection**
   1. Clinical signs and symptoms:
      a. Generalized lymphadenopathy
      b. Chronic or recurrent diarrhea
      c. Hepatosplenomegaly
      d. Failure to thrive
      e. Parotitis
      f. Progressive neurological disease
      g. Recurrent invasive bacterial or fungal infection
      h. Opportunistic infections (see Table 17.1) (p 259)
   2. Diagnostic tests: Children with HIV infection usually have detectable HIV antibody 6–12 weeks after exposure (exception: infants of HIV positive mothers: see section B.4)
      a. Enzyme-linked immunoabsorbent assay (ELISA) screening test to detect HIV-specific antibodies present in serum.
      b. Western blot: detects serum antibody bound to specific HIV antigens.
      c. Immunofluorescence assays.

    d. Assays being developed and tested in research centers include:
      1) HIV-specific IgA antibodies
      2) HIV culture
      3) Specific p24 viral coat antigen
      4) Amplification of viral genome with the polymerase chain reaction (PCR)

3. Results of tests of humoral and cellular immunity consistent with HIV infection
    a. Low absolute lymphocyte number
    b. Reduced T helper (CD4) cell/ T suppressor (CD8) cell ratio
    c. Polyclonal hypergammaglobulinemia
    d. Decreased CD4 cell number or percentage
      1) Calculation of absolute CD4 cell number:
        a) Obtain simultaneous CBC with differential and T cell subsets including %CD4 cells.
        b) Total lymphocytes = white blood cell count (WBC) × % lymphocytes
        c) Total number CD4 cells = total lymphocytes × % CD4

4. Infants of HIV seropositive mothers: Difficult diagnosis in the first 15 months of life due to presence of maternal antibody. For these infants, follow clinical exam and tests of immune function, and treat appropriately for HIV and opportunistic infections (see below).
    a. Infant is **HIV indeterminate** if <15 months of age and asymptomatic. Follow clinical examination, absolute lymphocyte number, CD4 cell counts, CD4/CD8 ratios, and immunoglobulins.
    b. Infant is **HIV positive** if any of the following conditions are satisfied:
      1) There are **positive antibody tests** with **laboratory evidence of immune deficiency** and **symptoms associated with HIV infection** (see section B1 or CDC classification [Red Book 1991, p.119]).
      2) The infant has a **positive viral culture** or a **positive PCR assay,** repeated and confirmed.
      3) **The infant has illness defined as AIDS** (see Table 17.1).

TABLE 17.1.
Indicator Diseases for the Diagnosis of AIDS*

Disease	Category
Candida esophagitis	A, B
Candida of trachea, bronchi or lungs	A
Disseminated or extrapulmonary coccidiomycosis	C
Extrapulmonary cryptococcosis	A
Chronic intestinal cryptosporidiosis	A
CMV disease (other than liver,spleen,nodes), onset >1 mo of age	A
CMV retinitis with loss of vision	A, B
HIV encephalopathy	C
HIV wasting syndrome	C
Disseminated or extrapulmonary histoplasmosis	C
Chronic intestinal isosporiasis (>1 mo duration)	C
HSV ulcer, chronic (>1 mo duration)	A
HSV pneumonitis or esophagitis (onset >1 mo of age)	A
Kaposi sarcoma	A, B
Lymphoid interstitial pneumonitis	A, B
Primary brain lymphoma	A
Burkitt's lymphoma or immunoblastic sarcoma	C
Multiple or recurrent bacterial infections	C
Disseminated or extrapulmonary *Mycobacterium avium* complex or *M. kansasii*	A
Disseminated or extrapulmonary *M. tuberculosis* or acid fast infection	C
Pneumocystis carinii pneumonia	A, B
Progressive multifocal leukoencephalopathy	A
Toxoplasmosis of brain, onset at >1 mo of age	A, B

*AIDS is diagnosed if:
    a. There is a definite diagnosis of a disease from category A (e.g., biopsy or culture),
and
    b. There is no other cause for immunodeficiency.
or
    a. There is laboratory evidence of HIV infection,
and
    b. There is a presumptive diagnosis of a disease from category B.
or
    a. A disease from category C is present,
and
    b. There is laboratory evidence of HIV infection.

Ref: Adapted from The Red Book, 1991:117.

c. **HIV-negative** infants initially may test antibody-positive but will seroconvert by age 15 months.

5. HIV infection in children

C. **Prophylaxis for *Pneumocystis carinii* Pneumonia (PCP):** Most common opportunistic infection in children.

1. Initiate prophylaxis for children >1 month of age who are
   a. HIV seropositive **or**
   b. HIV infected **or**
   c. <12 months with HIV-positive mother

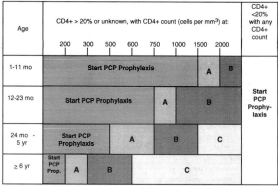

A: No prophylaxis recommended at this time; recheck CD4+ count in 1 month.
B: No prophylaxis recommended at this time; recheck CD4+ count at least every 3-4 months.
C: No prophylaxis recommended at this time; recheck CD4+ count at least every 6 months.

FIG 17.1.
Recommendations for the Initiation of PCP Prophylaxis (MMWR, 1991 40:RR–2)

2. Start prophylaxis for any child with a history of PCP.
3. Prophylactic regimen:
   a. Trimethoprim (TMP)-sulfamethoxasole (SMX): 150 mg TMP/m^2 and 750 mg SMX/m^2/day divided BID for 3 consecutive days of the week (max, 320 mg TMP daily).

b. Consider monthly regimen of aerosolized pentamidine in older children and adolescents if TMP-SMX is contraindicated. Doses vary for different preparations. The use of IV pentamidine is being studied.

c. Dapsone: 1 mg/kg (max, 100 mg) PO daily is an alternative in older children.

D. Antiviral Therapy

1. Zidovudine (AZT), a thymidine analogue, is currently recommended for use in children. See Formulary for details (Chapter 25).

2. Guidelines for starting AZT therapy:

Age (yr)	CD4 Count (Cells/mm^3)	**or**	%CD4
<1	<1750		<30
1–2	<1000		<25
2–6	<750		<20
>6	<500		<20

Ref: HIV Resource Center, Workshop on Retroviral Therapy, 1992.

3. Dideoxyinosine (ddI) has been approved for use in children.

E. Immunizations: Specific guidelines are discussed in Immunoprophylaxis, Chapter 16.

II. SEXUALLY TRANSMITTED DISEASES (STDs)
Note: Several organisms are primarily transmitted through sexual contact, including HIV and syphilis; these often coexist and must be considered in any patient diagnosed with an STD. Please refer to The Medical Letter (1991, 33:70–81), or current editions of the Red Book for detailed discussions of those STDs not covered here.

A. Vaginitis, Cervicitis, and Pelvic Inflammatory Disease

1. Organisms
   a. *Trichomonas vaginalis*
   b. *Gardnerella vaginalis, Mycoplasma hominis,* and anaerobic bacteria contribute to bacterial vaginosis (not necessarily sexually acquired).
   c. *Candida* (though not sexually transmitted)

2. Evaluation
    a. Microscopic
        1) Saline prep: for trichomonas, vaginosis (clue cells), leukocytes.
        2) KOH prep for yeast.
    b. Cervical cultures for *N. gonorrhoeae* and *C. trachomatis*.
    c. Cervical gram stain to look for presence of large numbers of polymorphonuclear cells (indicative of cervicitis), or gram-negative intracellular diplococci *(N. gonorrhoeae)*.

B. Urethritis and Acute Epididymitis: Most common organisms: *C. trachomatis, N. gonorrhoeae* or *Ureaplasma urealyticum*. Culture discharge as indicated. Asymptomatic partners of patients with known infection should be treated.

C. Sexual Abuse: Evaluate victims of sexual abuse for STDs and consider treatment. All children:
1. Throat, rectal, vaginal and/or endocervical cultures for *N. gonorrhoeae* and *C. trachomatis*.
2. Darkfield exam of any chancres for syphilis. Serological tests for syphilis.
3. Consider evaluation for HIV, hepatitis B, herpes simplex, and other STDs as indicated.
    Ref: Red Book 1991; p.107.

III. SYPHILIS: Disease caused by the spirochete *Treponema pallidum*. May be acquired through sexual contact, or may be congenitally transmitted.

A. Diagnosis
1. Clinical presentation: 3 stages
    a. Primary: Indurated, painless ulcers of skin and mucous membranes, most commonly genitalia.

Treatment

Type of Infection	Therapy of Choice	Alternative Regimen[†]
Pelvic inflammatory disease		
Inpatient	Either Cefoxitin 2 gm IV Q6h **or** Cefotetan 2 gm IV Q12h **plus** Doxycycline* 100 mg IV Q12h until improved **then** Doxycycline* 100 mg PO BID to complete 10–14 days	Clindamycin 900 mg IV Q8h **plus** Gentamicin 2 mg/kg IV once **then** Gentamicin 1.5 mg/kg IV Q8h until improved **then** Doxycycline*·§ 100 mg PO BID to complete 10–14 days.
Outpatient	Cefoxitin 2 gm IM once **and** Probenicid 1 gm PO once **or** Ceftriaxone 250 mg IM once (without probenicid) **or** Cefixime 400 mg PO once **then** Doxycycline* 100 mg PO BID for 10–14 days	
Trichomoniasis	Metronidazole† 2 gm PO once	Metronidazole† 500 mg PO BID for 7 days
Bacterial vaginosis	Metronidazole† 500 mg PO BID for 7 days	Clindamycin 300 mg PO BID for 7 days
Gonorrhea in children <45 kg (proctitis, pharyngitis, urogenital infection)	Ceftriaxone 125 mg IM once	Amoxicillin 50 mg/kg PO once **plus** Probenecid 25 mg/kg PO once (max, 1 gm) **or** Spectinomycin‡ 40 mg/kg IM once (without probenicid).

*Doxycycline contraindicated in pregnancy. Use erythromycin (not estolate), 500 mg PO QID for 10–14 days.
†Contraindicated in first trimester of pregnancy.
‡Not useful in pharyngitis.
§Or clindamycin 450 mg PO QID to complete 14 days.

Ref: The Medical Letter 1991, 33: pp. 70–81.

      b. Secondary: May have rash, usually maculopapular involving palms and soles, or mucous membrane involvement (condyloma lata, mucous patches). May have fever, malaise, arthralgias, generalized lymphadenopathy.

      c. Tertiary: Usually not in children; usually >15 years after primary.

         1) Neurosyphilis

         2) Aortitis

         3) Gummas of skin, bone, and/or viscera

  2. Laboratory tests

      a. Nontreponemal serologic tests are quantitative assays for antibody directed against antigen resulting from host tissue interaction with the trepenome. Useful for screening, assessing treatment adequacy, or detecting relapse. False positives may occur in people with infections such as EBV or in people with autoimmune disorders.

         1) Venereal disease reference laboratory (VDRL) slide test

         2) Rapid plasma reagin (RPR) card test, and

         3) The automated reagin test (ART)

      b. Treponemal assays measure antibody directed against specific spirochetal antigens: nonquantitative, confirmatory tests. Reactive tests remain positive for life, therefore not useful for identifying disease recurrence:

         1) Fluorescence treponemal antibody (FTA) test

         2) Fluorescence treponemal antibody absorbed (FTA-ABS) test

         3) Microhemagglutination test for *T. pallidum* (MHA-TP)

         4) *T. pallidum* immobilization test

      c. Direct fluorescence antibody staining (DFA) of organisms from tissue.

B. Congenital Syphilis

  1. Evaluation

      a. All pregnant women should be screened serologically early in pregnancy and early in the third trimester. Treat if evidence of infection.

b. Evaluate any infant with clinical evidence of syphilis who has a reactive cord blood test or who is born to a serologically positive mother. Determine adequacy of maternal treatment. Consider treatment inadequate if:

1) Untreated
2) Treatment record poorly documented
3) Incomplete doses or length of treatment
4) Treated with non-penicillin regimen
5) Treated <1 month before delivery
6) Maternal antibody has not decreased 4-fold or more in 3 months with course of treatment.

2. Further evaluation

a. Physical examination: e.g., rash (vesicobullous), hepatomegaly, generalized lymphadenopathy, persistent rhinitis.

b. Serologic test on infant's venous blood (cord blood may give false positive results).

c. Examine CSF for possible neurosyphilis: protein and cell count (may be elevated) and VDRL (do not use RPR or FTA-ABS [high false positive rate]).

d. Radiographic studies: long bone films for diaphyseal periostitis, osteochondritis.

e. HIV antibody test: high incidence of co-infection with HIV and *T. pallidum*.

C. Treatment

1. Congenital Syphilis

a. Treat 10–14 days with IV penicillin if evidence of syphilis, or maternal treatment was inadequate. Treat infants suspected of syphilis regardless of CSF results. (See Red Book for specific recommendations.) Dose: aqueous penicillin G, 50,000 units/kg/dose IV or IM q8–12 hours; **or** procaine penicillin G, 50,000 units/kg IM daily for 10–14 days. Follow nontreponemal tests at 3, 6, and 12 months posttreatment until nonreactive.

b. Asymptomatic infants born to serologically positive mothers with adequate maternal therapy and with no clinical, radiographic, or laboratory evidence of disease may be discharged with follow up. Check nontreponemal assays at 1, 2, 3, and 6 months of age. If follow up cannot be assured, treat with a single dose of benzathine penicillin G, 50,000 units/kg IM.

2. Early Acquired Syphilis: Treat with benzathine penicillin G 50,000U/kg, IM (Max = 2.4 million U) tetracycline 500mg PO QID or doxycycline (100 mg PO BID) for 2 weeks in penicillin allergic non-pregnant adolescents, children >9 years old. Alternatively, erythromycin 500 mg QID for 2 weeks in penicillin-allergic patients.

IV. TUBERCULOSIS
A. Recommended Tuberculosis Testing

1. Testing schedule
   a. Test in low-risk children at health visits. Recommend test at time of MMR vaccine, 12–15 months of age, 4–6 years of age, 14–16 years of age.
   b. Annual tuberculin testing in high-risk children.
   c. Test children exposed to someone with known active disease. If initial test is negative, repeat 8–10 weeks after separation from contact.

2. Standard tuberculin test: Mantoux test 5 TU-PPD (0.1 ml)
   a. Inject intradermally on volar aspect of forearm to form 6–10 mm wheal. Read at 48–72 hours.
   b. In adults, clinical disease associated with tuberculin reaction of ≥15 mm or ≥10 mm in high-risk populations. Children with disease may have smaller reactions, therefore clinically evaluate those with reactions 5 to 9 mm.
   c. Consider reaction of ≥5 mm as positive in children with:
      1) Clinical or radiographic evidence of TB
      2) HIV seropositivity
      3) Immunosuppressed individuals in close contact with someone with AFB-positive sputum.
   d. Consider skin reactions of ≥10 mm as positive in BCG recipients unless low risk of exposure or recent BCG vaccination can be demonstrated.

B. Drug Therapy

1. Prophylaxis and treatment of tuberculosis

Infection/Disease	Regimen	Comments
Asymptomatic infection (positive skin test, no disease)		Give at least 6 mo with good patient compliance
Isoniazid susceptible	Isoniazid daily for 9 mo†	
Isoniazid resistant	Rifampin daily for 9 mo	If daily therapy not possible, 9 mo of twice weekly therapy*
Pulmonary and hilar adenopathy **or** Extrapulmonary other than meningitis, disseminated (miliary), or bone/joint	Standard—6 mo Isoniazid, rifampin, and pyrazinamide daily for 2 mo, then isoniazid and rifampin daily for 4 mo **or** Isoniazid, rifampin and pyrazinamide daily for 2 mo, then isoniazid and rifampin twice weekly for 4 mo Alternative—9 mo (low incidence of drug resistance) Isoniazid and rifampin daily for 9 mo **or** Isoniazid and rifampin daily for 1 mo, then isoniazid and rifampin twice weekly* for 8 mo	If drug resistance possible, add streptomycin or ethambutol to initial therapy until susceptibility is known For hilar adenopathy: 6 mo of isoniazid and rifampin daily has been shown to be sufficient if drug resistance unlikely
Meningitis, disseminated (miliary) and bone/joint	Isoniazid, rifampin, pyrazinamide, and streptomycin daily for 2 mo, then isoniazid and rifampin daily for 10 mo **or** Isoniazid, rifampin, pyrazinamide, and streptomycin daily for 2 mo, then isoniazid and rifampin twice weekly* for 10 mo	Give streptomycin in initial therapy until drug susceptibility known If resistance to streptomycin possible, may use capreomycin (15–30 mg/kg/24h) or kanamycin (15–30 mg/kg/24h) instead of streptomycin

*If noncompliance possible, twice weekly dosing under direct supervision of health care provider recommended. Dosing differs from daily regimen.
†A minimum of 12 months for HIV-infected children.

Adapted from Red Book 1991; 493–499, and Pediatrics 1992;89:161.

2. Drug regimens

Drug	Daily Dose (mg/kg/24h)	Twice Weekly Dose (mg/kg/Dose)	Maximum Dose
Isoniazid	10–15	20–40	Daily: 300 mg Twice weekly: 900 mg
Rifampin	10–20	10–20	600 mg/24g
Pyrazinamide	20–40	50–70	2 g/24h
Streptomycin	20–40 (IM)	20–40 (IM)	2 g/24h
Ethambutol	15–25	50	2.5 g/24h

Adapted from Red Book, 1991. p 500.

C. Managment of Infants of TB-infected Mother or Other Household Contact

	Mother (Contact)	Newborn	Comments
I	Positive PPD, no evidence of infection.	No therapy if no evidence of contact or exposure; consider INH (10/mg/kg/day) until all contacts cleared of active infection	PPD to infant at 4–6 wk, 3–4 mo
II	Newly diagnosed TB minimal disease or treatment >2 wk **and** noncontagious at delivery	INH until negative PPD at 3–4 mo and no active cases in household; BCG vaccine if compliance not assured, and mother with AFB-positive smear	Report to Health Department; refer mom for treatment; examine infant monthly, check PPD, chest x-ray on infant at 4–6 wk, 3–4 mo, 6 mo; may breastfeed
III	Contagious TB infection	INH as II; BCG as II	Same as II, except isolate mother from infant until mom no longer contagious
IV	Hematogenous spread of TB	A. INH and rifampin if congenital TB not suspected; repeat PPD at 6 mo; if positive continue INH until age 12 mo B. If congenital TB suspected, treat with INH, rifampin, pyrazinamide, and streptomycin; if positive diagnosis, treat with INH and rifampin using regimen for TB meningitis	Same as II; infant at risk for congenital TB; do CXR and PPD at birth; if no congenital TB, isolate mom until no longer contagious

D. **Bacillus Calmette-Guerin (BCG):** Live attenuated viral vaccine
1. Indications
   a. Skin test-negative children repeatedly exposed to someone with sputum-positive TB or with TB resistant to INH or rifampin.
   b. Children in groups with a high rate of new infections.
   c. Infants of TB-infected mothers where compliance cannot be assured (may have inadequate response to the vaccine). Test PPD 2–3 months after vaccination; if negative, repeat BCG.
   d. Consider in uninfected children only with unavoidable risk of exposure and other means of prevention have failed or not feasible.
2. Contraindications: Children with the following:
   a. Burns
   b. Skin infections
   c. Immunodeficiencies
   d. Symptomatic HIV infection
   e. Immunosuppression

V. ISOLATION TECHNIQUES FOR SELECTED ILLNESSES

Note: Use universal precautions during all patient encounters to reduce the risk of transmission of blood-borne pathogens. Minimize contact with blood and body fluids* of all patients as follows:

Needles and sharps: Do not recap needles; dispose of needles in needle containers only.

Gowns and gloves: Wear when contact with blood and body fluids is likely.

Protective eyewear and mask: Wear when splashing is likely.

Isolation Precautions

Strict	Respiratory	AFB	Contact With Mask	RSV	Contact	Enteric
Disseminated zoster	Rubeola	Tuberculosis	Congenital rubella[1, 3]	Bronchiolitis, etiology unknown in children <2 yr	Extensive wound infection, other than staphylococcal	Cholera
Localized herpes zoster, lesions *cannot be* covered	Pertussis		Influenza			Clostridium difficile colitis
Meningococcal pneumonia[2]			Invasive *H. influenzae*[2]	Respiratory syncytial virus	Gas gangrene	Diarrhea, infectious (suspected or confirmed)
Staphylococcal burn wound infection, extensive			Mumps		Herpes simplex, neonatal	Hepatitis A
Varicella			Meningococcemia[2]		Localized herpes zoster, lesions can be covered[4]	Meningitis, enteroviral
			Meningitis, *H. influenzae* or *N. meningitidis*[2]		Staphylococcal wound or skin infection, contained by dressing	Salmonellosis (typhoidal or nontyphoidal)
			Rabies[3]		Syphilis, congenital[2]	Yersiniosis
			Parainfluenza			
			Rubella, primary infection[1, 3]			
			Staphylococcal pneumonia			
			Staphylococcal wound or skin infection, extensive			

Explanation of Isolation Precautions

	Strict	Respiratory	AFB	Contact With Mask	Contact	RSV	Enteric
Single room	Yes, door closed	Yes, door closed	Yes, door closed	Preferred	Preferred	Preferred; roommates must be without congenital heart disease, chronic lung disease, or immune suppression	Yes, when soiling with feces/urine likely
Gown	Yes	No	No	Yes, contact with patient	Yes, contact with patient	Yes, contact with patient	Yes, when soiling with feces/urine likely
Mask	Yes	Yes	Yes, high filtration	Yes, at bedside	No	Yes, at bedside	No
Gloves	Yes	No	No	Yes, contact with infective material	Yes, contact with infective material	Yes, to enter room	Yes, contact with feces/urine or contaminated articles

*Blood; all fluids containing visible blood; CSF; vaginal secretions; semen; and synovial, pericardial, amniotic, peritoneal, and pleural fluid.

[1]Susceptible pregnant women should avoid contact

[2]Until 24 hours after effective treatment is begun

[3]Private room required

[4]Roommates must be immune

Ref: The Johns Hopkins Hospital, Infection Control Department, personal communication.

MICROBIOLOGY   *18*

I. STAINING TECHNIQUES
A. Background
1. Microorganisms that are well-stained are more easily identified under the microscope, and more readily differentiated from other microorganisms. The Gram stain, acid-fast stain, and India ink stain are the stains most commonly used.
2. Remember
   a. *Thin* smears give the best results.
   b. Always allow smears to air dry before they are fixed; heating wet smears usually distorts organisms and cells.
   c. Fix smears with gentle heat by quickly passing slide through a flame (no more than 4 times). Test temperature by tapping slide on the back of your hand; it should feel warm. Allow slide to cool before staining.

B. Gram Stain
1. Flood slide with **gentian (Crystal) violet** for 1 min. Wash with gently running water.
2. Flood with **iodine solution** for 1 min. Wash with gently running water.
3. Decolorize with **acetone/alcohol** for 3–4 sec. Wash with water immediately.
4. Counterstain with **safranin** for 30 sec. Wash with water.
5. Alternatively, use **rapid method.** Follow same sequence as above, but have each agent on smear for only 10 sec. Acetone/alcohol still only 3–4 sec.

C. Acid Fast Stain
1. Flood slide with **Kenyoun's stain** for 5 min. Wash with water.
2. Decolorize with **acid alcohol** for 2 min. Wash with water.
3. Counterstain with **0.5% methylene blue** for 2 min. Wash with water.

D. India Ink: Used mainly for identification of *Cryptococcus*. Mix one drop of test fluid and one drop of India ink, cover with coverslip, and press out excess fluid. Ring with Vase-

line. Look for organisms: round refractile images against black background. If index of suspicion is high, incubate preparation at 37° C and reexamine in 24–48h.

II. CULTURE TECHNIQUES

A. **Bacterial Culture:** When immediate culturing is not available through the hospital laboratory, culture as follows:

1. **Blood:** Optimally, the sample volume should equal l0% of the volume of the culture medium. When patient is treated with penicillin consider using penicillinase-containing broth (although value of penicillinase media is questionable).

2. **CSF:** Innoculate chocolate blood agar (place in CO_2 jar), 5% sheep blood agar, MacConkey agar, and thioglycollate broth.

3. **Cavity Fluid:** Culture the same as CSF. Peritoneal and abscess cultures should be placed in special anaerobic containers.

4. **Nasopharynx, eye, and ear** (in order of plating): Chocolate blood agar, 5% sheep blood agar, MacConkey agar (or Thayer-Martin in infants). Place swab in transport medium.

5. **Throat** (in order of plating): 5% sheep blood agar and MacConkey agar. Place swab in transport medium.

6. **Vagina and urethra** (in order of plating): Chocolate blood agar, Thayer-Martin agar, broth (institution specific). Always culture immediately, and always do Gram stain.

7. **Skin** (in order of plating): 5% sheep blood agar, MacConkey agar, thioglycollate broth. Place swab in transport medium.

B. **Fungal Microscopic Examination:** Using a scalpel, scrape edges of lesion in which fungus is suspected onto a glass slide. Cover scrapings with l0% to 20% KOH or NaOH and apply a coverslip. Warm over light bulb for a few minutes (15 minutes is ideal). Examine for fragments of mycelia and spores.

C. *Chlamydia trachomatis* **Culture**

1. Send specimens in *Chlamydia* transport media if available from the hospital laboratory. If swabs are used to collect the specimen, extract them immediately into the transport medium and discard them. Extract by pressing and rotating the swab against the wall of the specimen container.

Use Dacron swabs. Cotton-wool swabs and calcium alginate swabs are unacceptable.
2. If cell culture inoculation is delayed:
   a. If <24h: refrigerate specimen at 4° C.
   b. If >24h: freeze specimen at −70° C in mechanical freezer.
D. Viral Cultures
1. Send pharyngeal, nasopharyngeal, and rectal swabs in viral culture media. CSF, blood, bone marrow, and urine may be sent in sterile containers.
2. For optimal culture results, specimens should be cultured within 1 hour after collection.

III. TZANCK PREP: Used to identify multinucleated giant cells in lesions infected with herpes simplex, herpes zoster, or varicella infections. The lesions tested must be vesicular or bullous. Unroof vesicle or bulla, blot off fluid, and gently curette base with blunt end of scalpel. Spread scraping on a glass slide, fix in methyl alcohol, then stain with Giemsa or Wright stain.

IV. ANTIGEN/ANTIBODY DETECTION TESTS: A variety of antigen and antibody detection tests are available using immunofluorescence, ELISA, latex agglutination, and other techniques to identify bacteria, *Chlamydia,* virus, fungi, and protozoa. These tests vary in their sensitivity and specificity, and many are available for office use. Refer to your processing laboratory for test availability and specimen handling.

V. SCABIES VISUALIZATION: Scabies is an eczematous eruption caused by hypersensitivity to the arthropod *Sarcoptes scabiei,* is characterized by pruritic papules, vesicles, pustules, and burrows, often occuring on the hands, buttocks, genitals, in the axillae, on the flexure surfaces of the arms, and in infants on the palms, soles, head, and neck. A simple diagnostic test that is highly predictive but not extremely sensitive is to scrape a burrow or unscratched papule with a sharp instrument that has been covered with mineral oil. Deposit the scrapings onto a glass slide, and examine for mites, ova, or feces.

NEONATOLOGY   *19*

I. **FETAL ASSESSMENT**
A. **Genetic Diagnosis and Fetal Anomaly Screening**
  1. Maternal Serum Alpha-Fetoprotein Screening (MSAFP)
    a. Performed at 15–20 weeks gestation. Measures amount of fetal protein in maternal circulation.
    b. Low values are associated with an increased risk of trisomy 21, 13, and 18.
    c. Elevations will identify nearly 100% of pregnancies with anencephaly, 70–85% with open spina bifida, and 70% with ventral wall defects. Other conditions associated with increased MSAFP include urogenital malformations, multiple gestation, fetomaternal hemorrhage, Turner's syndrome, cystic hygroma, and epidermolysis bullosa.
  2. Ultrasonography
    a. Approximately 80% of major fetal anomalies can be diagnosed with ultrasonography performed during the second trimester.
    b. Amniotic fluid volume can be estimated. Amniotic fluid volume is dependent upon fetal swallowing (500 ml/day at term), fetal micturition (26–43 ml/hr at term) and maternal/fetal exchange of amniotic fluid at the chorionic villi of the placenta.

Condition	Congenital Causes	Other Diagnoses
Polyhydramnios	Nervous system abnormalities (anencepahly, Werdnig-Hoffman, etc.) gastrointestinal anomalies (gastroschisis, duodenal atresia, diaphragmatic hernia), cystic adenomatoid malformation, trisomies	Chest anomalies, conjoined twins, chylothorax, fetal death, hydrops, maternal diabetes, various tumors
Oligohydramnios	Renal/urogenital abnormalities (agenesis, polycystic kidneys, posterior urethral valves), placental insufficiency, premature rupture of membranes (PROM), Potter syndrome	Lung hypoplasia, contractures, and limb deformities

Ref: Queenan JT, Management of High Risk Pregnancy, 2nd ed. Oradell, NJ; Medical Economic Books, 1985. p 239.

3. Prenatal Diagnosis: Fetal cells/tissue may be obtained by amniocentesis, chorionic villus sampling (CVS), or percutaneous umbilical blood sampling (PUBS) for chromosomal analysis and molecular genetic diagnosis, as well as for diagnosis of congenital infections, fetal blood type, etc.

Method	Timing in Gestation	Risk of SAB (%)
CVS	8–10 wk	1–5
PUBS	2nd trimester to term	< 1
Amniocentesis	15–17 wk	0.5–1.0

Ref: Queenan JT (ed) Management of High Risk Pregnancy, 2nd ed. Oradell, NJ; Medical Economic Books 1985:239. Wax J, Blakemore K, What can be learned from cordocentesis? Clinics in Laboratory Medicine 1992; 12(3):503-522.

4. Molecular Genetic Diagnosis
   See Genetics, Chapter 12, for specific diseases.

B. Fetal Maturity

1. Gestational dating: The most accurate method of estimating gestational age is by ultrasonographic measurements of crown-rump length during the first trimester. From the first trimester through 34 wks, the biparietal diameter is accurate to within10 days. Other measurements used in 2nd and 3rd trimester include fetal abdominal diameter and femur length.

2. Lung maturity

   a. Amniotic fluid can be tested for phospholipid components of fetal lung surfactant.

   b. The lecithin-to-sphingomyelin (L/S) ratio is the most widely used index. An L/S of >2.0 indicates fetal lung maturity in most cases. An L/S of <2 does not reliably exclude lung maturity.

   c. The presence of phosphatidylglycerol (PG), a late-appearing surfactant component, has greater positive predictive value than the L/S ratio in determining fetal lung maturity. However, PG has lower sensitvity. A positive PG is helpful when the L/S is marginal.

   Ref: Creasy G, Simon N. Am J Perinatol 1984; 1:302. Kulovitch M, Gluck L. Am J Obstet Gynecol 1979; 135:64. Kulovitch M, et al. Am J Obstet Gynecol 1979; 135:57.

C. Antepartum Fetal Monitoring

1. Nonstress test (NST): The fetal heart rate is continuously monitored with the mother at rest. Normal or reactive nonstress test: At least two accelerations in fetal heart rate >15 beats/minute above baseline, lasting 15 seconds or more, occurring within a 10 minute period. A nonreactive pattern does not meet these criteria. The NST is less specific when assessing fetuses <32 weeks gestation.

2. Biophysical profile: Ultrasonography is used to assess fetal activity over a 30 minute period, and to estimate amniotic fluid volume. The parameters examined include fetal breathing movements, gross body movements, tone, heart rate, and quantitative amniotic fluid volume. Scores are 2 if normal or 0 if abnormal. Low scores may reflect fetal distress, fetal prematurity.

3. Doppler: Pulsed-wave doppler is used to assess flow velocity waveforms in maternal and fetal vessels, most commonly the umbilical artery. Both the systolic/diastolic (S/D) ratio and pulsatility index (PI) may be described. The S/D ratio should be ≤3 after 28–30 weeks, the PI should be ≤1. Elevated values suggest increased placental resistance.

4. Contraction Stress Test (CST): Fetal heart rate and maternal uterine contractions are monitored continuously while uterine contractions are induced either by breast stimula-

tion or intravenous oxytocin administration. A negative but reassuring test has no persistent fetal HR decelerations following the contractions. A positive but nonreassuring test has persistent late fetal HR decelerations indicating uteroplacental insufficiency.

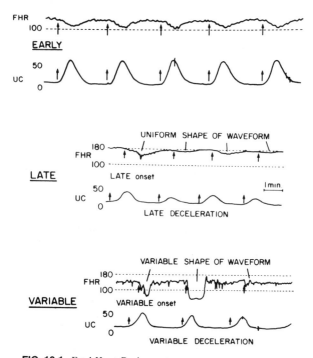

FIG 19.1. Fetal Heart Racings Ref : Taeusch H et al. (eds). Schaffer and Avery's Diseases of the Newborn, 6th ed. Philadelphia: WB Saunders, 1991.

D. Intrapartum Fetal Monitoring

1. Fetal heart rate (FHR) monitoring

   a. Normal baseline FHR is 120–160 beats per minute (bpm). Isolated accelerations >160 bpm suggest a good prognosis. Mild bradycardias (100–120 bpm) are usually benign.

   b. A normal tracing includes both short term "beat to beat" variability (amplitude 10–25 bpm), and slower oscillations in heart rate (frequency 3–10 cycles per minute). Loss of variability suggests fetal distress. Drugs, smoking, fetal sleep, prematurity, and other factors also can decrease variability.

   c. Early decelerations represent head compression and are benign.

   d. Variable decelerations represent cord compression and do not always indicate fetal distress.

   e. Late decelerations are caused by uteroplacental insufficiency and indicate fetal distress.

   f. A sinusoidal or undulating FHR pattern may be a sign of severe fetal compromise and is associated with a high rate of perinatal loss.

   Ref: For references on fetal monitoring see Petre, R (ed): Clin Perinatol 1982:9(2). Polin J, Frangipane W. Ped Clin North Amer 1986; 33:621; Yeomans E, et al: Am J Obstet Gynecol 1985; 151:798.

E. Perinatal Blood Gas Evaluation

Normal Values

Site	pH	PO_2	PCO_2
Scalp	7.25–7.35	20–25	40–45
Umbilical vein	7.35±0.15	30±15	35±8
Umbilical artery	7.28±0.15	15±10	45±15

Ref: Adapted from Polin J, Frangipane W. Ped Clin North Amer 1986; 33:621.

II. NEWBORN ASSESSMENT

A. Apgar scores: Rapid clinical assessment of infant performed at 1 and 5 min after birth. If the infant is compromised, assessment repeated at 10 and 20 min.

	Score		
	0	1	2
Heart rate	Absent	<100	>100
Respiratory effort	Absent, irregular	Slow, crying	Good
Muscle tone	Limp	Some flexion of extremeties	Active motion
Reflex irritability (nose suction)	No response	Grimace	Cough or sneeze
Color	Blue, pale	Extremities blue	Completely pink

Ref: Adapted from Apgar V. Anesth Analg 1953; 32:260.

B. Gestational Age

   1. Anterior lens vessels examination

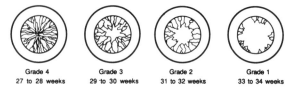

| Grade 4 | Grade 3 | Grade 2 | Grade 1 |
| 27 to 28 weeks | 29 to 30 weeks | 31 to 32 weeks | 33 to 34 weeks |

FIG 19.2. Anterior Lens Vessels Ref: Hittner, H et al. J Pediatr 1977; 91:455

   2. Neuromuscular and physical maturity (Ballard)
      a. Neuromuscular maturity
         1) Posture: Observe infant quiet, supine. Score 0: arms, legs extended; 1: beginning flexion of hips and knees, arms extended; 2: stronger flexion of legs, arms extended; 3: arms slightly flexed, legs flexed and abducted; 4: full flexion of arms, legs.
         2) Square window: Flex hand on forearm enough to obtain fullest possible flexion without wrist rotation. Measure angle between the hypothenar eminence and the ventral aspect of the forearm.

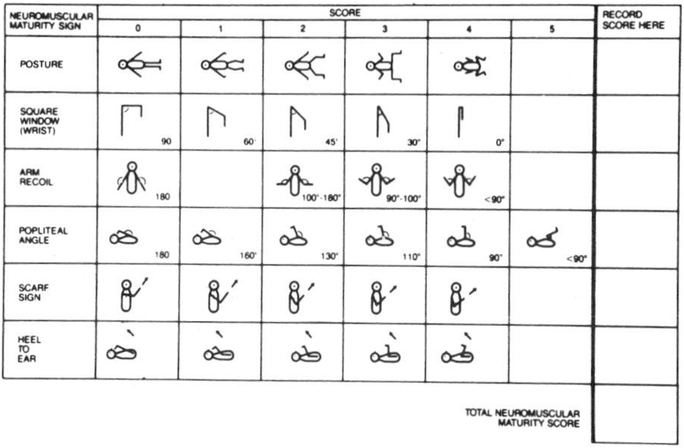

NEUROMUSCULAR MATURITY SIGN	SCORE						RECORD SCORE HERE
	0	1	2	3	4	5	
POSTURE							
SQUARE WINDOW (WRIST)	90°	60°	45°	30°	0°		
ARM RECOIL	180°		100°-180°	90°-100°	<90°		
POPLITEAL ANGLE	180°	160°	130°	110°	90°	<90°	
SCARF SIGN							
HEEL TO EAR							
					TOTAL NEUROMUSCULAR MATURITY SCORE		

FIG 19.3.
Neuromuscular Maturity (Ballard)

3) Arm recoil: With infant supine, flex forearms for 5 sec, then fully extend by pulling on hands, then release. Measure the angle of elbow flexion to which the arms recoil.

4) Popliteal angle: Hold infant supine with pelvis flat, thigh held in the knee-chest position. Extend leg by gentle pressure and measure the popliteal angle.

5) Scarf sign: With baby supine, pull infant's hand across the neck toward the opposite shoulder. Determine how far the elbow will go across. Score 0: Elbow reaches opposite axillary line; 1: past midaxillary line; 2: past midline; 3: elbow unable to reach midline.

6) Heel-to-ear maneuver: With baby supine, draw foot as near to the head as possible without forcing it. Observe distance between foot and head, and degree of extension at the knee. Knee is free and may be down alongside abdomen.

Ref: Ballard J, et al. J Pediatr 1979; 95: 769-774.

B. Physical Maturity

Physical Maturity Sign	Score					Record Score Here
	0	1	2	3	4	5
Skin	Gelatinous, red, transparent	Smooth, pink, visible veins	Superficial peeling, and/or rash, few veins	Cracking; pale area; rare veins	Parchment; deep cracking; no vessels	Leathery, cracked, wrinkled	
Lanugo	None	Abundant	Thinning	Bald areas	Mostly bald		
Plantar creases	No crease	Faint red marks	Anterior transverse crease only	Creases anterior 2/3	Creases cover entire sole		
Breast	Barely perceptible	Flat areola, no bud	Stippled areola, 1–2 mm bud	Raised areola, 3–4 mm bud	Full areola, 5–10 mm bud		
Ear	Pinna flat, stays folded	Slightly curved pinna; soft with slow recoil	Well-curved pinna; soft but ready recoil	Formed and firm with instant recoil	Thick cartilage; ear stiff		
Genitals (male)	Scrotum empty; no rugae		Testes descending; few rugae	Testes down; good rugae	Testes pendulous; deep rugae		
Genitals (female)	Prominent clitoris and labia minora		Majora and minora equally prominent	Majora large, minora small	Clitoris and minora completely covered		
					Total physical maturity score		

C. **Maturity Rating:** Add scores for neuromuscular and physical maturity assessment. The Ballard is most accurate when performed between 30 and 42 hours of age.

Score	5	10	15	20	25	30	35	40	45	50
Weeks	26	28	30	32	34	36	38	40	42	44

III. MANAGEMENT OF THE PRETERM INFANT
A. Fluid Management

1. Fluid balance is determined by insensible water losses (evaporation through skin and alveoli), stool water loss, renal water loss, water loss due to metabolism. Preterm infants experience increased insensible losses through the skin, due to increased surface area per unit body mass, and immaturity of the skin. The degree of loss is determined by the body weight and gestational age.

Estimates of Insensible Water Loss at Different Body Weights*

Body Weight (g)	Insensible Water Loss (ml/kg/day)
<1,000	60–70
1,000–1,250	60–65
1,251–1,500	30–45
1,501–1,750	15–30
1,751–2,000	15–20

*AGA infants in a thermonueutral environment during the first week of life.

Ref: Veille JC, Clinics in Perinatology 1988; 15(4):863

Assessment of Fluid Status

Body weight	Hematocrit
Blood pressure	Urine output
Heart rate	Serum sodium
Urine specific gravity/osmolality	Blood urea nitrogen/creatinine
Skin turgor/peripheral perfusion	Fractional excretion of sodium

Water Requirements (ml/kg/24h) of Newborns

Birthweight (g)	Age		
	1–2 Days	3–7 Days	7–30 Days
< 750	100–250	150–300	120–180
750–1000	80–150	100–150	120–180
1000–1500	60–100	80–150	120–180
> 1500	60–80	100–150	120–180

Ref: Adapted from Schaffer and Avery, ed. Diseases of the Newborn, 6th ed.
1991;WB Saunders, Philadelphia. p 710.

2. Glucose requirements
   a. Neonates require about 6 mg/kg/min of glucose to maintain euglycemia (40–100 mg/dl). Excess administration may cause hyperglycemia and subsequent osmotic diuresis. Frequent blood glucose determinations allow appropriate changes to be made.
   b. Formula to calculate rate of glucose infusion:

$$\frac{(\% \text{ glucose in solution} \times 10) \times (\text{rate of infusion})}{60 \times \text{weight (kg)}} = \text{mg/kg/min glucose}$$

Ref: Cornblath M, Schwartz R., Disorders of Carbohydrate Metabolism in Infancy,
3rd ed. 1991; Blackwell Scientific Publiciations.

3. Electrolyte requirements: Serum Na and K levels should be monitored frequently, with therapy adjusted accordingly.
   a. Sodium
      1) None required in the first 72 hours of life, unless the serum Na is less than 135 and there is no evidence of volume overload.
      2) After 72 hours of life, term infants require 2–3 mEq/kg/day of sodium and preterm infants require 3–5 mEq/kg/day of sodium.
   b. Potassium should be added to fluids after good urinary output is established and potassium is < 4.5. K requirements are 1–2.5 mEq/kg/day.
   c. Common electrolyte abnormalities in small premature infants include hyponatremia, hypernatremia, hyperkalemia, hyperglycemia, and hypocalcemia.

B. Neutral Thermal Environmental Temperatures

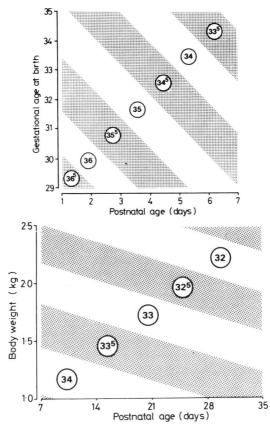

FIG 19.4. Neutral Thermal Environmental Temperatures Ref: Nelson, N (ed). Current Therapy in Neonatal-Perinatal Medicine-2. Philadelphia: BC Decker, Inc. 1990, p. 368.

C. **Nutrition**
   1. Caloric requirements

Term, healthy, enterally fed	100–120 kcal/kg/day
Premature	115–130 kcal/kg/day
IUGR (parenterally fed)	79–100 kcal/kg/day

   Note: Caloric requirements may be increased in neonates with IUGR, congenital heart disease, BPD, or "short gut" syndrome. Monitor nutritional status by following electrolytes, calcium, phosphorus, alkaline phosphatase and complete blood counts frequently. Patients on parenteral nutrition should receive frequent magnesium, ALT, AST, bilirubin, albumin, and triglyceride determinations.

   2. Protein requirements

Preterm	3.5–4.5 g/kg/day
Term	1–2 g/kg/day

   3. Mineral requirements
      a. Premature infants have a higher calcium and phosporus requirement and, therefore, need special formulas or human milk fortifier. Milk fortifier should not be added until after the second week, due to the risk of excessive calcium/phosphorus intake (since early breast milk is high in these minerals).
      b. Iron: Enterally fed premature infants who are not receiving multiple transfusions require supplements of 2 mg/kg/day of elemental iron.
   4. Indications for parenteral nutrition
      a. Very low birthweight infants
      b. Respiratory disease
      c. Necrotizing enterocolitis (NEC)
      d. Gastrointestinal anomalies
      Ref: Schaffer and Avery, ed. Diseases of the Newborn, 6th ed. 1991;WB Saunders, Philadelphia.

D. Respiratory Management

1. Respiratory distress syndrome (RDS), due to lung immaturity and deficiency of surfactant production, is marked by tachypnea, retractions, grunting, and increasing cyanosis within minutes of birth. Chest x-ray reveals diffuse fine reticulogranular markings.

   a. Exogenous surfactant may be administered immediately after birth (prophylactic), or when the infant demonstrates clinical RDS (rescue). See Formulary (Chapter 25) for dosing and administration.

   b. Conventional mechanical ventilation is employed to support the infant's air exchange.

      1) Indications for assisted ventilation:

         a) Respiratory acidosis with a pH of $<7.2 - 7.25$

         b) Severe hypoxemia (PaO_2 $<50 - 60$ mm Hg) despite high FiO_2 ($70 - 100\%$)

         Ref: Waldermar, A, Martin R. Ped Clin North Am 33(1):227-230.

   c. Therapies for infants failing conventional ventilation

      1) High-frequency oscillation

      2) High-frequency jet ventilation

      3) Extracorporeal membrane oxygenation (ECMO): only indicated after 34 weeks gestation due to risk of IVH.

      Ref: Short B, Miller M, Anderson K, Clinics in Perinatology 1987; 14(3):737,581.

2. Apnea and bradycardia

   a. Cessation of breathing for ≥ 20 seconds with decrease in heart rate. Apnea may be **central** (no diaphragmatic activity), **obstructive** (upper airway obstruction with continuuous diaphragmatic activity), or **mixed** (a combination of the above).

   Incidence (Age)

≤28 wk	~100%
30 wk	50%
34 wk	<7%

   b. A pathologic cause for apnea/bradycardia should be considered when there is an abrupt increase in the frequency or severity of episodes, when apnea develops after one week of life in an infant who did not have RDS, or when apnea occurs in a term infant.

  c. Treatment of apnea of prematurity

    1) Methylxanthines: caffeine and theophylline (see Formulary, Chapter 25, for dosing).

    2) Nasal CPAP (continuous positive airway pressure) with room air flow if the infant does not require supplemental oxygen for another reason.

Ref: Jones D, et al. Hospital Care of the Recovering NICU Infant. Baltimore, Williams & Wilkins, 1981.

E. Hyperbilirubinemia

1. Bilirubin levels should be followed in all jaundiced infants as well as in all premature infants, infants with ABO incompatibility and/or positive direct Coombs test, and infants with sepsis. **Institution of phototherapy and exchange transfusion remain controversial.** The decision to institute therapy should be based on the level of bilirubin as well as the infant's clinical condition, including degree of bruising, instability, etc.

2. Management

  a. Flourescent bulb phototherapy (consider 10% increase in fluid requirements) intensity 6–12 microwatts/cm^2 nm

  b. Fiberoptic blanket phototherapy (no increase in fluid requirements) intensity 50 microwatts/cm^2 nm

  c. Exchange transfusion (see Chapter 4, Procedures)

Ref: Ennever JF, Clinics in Perinatology 17(2):478

F. Necrotizing Enterocolitis (NEC)

1. Incidence 1–5%, most in infants < 1500 g. 10% of cases occur in full-term infants.

2. Clinical staging system for NEC:

Stage	Clinical Findings	Radiographic Findings	Treatment	Survival (percent)
I (suspected NEC)	Mild abdominal distention; poor feeding; vomiting	Mild ileus	Medical, including workup for sepsis	100
II (definite NEC)	The above, plus: marked abdominal distention and GI bleeding	Significant ileus; pneumatosis intestinalis; portal vein gas (9% of cases)	Medical	96
III (advanced NEC)	The above, plus deterioration of vital signs; septic shock	The above, plus pneumo-peritoneum (60% of cases)	Surgical	50

3. Medical Managment
   a. Decompression of GI tract
   b. Broad spectrum antibiotics
   c. Fluid resuscitation
   d. Frequent clinical, laboratory, and radiographic assessment for development of gangrene or perforation
      Ref: Kosloske A, Musemeche CA, Clinics in Perinatology 1989; 16(1):103

IV. OTHER MAJOR COMPLICATIONS OF PREMATURITY

A. Patent Ductus Arteriosus: Incidence: 15–36% of preterm infants; more common with earlier gestational age.

B. Retinopathy of Prematurity

Stage 1	Demarcation line separates avascular from vascularized retina
Stage 2	Ridge forms along demarcation line
Stage 3	Extraretinal, fibrovascular proliferation tissue forms on ridge
Stage 4	Retinal detachment
Plus disease	Posterior tortuosity and engorgement of blood vessels that may be present at any stage
Pre-threshold	Zone 1, any stage
	Zone 2, stage 2 and plus disease
	Zone 2, stage 3
Threshold	A level of severity at which the risk of blindness predicted approaches 50%; 5 contiguous or 8 total 30° sectors of stage 3 in zone 1, or Zone 2 with plus disease

Ref: Ben-Sira I, et al. Pediatrics 1984; 74:127.

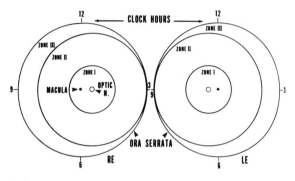

FIG 19.5.
Zones of the Retina

C. Intraventricular Hemorrhage (IVH)

1. Incidence: 30% of infants < 30 wk will have some degree of IVH.
2. Classification by head ultrasound

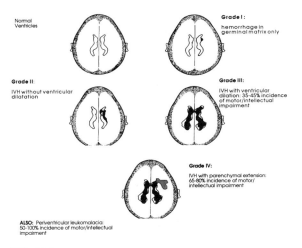

Normal Ventricles

Grade I: hemorrhage in germinal matrix only

Grade II: IVH without ventricular dilatation

Grade III: IVH with ventricular dilation: 35-45% incidence of motor/intellectual impairment

Grade IV: IVH with parenchymal extension: 65-80% incidence of motor/intellectual impairment

ALSO: Periventricular leukomalacia: 50-100% incidence of motor/intellectual impairment

FIG 19.6.

Intraventricular hemorrhage classification

Ref: Papile, L et al. J Pediatr 1978; 92:529. Partridge J, et al. J Pediatr 1983; 102:287. Personal communication, Marilee Allen, M.D., Johns Hopkins Hospital. Harrison H, The Premature Baby Book. New York, St. Martin's Press, 1983:97.

NEPHROLOGY 20

I. **URINALYSIS:** A "liquid biopsy of the urinary tract." Evaluate specimen within 1 hour after void, ideally collecting the first morning void.

A. **General Characteristics**

1. Appearance

a. Color

Red	Adriamycin, methyldopa, beets, blackberries, desferoximine (with elevated serum iron), phenytoin, food-coloring, hemoglobin, phenazopyridine (acid urine), phenolphtalein (alkaline urine), phenothiazines, porphyrins, Povan, red blood cells, red diaper syndrome (nonpathogenic *Serratia marcescens*), urates.
Yellow-brown	Antimalarials (pamaquine, primaquine, quinicrine), azulfidine (alkaline urine), B-complex vitamins, bilirubin, carotene, cascara, metronidazole, nitrofurantoin, sulfonamides.
Brown-black	Hemosiderin, homogentisic urine (alkaptonuria), melanin (especially in alkaline urine), myoglobin, old blood, quinine.
Purple-brown	Porphyrins (old urine)
Deep yellow	Riboflavin
Orange	Phenazopyridine, rifampin, urates, warfarin
Blue-green	Adriamycin, amitriptyline, blue diaper syndrome (familial metabolic disease nephrcalcinosis), biliverdin (seen in chronic obstructive jaundice), indomethicin, methylene blue, *Pseudomonas* UTI (rare), riboflavin.

b. Clarity: Turbidity usually is normal; most often due to crystal formation at room temperature. Uric acid crystals form in acidic urine, phosphate crystals in alkaline urine. Cellular material and bacteria can also cause turbidity.

2. Specific Gravity

a. Hydrometer/urinometer: Requires at least 15 ml of urine at room temperature. Device must be free-floating in the sample.

b. Refractometer: Requires only one drop of urine. Based on the principle that the refractive index (RI) of a solution is related to the content of dissolved solids present. The RI varies with but is not identical to specific gravity. The refractometer measures RI but is calibrated for specific gravity. Glucose, abundant protein, and iodine-containing contrast material can give falsely high readings.

3. pH: Estimated using indicator paper or dipstick. To improve accuracy, use freshly voided specimen and pH meter.

B. Chemical Determinations

1. Protein

a. Tests for protein

1) Dipstick: Easiest method. Significant if 1+ (30 mg/dl) on 2 of 3 random samples 1 week apart if urine specific gravity is <1.015 or 2+ (100 mg/dl) on similarly collected urine if specific gravity is >1.015. Confirm with a 24 hour collection. False positives can occur with highly concentrated or alkaline urine, quaternary ammonium cleansers, phenazopyridine therapy.

2) Sulfosalicylic acid (SSA) test: Add 0.5–0.8 ml (5–8 drops) of 20% SSA to 5 ml of urine (pH should be 4.5–6.5) and examine for turbidity. Barely evident turbidity is graded ±; increasing amounts of turbidity are grades 1–4+. False positives result from cephalosporins, concentrated urine, gross hematuria, IV contrast, PAS, penicillins, phosphates, sulfonamides, tolbutamide.

3) Protein/creatinine ratio; Determine ratio of protein (mg/dl) and creatinine concentrations (mg/dl) in urine collected randomly during normal ambulation. Ratio ≥0.2 suggests significant proteinuria. Confirm with 24-hour urine collection.

Ref: Ginsberg JM et al. New Engl J Med 1983, 309:1543

4) 24-hour urine collection (see Method section II.A.1.b.): Most quantitative method.

a) Urine protein (mg/m^2/hours of collection):

0	4		40
∧-Normal	-∧∧-	Abnormal	-∧∧-Nephrotic->

Ref: Norman ME. Ped Clinic of North America 1987; 34:553

b. Types of proteinuria
    1) Transient proteinuria: Most common in children. Associated with exercise, postural changes, cold exposure, fever, emotional stress. Not transient in true renal disease. Diagnosis made when serial urines negative for protein.
    2) Orthostatic proteinuria: Also common. Not associated with renal pathology. Orthostatic proteinuria is confirmed if samples 1 and 5 contain protein and samples 3 and 4 do not. Sample 2 may contain some protein. To diagnose:
        a) Make strictly NPO after 9 PM and until test is completed.
        b) Have patient void immediately before retiring; label this sample 1.
        c) Have patient void without rising at midnight and at 5 AM (samples 2 and 3).
        d) Have patient void at 7 AM. May rise to void. (sample 4).
        e) Have patient walk actively from 7–9 AM (still NPO) and void at 9 AM (sample 5).
        f) For each specimen record specific gravity and protein content.
    3) Persistently abnormal or nephrotic range proteinuria requires evaluation for renal disease. Suggested workup should include:
        a) Blood electrolytes, BUN, creatinine serum proteins, cholesterol.
        b) C3, C4, ASO titer, ANA.
        c) Renal ultrasound (other radiologic studies as indicated).
        d) Referral to pediatric nephrologist.
            Ref: Norman ME. Ped Clinics of North America 1987;34:556

2. Sugars: Normally, urine does not contain sugars. Glucosuria is suggestive but not diagnostic of diabetes mellitus or proximal renal tubular disease (see section II.B.1.b.). The presence of other reducing sugars can be confirmed by chromatography.

   a. Dipstick: Easiest method but specific for glucose. False negative with a high level of ascorbic acid (used as a preservative in antibiotics) in urine.

   b. Clinitest tablets (Ames Co.): Identifies all reducing substances in urine including: reducing sugars (glucose, fructose, galactose, pentoses, lactose), amino acids, ascorbic acid, chloral hydrate, chloramphenicol, creatinine, cysteine, glucuronates, hippurate, homogentisic acid, isoniazid, ketone bodies, nitrofurantoin, oxalate, PAS, penicillin, salicylates, streptomycin, sulfonamides, tetracycline, uric acid. Since sucrose is not a reducing sugar it is not detected by clinitest or dipstick.

      1) Method: Use 5 drops of urine, 10 drops of water, 1 tablet. Compare with standard scale.

Color	% Reducing Substance
Blue	Negative
Greenish blue	Trace
Green	0.5
Greenish brown	1.0
Yellow	1.5
Brick red	2.0

3. Ketones: Except for trace amounts, ketonuria suggests ketoacidosis, usually from either diabetes mellitus or catabolism induced by inadequate intake. Neonatal ketoacidosis may occur with a metabolic defect, such as propionic acidemia, methylmalonic aciduria, or a glycogen storage disease.

   a. Dipstick: Detects acetoacetic acid best, acetone less well. Does not detect beta-hydroxybutyrate. False positives may occur after phthalein administration or with PKU.

   b. Acetest tablets (Ames Co.): detects only acetoacetic acid and acetone.

4. Hemoglobin and myoglobin: Centrifuged urine usually contains fewer than 5 RBCs/hpf. Significant hematuria is 5–10 RBCs/hpf and corresponds to a Chemstrip reading of 50 RBCs/hpf or Labstix reading "trace hemolyzed" or "small".

   a. Dipstick: Positive with intact RBCs, hemoglogin, and myoglobin; can detect as few as 3–4 RBCs/hpf. False positives are caused by the presence of peroxidase (released from some bacteria), high ascorbic acid concentrations, and Betadine (i.e., from fingers of medical staff).

   b. Microscopy: Used to differentiate hemoglobinuria or myoglobinuria from hematuria (intact RBCs). In addition, examination of RBC morphology by phase contrast microscopy may help localize source of bleeding.

   c. Differentiation of hemoglobinuria and myoglobinuria.

      1) History: Hemoglobinuria is seen with intravascular hemolysis or in hematuric urine that has stood for an extended period. Myoglobinuria is seen in crush injuries, vigorous exercise, major motor seizures, fever and malignant hyperthermia, electrocution, snakebite, ischemia, and some muscle and metabolic disorders.

      2) Laboratory studies: Clinical laboratories may use many techniques to directly measure hemoglobin or myoglobin. Other laboratory data may also be used to identify indirectly the source of urinary pigment. For example, in nephropathy from myoglobinuria, BUN/creatinine ratio is low (creatinine is released from damaged muscles) and CPK is high.

   d. Suggested work-up of persistent hematuria:

      1) Urine culture, sickle cell screen, urine calcium:creatinine ratio

      2) Blood electrolytes, BUN, creatinine, serum

      3) Proteins

      4) ASO titers, C3, C4, ANA

      5) Renal ultrasound and other indicated radiologic studies

      6) Referral to pediatric nephrologist

   Ref: Norman ME. Ped Clinics of North America 1987;34:550.

5. Bilirubin/Urobilinogen
   a. Dipstick: Measures each individually. Both are normally present in the urine in only very small amounts.
   b. Correlating the results of both tests can provide very helpful diagnostic information.

	Normal	Hemolytic Disease	Hepatic Disease	Biliary Obstruction
Urine urobilogen	Normal	Increased	Increased	Decreased
Urine bilirubin	Negative	Negative	±	Positive

Ref: Modern Urinalysis, Ames Company 1974:51.

C. Sediment
1. Light microscopy: Used to examine unstained, centrifuged urine for formed elements, including casts, cells, and crystals. Centrifuge 10 ml for 5 minutes, then decant 9 ml of

The Art of the Urine Microscopic Examination

	Color Plate
Yeast forms: look for hyphae, budding forms	1, 2, 3
Fresh RBCs do not take stain, are uniform in shape and size. (Note squamous cell for size comparison.)	4
Polymorphonuclear neutrophils (nuclei stain light pink on gram stain)	5
Squamous epithelial cells	6 (A)
Bladder cells (appear in large numbers in patients with cystitis)	6 (B)
Polymorphonuclear cells	6 (C)
Trichomonas	7
Urate crystals (often brown-green, multiple shapes)	8
Oxalate crystals (normal, any pH, multiple shapes)	9
Phosphates (normal, limited to alkaline urine, multiple shapes)	10
Hyaline cast (1–2 RBCs diameters in width; may be found in the absence of kidney disease)	11 (A)
Granular cast (4 RBC diameters, containing disintegrated cells; suggestive of kidney disease)	11 (B)
RBC cast (usually diagnostic of glomerulonephritis or acute tubular necrosis or may occur following *severe* exercise.)	12
Waxy cast (originate from RBC casts trapped in the nephron for long periods; usually 8–10 RBC diameters; usually brittle.)	13

Ref: Shapter RK, Pharmaceuticals Division, CIBA-GEIGY, New Jersey, 1976.

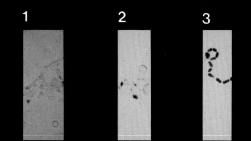

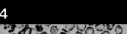

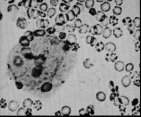

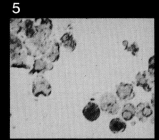

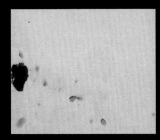

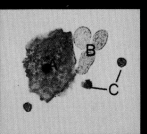

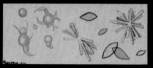

8

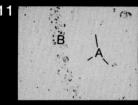

11

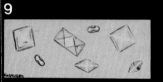

9

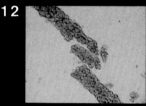

12

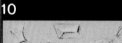

10

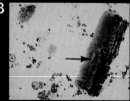

13

supernatant. Resuspend sediment in remaining 1 ml of urine. Place drop on glass slide; use coverslip. Best results with subdued light. Focus particularly on edge of coverslip since formed elements collect there. See color plates for illustration of urine sediment.

Ref: Henry JB. Clinical Diagnosis and Management by Laboratory Methods. Philadelphia: WB Saunders 1984;380. Greenhill A, et al. Pediatric Clin North Am 1976;23:661

D. Screening Tests for Urinary Tract Infections (UTIs)
Note: All tests must be confirmed with a urine culture.
1. Dipstick
   a. Nitrite test: Detects nitrites produced by reduction of dietary nitrates by urinary bacteria. (especially *E. coli., Klebsiella, Proteus*). A positive test is virtually diagnostic of bacteriuria. False negatives can occur with inadequate dietary nitrates, insufficient time for bacteria proliferation or conversion of nitrates to nitrites, inability of bacteria to reduce nitrates to nitrites (many gram positive organisms as well as *Enterococcus, Mycobacterium,* fungi), and large volume of dilute urine.
   b. Leukocyte esterase test: Detects esterases released from broken-down leukocytes. This is therefore an indirect test for WBCs that may or may not be present with a UTI.
   c. Bac-T screen: Colorimetric test that traps bacteria in filter and stains them with a safrinine dye. Does not require bacterial growth. Reportedly 93–97% sensitive.
2. Urine gram stain: Used to screen for UTIs. One organism/hpf in uncentrifuged urine represents at least 10 to the fifth colonies/ml.

   Ref: Feigin RD, Cherry JD. Pediatric Infect Dis, 1992;483.

II. RENAL FUNCTION TESTS
A. Tests of Glomerular Function
1. Creatinine clearance (Ccr): (timed specimen)
   a. Purpose: Standard measure of glomerular filtration rate (GFR); closely approximates inulin clearance in the normal range of GFR. When GFR is low, Ccr is greater than inulin clearance. Inaccurate in children with obstructive uropathy.

b. Method: Collect urine over any time period; record interval to the nearest minute. Have patient empty bladder (discard specimen) before beginning collection. Collect all urine during time interval, including urine voided at the end of the collection period. If the patient's renal function is stable, draw blood sample once during test period. (If function is changing rapidly, draw blood sample at beginning and end of period and use the average.)

c. Calculation:

$$Ccr = U \ V \ / \ P \ x \ 1.73/S.A. = ml/min/1.73M^2$$

U (mg/dl) = urinary creatinine concentration

V (ml/min) = total urine volume (ml) divided by length of collection interval (min). Note that 24 hours = 1440 min.

P (mg/dl) = serum creatinine concentration (may average two levels).

S.A. (m^2) = surface area.

d. Normal values (measured by inulin clearance)

Age	GFR (Mean)
Newborns (<24 hr) (fairly constant for 27–43 wk gestation	1.07 ± 0.12 ml/min/kg
Premature infants (>24 hr)	No reference values (varies with gestational age)
5–7 days	50.6 ± 5.8 ml/min/m^2
1–2 mo	64.6 ± 5.8 ml/min/m^2
3–4 mo	85.8 ± 4.8 ml/min/m^2
5–8 mo	87.7 ± 11.9 ml/min/m^2
9–12 mo	86.9 ± 8.5 ml/min/m^2
1–5 yr-adolescent	
Males	124.0 ± 25.8 ml/min/m^2
Females	108.8 ± 13.5 ml/min/m^2
Adults (postpubertal)	
Males	105.0 ± 13.9 ml/min/m^2
Females	95.4 ± 8.0 ml/min/m^2

Ref: Robillard JE et al. Pediatrics Update-Review for Physicians. New York: Elsevier North Holland, 1980; 168–69; Schwartz GJ et al.: J Pediatr 1984; 104:849; Fobias GJ et al. N Engl J Med 1962;

2. Creatinine Clearance: Spot Urine
   a. Purpose: Useful when a timed specimen cannot be collected; correlates well with standard creatinine clearance for children with relatively normal body habitus. If habitus markedly abnormal than more standard methods of measurement of Ccr must be used.
   b. Calculation:
      Estimated Ccr = kL / Pcr
      k = proportionality constant
      L = height (cm)
      Pcr = plasma creatinine (mg/dl)

k Values	
LBW during first year of life	0.33
Term AGA during 1st year of life	0.45
Children and adolescent girls	0.55
Adolescent boys	0.70

Ref: Schwartz, GJ et al. Pediatric Clinics of North America, 1987;34:571.

3. Glomerular function as determined by nuclear medicine scans. See Radiology, Chapter 24.

B. Tests of Tubular Function
1. Proximal tubule
   a. Proximal tubule reabsorption: Proximal tubule is responsible for resorption of electrolytes, glucose, and amino acids. Studies to determine proximal tubular function compare urine and blood levels of specific compounds arriving at percent tubular resorption (Tx):

$$Tx = 1 - \frac{Ux/Px}{Ucr/Pcr} \times 100\%$$

Ux = concentration of compound in urine
Px = concentration of compound in plasma
Ucr = concentration of creatinine in urine
Pcr = concentration of creatinine in plasma
This formula is also used for amino acids, electrolytes, calcium and phosphorus.

b. Glucose reabsorption: Glucose threshold is plasma glucose concentration at which significant amounts of glucose appear in the urine. The presence of glycosuria must be interpreted in relation to simultaneously determined plasma glucose concentration. If plasma glucose concentration is < 120 mg/dl, and glucose is present in the urine, this implies incompetent tubular reabsorption of glucose and proximal renal tubular disease. (For discussion of normal values and further studies of proximal tubule function consult Holliday MA et al. Pediatric Nephrology. Baltimore, MD: 1987.)

c. Urine calcium: Hypercalciuria is seen with RTA, vitamin D intoxication, hyperparathyroidism, steroids, immobilization, excessive calcium intake, and loop diuretics. May be idiopathic (associated with hematuria and renal stones). Diagnosis:

1) 24 hr urine: Calcium >4 mg/kg/24h
2) Spot urine: Determine Ca/Cr ratio (mg). Normal, < 0.21; mean, 0.08 (boys); 0.06 (girls); no standards for premature infants.

Ref: Moore ES et al. J Pediatr 1987; 92:906; Stapleton FB et. al. N Engl J Med 1984;310:1345.

2. Distal tubule

a. Urine acidification: A urine acidification defect should be suspected when random urine pH values are > 6 in the presence of systemic metabolic acidosis. Acidification defect should be confirmed by simultaneous venous or arterial pH, plasma bicarbonate concentration, and pH meter (not dipstick) determination of pH of fresh urine.

1) Technique
   a) Perform test in consultation with a nephrologist.
   b) Proceed only if child is well hydrated.
   c) Give ammonium chloride 75 mEq/m^2
   d) Measure urine pH with pH meter every hour for 5h.
   e) Measure plasma bicarbonate concentration 3h after ingestion of ammonium chloride.

2) Results: The urine pH should fall below 5.5 and plasma bicarbonate should fall 4–5 mEq/L. If urine pH is not lower than 5.5 and the plasma bicarbonate is not below 20 mEq/L (18 for infant), larger doses of ammonium chloride may be necessary to produce plasma bicarbonate concentration below an abnormal renal bicarbonate reabsorption threshold. Extreme care should be taken when using larger doses of ammonium chloride.

Ref: Edelmann CM et al. Pediatr Res 1967; 1452.

3) Interpretation: normal response as noted.

   a) Type 1 renal tubular acidosis (RTA) (defect in distal tubular excretion of hydrogen ion): Fall in plasma bicarbonate concentration; urine pH remains above 6.0.

   b) Type 2 RTA: (defect in proximal tubular reabsorption of bicarbonate): Fall in plasma bicarbonate concentration; fall in urine pH below 5.5.

   c) Type 3 RTA: (probable variant of type 1 RTA): Defect in distal tubular hydrogen ion excretion plus bicarbonaturia (bicarbonate leak subsides after adolescence).

   d) Type 4 RTA: Associated with hyperchloremic acidosis and hyperkalemia. Has five subtypes. Seen with adrenal insufficiency, obstructive uropathy, diabetic neuropathy, pyelonephritis, and other disorders.

   Ref: McSherry E. Kidney Int 1981;20:799; Chan JCM. J Pediatr 1983; 102:327.

b. Urine concentration: A random urine specific gravity of 1.023 or more indicates intact concentrating ability within the limits of clinical testing; no further tests are indicated. A first-voided specimen following overnight fast is adequate to test concentrating ability. For more formal testing, see water deprivation test (Endocrinology, Section III.C.9).

Ref: Edelmann CM, et al. Am J Dis Child 1967; 114:639.

III. OLIGURIA

A. BUN/Cr ratio (both in mg/dl)

1. Normal: 10–15
2. >20: prerenal azotemia or GI bleeding
3. <5: liver disease, starvation, inborn error of metabolism

   Ref: Greenhill A et al. Pediatr Clin North Am, 1976; 23:661.

B. Laboratory Differentiation (numbers in parentheses are for neonates)

Test	Prerenal Oliguria		Low Output Failure		ADH Secretion
Urine sodium	<20	(<40)	>40	(>40)	>40
Specific Gravity	< 1.020	(1.015)	< 1.010	(< 1.015)	> 1.020
Osmolality (mOsm/L)	> 500	(> 400)	< 350	(< 400)	>500
Urine/plasma osmolality ratio	>1.3		< 1.3		>2
Urea nitrogen	>20		< 10		>15
Creatinine	>40	(> 20)	< 20	(< 15)	>30
RFI*	<1	(< 3)	> 1	(> 3.0)	>1
FE (Na)†	<1	(< 2.5)	> 1	(> 3.0)	Close to 1

*RFI (renal failure index) = $(U_{Na} \times 100)/U_{Cr}P_{Cr}$.
†FE (Na) (fractional excretion of sodium) = $(U_{Na}/P_{Na})/(U_{Cr}/P_{Cr}) \times 100$.

Ref: Adapted from Rogers, et al: Textbook of Pediatric Intensive Care, Williams and Wilkins, Baltimore: 1992;1198.

IV. ACUTE DIALYSIS

A. Indications

1. Metabolic or fluid derangements not controlled by aggressive medical management alone. Generally accepted criteria include:

   a. Volume overload with evidence of pulmonary edema or hypertension which is refractory to therapy.

   b. Hyperkalemia >6.0 mEq/L if hypercatabolic, or >6.5 mEq/L despite conservative measures.

   c. Metabolic acidosis with pH <7.2 or HCO^3 <10

   d. BUN >150; lower if rising rapidly.

   e. Neurologic symptoms secondary to uremia or electrolyte imbalance.

   f. Calcium/phosphorus imbalance, e.g. hypocalcemia with tetany or seizures in the presence of a very high serum phosphate.

2. Dialyzable toxin or poison (i.e. lactate, ammonia): For list of dialyzable poisons see Poisoning, Section III.B.2.

B. Techniques

1. Peritoneal dialysis (PD): Requires catheter to access the peritoneal cavity. May be used acutely as well as chronically as in continuous ambulatory peritoneal dialysis (CAPD).

   a. Available fluids and additives

   1) The most commonly used commercial dialysate (Baxter) contains 132 mEq Na, 3.5 mEq Ca, 0.5 mEq Mg, 96 mEq Cl, 40 mEq lactate, in each liter.

   2) This solution is available with 1.5%, 2.5%, or 4.25% dextrose. Dextrose content is selected depending on the amount of ultrafiltrate desired. Fluid is removed more rapidly with higher dextrose concentrations. Excessive use of higher osmolar solutions may result in hypovolemia and hypotension.

   3) Heparin is added (100–500 units/L) to initial dialysate to prevent clots from forming; this can be discontinued when outflow is clear.

   4) Cephalothin (250–500 mg/L) may also be added to the dialysate as the situation warrants.

   5) If serum potassium is <3.5 mEq/L, then potassium may be given IV or added to the dialysis fluid (3–4 mEq/L).

2. Hemodialysis (HD): Requires placement of special vascular access devices. May be the method of choice for certain toxins (i.e., ammonia, uric acid, or poisons.) or when there are contraindications to peritoneal dialysis.

   Ref: Rogers MC. Textbook of Pediatric Intensive Care. Baltimore: Williams & Wilkins, 1992:1205-1212.

3. Continuous arteriovenous hemofiltration (CAVH): Cleanses blood through principle of convective solute transport (analogous to basement membrane of glomerulus) instead of by diffusion as in conventional dialysis. Also requires special vascular access devices. Indications include: isolated fluid management, renal failure with profound hemodynamic instability, electrolyte disturbance(s), intoxications of substances that are freely filtered across particular ultrafiltration membrane utilized.

C. Peritoneal Dialysis (PD) vs. Hemodialysis vs. CAVH

	PD	HD	CAVH
Benefits			
Fluid removal	+	+ +	+ +
Urea and creatinine clearance	+	+ +	+
Potassium clearance	+ +	+ +	+
Complications			
Need for heparinization	−	+	+
Bleeding	−	+	+
Disequilibrium	−	+	−
Peritonitis	+	−	−
Pancreatitis	+	−	−
Thrombocytopenia	−	+	−
Neutropenia	−	+	−
Protein loss	+ +	−	−
Hypotension	+	+ +	+
Increased cardiac output	+	+	+
Respiratory compromise	+	Possible	−
Vessel thrombosis	−	+	+
Hyperglycemia	Possible	−	−
Lactic acidosis	Possible	−	Possible
Other infection	−	+	+
Inguinal hernia	+	−	−
Electrolyte imbalance	+	+	+
Abdominal pain	+	−	−

Ref: Adapted from Rogers MC. Textbook of Pediatric Intensive Care. Baltimore: Williams & Wilkins, 1992:1209.

NEUROLOGY ***21***

"If I only had a brain…,"
the Scarecrow; *Wizard of Oz*.

I.   NEUROLOGIC EXAMINATION

A.   Mental Status: Alertness, orientation, attention, memory, abstraction, language, behavior.

B.   Cranial Nerves

	Name	Screening Tests	Specific Signs of Dysfunction
I	Olfactory		Abnormal smell
II	Optic	Acuity, visual fields, fundus	
III	Oculomotor	Extraocular movements, accomodation, light response	Abnormal saccades or pursuits
IV	Trochlear		
VI	Abducens		Head tilt, disconjugate gaze
V	Trigeminal	Facial sensation Jaw movement	Corneal reflex (sensory component)
VII	Facial	Facial strength, symmetry, taste (anterior 2/3 of tongue)	
VIII	Vestibulocochlear	Hearing acuity, balance	
IX	Glossopharyngeal	Gag, speech quality, uvula movement	Dysarthria, nasal voice
X	Vagus		
XI	Accessory	Head turn, shoulder shrug	
XII	Hypoglossal	Tongue strength, symmetry	Dysarthria

C.   Motor

1. Muscle bulk
2. Tone
   a. Resistance to passive movement
   b. Stiffness with active skills (running, jumping, arising from the floor, or climbing onto the exam table)

3. Strength (maximum power)

    0/5 = no movement

    1/5 = palpable tightening of tendon without limb movement

    2/5 = movement in a gravity-neutral plane

    3/5 = movement against gravity

    4/5 = subnormal strength

    5/5 = normal strength

D. Sensory: Primary disorders of sensation are rare in children. Specific evaluation of light touch, temperature, proprioception, vibration, and higher cortical function require significant time, attention, cooperation, and intelligence. The Romberg test evaluates both position sense and spinal cord function. See Figure 21.1.

E. Coordination: Evaluate general coordination while watching activity including gross motor skills, as well as dressing or playing video games. Specific tests:

1. Rapid alternating and rapid repetitive movements
2. Finger-to-nose and heel-to-shin
3. Gait

F. Deep ("Tendon") Reflexes

Reflex	Site	Nerve
Jaw reflex	Pons	Trigeminal
Biceps	C_{5-6}	Musculocutaneous
Brachioradialis	C_{5-6}	Radial
Triceps	C_{6-8}	Radial
Superficial abdominal		
Above umbilicus	T_{7-9}	
Umbilicus and below	T_{10-12}	
Knee	L_{2-4}	Femoral
Ankle	S_{1-2}	Tibial

G. Development: Refer to Development, Chapter 8.

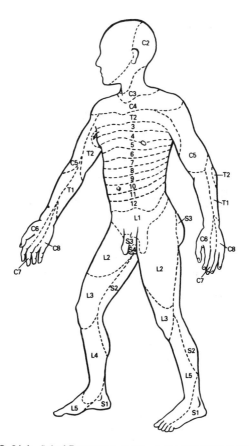

FIG 21.1. Spinal Dermatome. Ref: Examination of the Cranial and Peripheral Nerves Orrin Devinsky, Edward Feldmann; Churchill Livingstone, 1988:35, New York.

H. Spinal Pathways (Long Tracts)

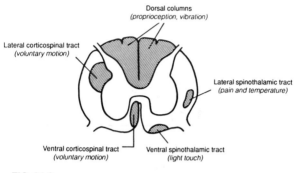

FIG 21.2.
Spinal Pathways

II. HEADACHES
A. Differential Diagnosis
1. Acute headaches
    a. Increased ICP: e.g., tumor, abscess, trauma, hydrocephalus, pseudotumor cerebri, blood.
    b. Decreased ICP: e.g., following LP or VP shunt, CSF leak (e.g. basilar skull fracture).
    c. Meningeal pain: e.g., meningitis, leukemia, blood.
    d. Vascular: e.g., vasculitis, hypertension, AVM.
    e. Bone.
2. Chronic Headaches
    a. Migraine (classic or common).
    b. Psychogenic: Depression, anxiety, conversion.
    c. Referred pain: Scalp, eyes, ears, sinuses, nose, teeth, pharynx, cervical spine.
    d. Non-specific: Tension or muscular.
B. Evaluation
1. History: Differentiate acute headaches from chronic or worsening headaches.

2. Physical examination: General careful neurologic and fundoscopic examination.

3. EEG only to differentiate migraine from complex partial seizures; MRI for focal neurologic symptoms, complicated migraine or chronic progressive headaches.

4. Other studies as clinically indicated (e.g., angiography).

C. Migraine Headache

1. Characteristics: Chronic, throbbing/pulsatile, unilateral (25–60%), bifrontal (young), early-car sickness (45%), relief with sleep, positive family history (>50%). Triggered by stress, menses, caffeine.

2. Associated symptoms: Nausea, vomiting, abdominal pain, photophobia. Complications: paresthesias, visual field cuts, aphasia, hemiplegia, ophthalmoplegia, basilar artery migraine, acute confusional state.

3. Classification
   a. Classic (≈33%) with aura, often fronto-temporal.
   b. Common: Lacks aura, "aching", often bilateral-frontal.

4. Treatment
   a. Acute: Symptomatic relief with darkroom/sleep, acetominophen, NSAIDs, ergotamine, propranolol, biofeedback.
   b. Prophylaxis: Dietary manipulation, remove food allergy.

   Ref: Singer H, Rowe S, Ped Annals; 21:6. 369-73.

III. PAROXYSMAL EVENTS
A. Differential Diagnosis

Diagnosis	Definition/Examples	Characteristics
Seizure	Paroxysmal discharge of neurons in brain resulting in alteration of function/behavior	± incontinence, ± postictal period.
Pseudoseizures	Paroxysmal, usually "dramatic" event appearing as a seizure, unassociated with ictal EEG changes.	May occur with suggestion; may be exacerbated by stress. No incontinence. No postictal period.

(Continued.)

Diagnosis	Definition/Examples	Characteristics
Head trauma	Loss of consciousness (LOC), post-traumatic seizures	± signs and symptoms of ICP.
Syncope	LOC due to dimished cerebral perfusion. May be due to hypovolemia, hypoxia, reduced cardiac output, arrhythmia, complicated migraine.	Typically, there is a precipitating event; patient may have blurred vision, nausea, and cold/clammy skin.
Breath-holding spells	Cyanosis and apnea, sometimes followed by a seizure, occuring in children age 6 mo to 5 years. Affect 4–5% of children. Occur in response to anger, fear, or frustration.	Cyanosis appears before the seizure. EEG not epileptiform during the event.
Sleep disorders	Nightmares, night terrors, narcolepsy	
Movement disorders	Paroxysmal, choreoathetosis, tic disorder	
Psychological/ behavioral	ADHD, panic attacks, daydreaming	
Gastrointestinal disorders	Sandifer syndrome, recurrent abdominal pain	Distractable, may be temporally associated with meals.
Drug or toxin-induced	Toxin-induced event	

Ref: Golden G, Pediatr Clin North Am 1992:715-25.

B. Paroxysmal Event Evaluation

1. History: Description, time course, and setting of event; history of illness, trauma, medication, toxins, fever; presence of postictal period, past history or family history of similar events. Try to get history from an eyewitness, before the story is altered by suggestion!

2. Physical examination: Careful general and neurologic examination, noting mental status, behavior, asymmetry, paralysis, cardiac abnormalities, phakomatosis, trauma.

3. Studies: Depends on clinical setting. Consider blood pressure (supine and upright) sodium, calcium, magnesium, BUN, creatinine, glucose, HCT, ECG, toxicology screen, head CT, MRI, lumbar puncture, and EEG with video monitoring.

C. Seizures

1. Epilepsy: Two or more non-febrile seizures.
2. Status epilepticus: Prolonged or recurrent seizure activity lasting over 30 minutes, without the patient regaining consciousness.
3. Classification: Helps to predict etiology and to determine an optimal therapeutic regimen.

	Seizure Type	Anticonvulsant Therapy*
Partial (focal)	Partial-simple (conscious), motor, sensory, autonomic	Carbamazepine, phenobarbital, phenytoin, valproic acid
	Partial-complex (consciousness impaired)	
	Partial with secondary generalization	
Generalized (nonfocal)	Tonic/Clonic	Carbamazepine, phenobarbital, phenytoin, valproic acid
Generalized (other)	Atonic	Valproic acid, clonazepam, benzodiazepines, methsuximide, ketogenic diet,† ACTH/corticosteriods
	Myoclonic	
	Atypical absence	
	Minor motor seizures	
	Absence	Ethosuximide, valproic acid
	Infantile spasms	ACTH, corticosteroids, valproic acid, benzodiazepines

*Please see Formulary, Chapter 25, for doses and side-effects.
†The ketogenic diet may be helpful in the management of intractable tonic and/or clonic and myoclonic seizures.

4. Etiology
   a. Partial onset and generalized tonic-clonic: Birth trauma, congenital defect, acquired cortical defect (stroke, neoplasm, infection).
   b. Generalized (other): genetic disordes, inborn errors of metabolism, congenital brain defect.
5. Treatment: Treatments of virtually all seizures should be directed to balance the probability and danger of more seizures against the probability of medication side effects. Generally, children with only one or a few scattered seizures should not receive medication until a pattern emerges. In all cases, monotherapy is the goal, with max-

imum tolerated doses of a single drug before changing to or adding a second drug.

D. Special Seizure Syndromes

1. Febrile seizure: Brief generalized seizure associated with rise of fever, but without any CNS infection or neurologic cause. Etiology seems to be immaturity of brain with lowered seizure threshold. No increased risk of mental retardation, cerebral palsy, other neurologic disorders, or death.

   a. Incidence: 3–4% of children, 6 months to 5 years of age

   b. Evaluation: Consider lumbar puncture or additional studies with any of the following:

      1) Seizures that last > 15 min
      2) Focal motor seizures
      3) Seizures that occur in child who is ill-appearing
      4) Seizures that occur in a child with an abnormal neurologic examination
      5) Seizures in a child pretreated with antibiotics
      6) Seizures that recur within 24 hours
      7) Seizures that occur 24 hours after the onset of fever

   c. Treatment: Anticonvulsant prophylaxis is not recommended for simple febrile seizures. **Educate parents and family members about fever and seizure management.**

   d. Outcome:

      1) Recurrence rate: 25–30% have second episode (typically within 6–12 months), 17% have third, 9% have >3 episodes.
      2) Risk of epilepsy: 2% (as compared to 0.5–1.0% of general population).
      3) Increased risk in children with 2 or more of the following:
         a) Complex febrile seizures
         b) Family history of nonfebrile seizures
         c) Previously abnormal development

         Ref: Freeman J, Pediatr Annals 21:6, 355-61.

2. Neonatal seizure: Various paroxsymal behaviors or electrical neuronal events tonic, myoclonic, clonic or subtle (blinking, chewing, pedaling or apnea) due to CNS immaturity.

a. Etiologies of neonatal seizures:

Etiology	Incidence (%)
Hypoxic-ischemic encephalopathy	35–40
Intracranial hemorrhage infarction	15–20
CNS infection	12–17
CNS malformation	5
Metabolic derangements: hypoglycemia, pyridoxine, inborn errors of metabolism, drug (toxin)	3–5
Other, idiopathic	5–20

b. Evaluation: Clinical criteria; as few as 40–50% have electrographic seizures on EEG.
c. Treatment: Treat underlying etiology; efficacy of standard anticonvulsants is poor; consider phenobarbital, benzodiazepines, phenytoin.
d. Outcome: Variable, depending on etiology of seizure. One study has documented long term neurologic sequelae in 30–50% of patients with neonatal seizures.

Ref: Ichord R, Pediatr Annals 21:6, 339-45

3. Infantile spasms: Clusters of "salaam motion" (head flexed, arms extended and legs drawn up) often after awakening, EEG with hypsarrhythmia (≈65%) in non-REM sleep.
   a. Etiologies
      1) Symptomatic (67%) causes include: congenital CNS malformation, asphyxia, neonatal seizures, tuberous sclerosis, metabolic, neonatal infection.
      2) Cryptogenic (33%).
   b. Treatment: ACTH, prednisone, valproic acid, benzodiazepines.
   c. Outcome: 33% of these patients will develop Lennox-Gastaut syndrome (mixed seizures, mental retardation, diffuse spike-wave on EEG), 10–25% will be intellectually normal with resolution of their infantile spasms.

IV. HYDROCEPHALUS: See "Coma/Increased Intracranial Pressure" in Chapter 2.

A. Diagnosis: Look for increasing head circumference, misshapen skull, bulging large anterior fontanelle, separated sutures with "cracked pot" sign, increased intracranial pressure, and developmental delay. Obtain head CT if increase in head circumference crosses percentiles or if patient is symptomatic. Differentiate hydrocephalus (enlarged ventricles) from megalencephaly (large brain) or hydrocephalus ex vacuo (loss of brain tissue).

B. Treatment

1. Medical

   a. Acute increase of intracranial pressure: See Chapter 2.

   b. Slowly progressive hydrocephalus: The following medications may be effective in children 2 weeks to 10 months of age with slowly progressive hydrocephalus:

      1) Acetazolamide: PO or IV: 25 mg/kg/24h, increase by 25 mg/kg/24h to maximum 100 mg/kg/day divided TID. Maximum 2 g/24h.

      2) Furosemide: 1 mg/kg/24h PO or IV divided TID.

      3) Polycitra: Titrate to maintain bicarbonate >18 mEq/L and normal Na and K. Usual dose is 8–10 mEq/kg/24h.

      4) Side effects: Mild lethargy, poor feeding, occasional tachypnea, transient diarrhea, increased susceptibility to dehydration (unable to concentrate urine).

      Ref: Shinnar S, et al. J Pediatr 1985, 107:31.

2. Surgical: Have shunt placed to drain CSF from cranium.

   a. Shunt types: Ventriculoperitoneal shunts are used most commonly. Ventriculoatrial and ventriculopleural shunts are associated with cardiac arrhythmias, pleural effusions, and higher rates of infection.

   b. Shunt components: Typically a shunt is composed of three parts: (a) proximal tubing, (b) a flushing device with a one-way valve, and (c) distal tubing.

   c. Shunt complications: Shunt dysfunction may be caused by infection, obstruction (clogging or kinking), disconnection, and migration of proximal and distal tips.

C. Acute Shunt Obstruction or Infection: Management

1. Test shunt function: Depress bulb and allow it to refill. Decreased bulb depression phase may be caused by distal shunt obstruction or a stiffened bulb. Poor refill suggests obstruction at the ventricular end, or excessive ventricular decompression.

2. Evaluate shunt integrity: Obtain shunt series (skull, neck, chest and abdominal films) to look for kinking or disconnection. Obtain head CT to evaluate shunt position, ventricular size and evidence of increased intracranial pressure.
3. Tap shunt: **This procedure should be performed by a neurosurgeon; however, if a neurosurgeon is unavailable or the patient is rapidly deteriorating, a shunt tap may be performed by any physician familiar with the procedure.**
   a. Cleanse the area over the shunt bulb using aseptic technique.
   b. Insert a long-nose 25-gauge butterfly needle into the flushing device, through the bulb diaphragm, into the proximal chamber. A stopcock attached to the butterfly tubing may help prevent air from entering the ventricular system. Measure the fluid pressure, and remove the minimum amount of fluid needed to achieve symptomatic relief.
   c. If blockage at the ventricular end is suspected and patient continues to deteriorate, insert a spinal needle (up to 18-gauge) through the burr hole through which the shunt was placed, and direct it toward the lateral ventricles. Measure the pressure and remove the minimal amount of fluid necessary for decompression.
   d. Send CSF for culture, cell count and differential, glucose, and protein.
4. Further management: Pursue medical and surgical management of hydrocephalus as outlined above.

NUTRITION 22

I. ENERGY REQUIREMENTS
A. RDA Protein and Energy

Category	Age (yr) or condition	Weight (kg)	Weight (lb)	Height (cm)	Height (in)	Protein (g)	Average Energy Allowance (kcal) (per kg)	Average Energy Allowance (kcal) (per Day)
Infants	0.0–0.5	6	9	60	24	13	108	650
	0.5–1.0	9	20	71	28	14	98	850
Children	1–3	13	29	90	35	16	102	1300
	4–6	20	44	112	44	24	90	1800
	7–10	28	62	132	52	28	70	2000
Males	11–14	45	99	157	62	45	55	2500
	15–18	66	145	176	69	59	45	3000
	19–24	72	160	177	70	58	40	2900
	25–50	79	174	176	70		37	2900
	51+	77	170	173	68		30	2300
Females	11–14	46	101	157	62	46	47	2200
	15–18	55	120	163	64	44	40	2200
	19–24	58	128	164	65	46	38	2200
	25–50	63	138	163	64		36	2200
	51+	65	143	160	63		30	1900
Pregnant	1st trimester					60		+0
	2nd trimester							+300
	3rd trimester							+300
Lactating	1st 6 mo					65		+500
	2nd 6 mo					62		+500

Hendricks, Kristy, Walker, Allan, Manual of Pediatric Nutrition, B.C. Decker Inc., Philadelphia, 1990: p. 62.

B.   Growth Failure/Caloric Requirements: After evaluation for the etiology of growth failure, one may calculate energy needs for catch-up growth using the formula:

$$\text{kcal/kg} = \frac{\text{RDA cal for weight-age* (kcal/kg)} \times \text{Ideal weight for actual age (kg)}}{\text{Actual weight (kg)}}$$

*Weight-age is the age at which the patient's current weight would be in the 50th percentile.

C.   Energy Requirements in Disease: More precise calculations of basal energy requirements are necessary to further define individual needs during periods of stress and disease. These calculations also help to identify those individuals at risk for

TABLE 22.1.
Basal Metabolic Rates: Infants and Children

Age 1 wk to 10 Mo		Age 11 to 36 Mo			Age 3 to 16 Yr		
	Metabolic Rate (kcal/hr)		Metabolic Rate (kcal/hr)			Metabolic Rate (kcal/hr)	
Weight (kg)	M or F	Weight (kg)	M	F	Weight (kg)	M	F
3.5	8.4	9.0	22.0	21.2	15	35.8	33.3
4.0	9.5	9.5	22.8	22.0	20	59.7	37.4
4.5	10.5	10.0	23.6	22.8	25	43.6	41.5
5.0	11.6	10.5	24.4	23.6	30	57.5	45.5
5.5	12.7	11.0	25.2	24.4	35	51.3	49.6
6.0	13.8	11.5	26.0	25.2	40	55.2	53.7
6.5	14.9	12.0	26.8	26.0	45	59.1	57.8
7.0	16.0	12.5	27.6	26.9	50	63.0	61.9
7.5	17.1	13.0	28.4	27.7	55	66.9	66.0
8.0	18.2	13.5	29.2	28.5	60	70.8	70.0
8.5	19.3	14.0	30.0	29.3	65	74.7	74.0
9.0	20.4	14.5	30.8	30.1	70	78.6	78.1
9.5	21.4	15.0	31.6	30.9	75	82.5	82.2
10.0	22.5	15.5	32.4	31.7			
10.5	23.6	16.0	33.2	32.6			
11.0	24.7	16.5	34.0	33.4			

Ref: Altman PL, Dittmer, DS, eds. Metabolism, Bethesda, MD: Federation of American Societies for Experimental Biology, 1968.

protein-energy malnutrition. To determine the requirements for particular patients, calculate the daily caloric requirement from the basal metabolic rate found in Table 22.1. Basal metabolic needs are increased 10–75% depending on the level of activity (10%, bed rest; 30%, limited activity; 50%, moderate activity; 75%, vigorous activity). Requirements for particular disease states are listed in Fig 22.1.

Example. A 1-year-old, 9-kg girl with a long bone fracture will require:

$$\text{BMR} = 21.2 \text{ kcal/hr} \times 24 \text{ hr} = 508.8 \text{ kcal/day}$$

$$\text{Long bone fracture} = 508.8 \text{ kcal/day} \times 1.3 \text{ (12–32\% increase)}$$
$$= 661 \text{ kcal/day}$$

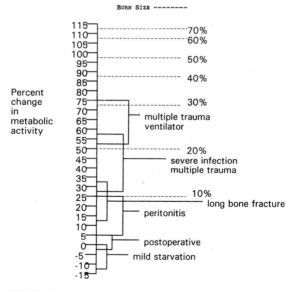

FIG 22.1.

Increased Energy Needs With Stress

From Dialogues in nutrition, 1979;3: 1–12. Adapted from Wilmore D. The metabolic management of the critically ill. New York: Plenum, 1977.

II. RECOMMENDED DAILY DIETARY ALLOWANCES[a]
A. Vitamins

Category	Age (yr) or Condition	Weight[b] (kg)	(lb)	Height[b] (cm)	(in)	Vitamin A (µg of RE)[c]	Vitamin D (µg)[d]	Vitamin E (mg of a-TE)[e]	Vitamin K (µg)	Vitamin C (mg)	Thiamin (mg)	Riboflavin (mg)	Niacin (mg of NE)[f]	Vitamin B6 (mg)	Folate (µg)	Vit B12 (µg)
Infants	0.0–0.5	6	13	60	24	375	7.5	3	5	30	0.3	0.4	5	0.3	25	0.3
	0.5–1.0	9	20	71	28	375	10	4	10	35	0.4	0.5	6	0.6	35	0.5
Children	1–3	13	29	90	35	400	10	6	15	40	0.7	0.8	9	1.0	50	0.7
	4–6	20	44	112	44	500	10	7	20	45	0.9	1.1	12	1.1	75	1.0
	7–10	28	62	132	52	700	10	7	30	45	1.0	1.2	13	1.4	100	1.4
Male	11–14	45	99	157	62	1000	10	10	45	50	1.3	1.5	17	1.7	150	2.0
	15–18	66	145	176	69	1000	10	10	65	60	1.5	1.8	20	2.0	200	2.0
	19–24	72	160	177	70	1000	10	10	70	60	1.5	1.7	19	2.0	200	2.0
Female	11–14	46	101	157	62	800	10	8	45	50	1.1	1.3	15	1.4	150	2.0
	15–18	55	120	163	64	800	10	8	55	60	1.1	1.3	15	1.5	180	2.0
	19–24	58	128	164	65	800	10	8	60	60	1.1	1.3	15	1.6	180	2.0
Pregnant						800	10	10	65	70	1.5	1.6	17	2.2	400	2.2
Lactating	1st 6 mo					1300	10	12	65	95	1.6	1.8	20	2.1	280	2.6
	2nd 6 mo					1200	10	11	65	90	1.6	1.7	20	2.1	260	2.6

[a]The allowances, expressed as average daily intakes over time, are intended to provide for individual variations among most normal persons as they live in the United States under usual environmental stresses. Diets should be based on a variety of common foods in order to provide other nutrients for which human requirements have been less well defined.

[b]Weights and heights of reference adults are actual medians for the U.S. population of the designated age, as reported by NHANESII. The median weights and heights of those <19 years of age were taken from Hamill et al. (1979). The use of these figures does not imply that the height-to-weight ratios are ideal.

[c]Retinal equivalents. 1 retinal equivalent = 1 microgram retinol or 6 microgram beta-carotene.

[d]As cholecalciferol. 10 micrograms cholecalciferol = 400 IU vitamin D.

[e]alpha-Tocopherol equivalents. 1 mg d-alpha tocopherol = 1 alpha-TE.

[f]1 NE (niacin equivalent) is equal to 1 mg of niacin or 60 mg of dietary tryptophan.

III. RECOMMENDED DAILY DIETARY ALLOWANCES
B. Minerals*

Category	Age (yr) or Condition	Weight (kg)	Weight (lb)	Height (cm)	Height (in.)	Calcium (mg)	Phosphorus (mg)	Magnesium (mg)	Iron (mg)	Zinc (mg)	Iodine (µg)	Selenium (µg)
Infants	0.0–0.5	6	13	60	24	400	300	40	6	5	40	10
	0.5–1.0	9	20	71	28	600	500	60	10	5	50	15
Children	1–3	13	29	90	35	800	800	80	10	10	70	20
	4–6	20	44	112	44	800	800	120	10	10	90	20
	7–10	28	62	132	52	800	800	170	10	10	120	30
M	11–14	45	99	157	62	1200	1200	270	12	15	150	40
	14–18	66	145	176	69	1200	1200	400	12	15	150	50
	19–24	72	160	177	70	1200	1200	350	10	15	150	70
F	11–14	46	101	157	62	1200	1200	280	15	12	150	45
	15–18	55	120	163	64	1200	1200	300	15	12	150	50
	19–24	58	128	164	65	1200	1200	280	15	12	150	55
Pregnant						1200	1200	320	30	15	175	65
Lactating	1st 6 mo					1200	1200	355	15	19	200	65
	2nd 6 mo					1200	1200	340	15	16	200	75

*The allowances, expressed as average daily intakes over time, are intended to provide for individual variations among most normal persons as they live in the United States under usual environmental stresses. Diets should be based up on a wide variety of common foods in order to provide other nutrients for which human requirements have been less well defined.

†Weights and heights of Reference Adults are actual medians for the U.S. population of the designated age, as reported by NHANES II. The median weights and heights of those under 19 years of age were taken from Hammill et al. (1979). The use of these figures does not imply that the height-to-weight ratios are ideal.

Ref: Food and Nutrition Board, National Academy of Sciences-National Research Council Recommended Dietary Allowances, Revised, 1989.

C. Infant Formula Analysis per 100 ml

Formula	kcal per oz	Protein gm	Protein % cal	Protein Type	Carbohydrate gm	Carbohydrate % cal	Carbohydrate Type	Fat gm	Fat % cal	Fat Type	Na (mEq)	K (mEq)	Ca (mg)	P (mg)	Fe (mg)	GI Solute Load (mOsm/L)
Human milk, mature	20	1.1	6	20% casein, 80% whey	7.2	42	Lactose	3.9	52	Human milk fat	0.8	1.3	28	14	0.03	290
Human milk, premature	22	1.7	9	20% casein, 80% whey	8	44	Lactose	3.9	48	Human milk fat	1.3	1.4	28	16	0.1	290
Alimentum	20	1.9	11	Hydrolized casein	6.9	41	Sucrose modified tapioca starch	3.8	48	MCT, 50%; safflower oil, 40%; soy oil, 10%	1.3	2.0	71	51	1.2	370
Carnation Good Start	20	1.6	9.8	Whey	7.4	44	Lactose 70%, maltdextrin	3.4	46	Palm olein, safflower, coconut	0.7	1.7	43	24	1.0	
Cow's milk, whole	20	3.3	21	80% casein, 20% whey	4.7	30	Lactose	3.3	49	Butterfat	2.1	3.9	79	40	0	260
Enfamil 20 (with Fe)	20	1.5	9	Nonfat cow's milk, demineralized whey	6.9	41	Lactose	3.8	50	Coconut, soy oil, palm olein, sunflower oil	0.8	1.8	46	31	0.11 (1.26)	300
Enfamil 24 (with Fe)	24	1.8	9	Nonfat cow's milk, demineralized whey	8.3	41	Lactose	4.5	50	Coconut, soy oil, palm olein, sunflower oil	1.0	2.2	55	38	0.13 (1.5)	360

Enfamil Premature Formula	20	2.0	Demineralized whey, nonfat milk solids	7.4	Corn syrup solids, lactose	44	3.4	MCT, 40%; soy 40%; coconut oil, 20%	44	1.1	110	55	0.17	244
Enfamil Premature Formula 24 (with Fe)	24	2.4	Demineralized whey, nonfat milk solids	9.0	Corn syrup solids, lactose	44	4.1	MCT, 40%; coconut and soy oils	44	1.4	132	68	0.2 (.15)	300
Evaporated milk-based formula*	20	2.8	80% casein, 20% whey	6.8	Lactose	40	3.2	Butterfat	43	1.9	111	87	0.08	
Human milk fortifier (per packet)	3.5 (kcal per cc)	0.2	Reduced mineral whey and casein	0.7	Corn syrup solids and lactose	77	0.0	0.0	3	0.0	22	11	0	120
Isomil	20	1.8	Soy protein isolate	6.8	Corn syrup and sucrose	40	3.7	Soy and coconut oil	49	1.3	71	51	1.21	240
MJ3232A	12.6	1.9	Casein hydrolysate	2.8	Tapioca starch, mono- and disaccharide-free	25	2.8	MCT, 40%; corn oils, 13%	57	1.3	63	42	1.26	250
Nursoy	20	2.1	Soy protein	6.9	Sucrose	40	3.6	Coconut, safflower, soy oils	48	0.9	63	44	1.2	266

*Denotes formula prepared as 19 oz of water and 2 tbsp sugar added to 13 oz can of evaporated milk. Vitamin and iron supplements are needed.

(Continued.)

326 *Diagnostic and Therapeutic Information*

Infant Formula Analysis per 100 ml (cont.).

Formula	kcal per oz	Protein gm	Protein % cal	Protein Type	Carbohydrate gm	Carbohydrate % cal	Carbohydrate Type	Fat gm	Fat % cal	Fat Type	Na (mEq)	K (mEq)	Ca (mg)	P (mg)	Fe (mg)	GI Solute Load (mOsm/L)
Nutramigen	20	1.9	11	Casein hydrolysate, amino acid premix	9.0	54	Corn syrup solids and corn starch	2.6	35	Corn oil	1.4	1.9	63	42	1.25	320
Protagen	20	2.3	14	Sodium caseinate	7.7	46	Corn syrup solids, sucrose, lactose	3.1	40	MCT, 85%; corn oil, 15%	1.6	2.1	63	47	1.25	220
Pregestimil	20	1.9	11	Casein hydrolysate cystine, tyrosine, and tryptophan	6.9	41	Corn syrup solids, dextrose, corn starch	3.8	48	MCT, 60%; corn oil, 20%; safflower oil, 20%	1.1	1.9	63	42	1.25	320
ProSobee	20	2.0	12	Soy protein isolate	6.7	40	Corn syrup solids	3.5	48	Coconut, soy oil, palm olein, sunflower oil	1.0	2.1	63	49	1.25	200
Ross carbohydrate-free	12	2.0	20	Soy protein isolate				3.6	80	Coconut and soy oil	1.3	1.9	70	50	0.15	74

Product															
Similac 20 (with Fe)	20	1.5	Nonfat cow's milk	9	7.2	Lactose	43	3.6	Coconut and soy oil	48	0.8	1.8	51	39	0.15 (1.2)	300
Similac 24 (with Fe)	24	2.2	Nonfat cow's milk	11	8.5	Lactose	42	4.3	Coconut and soy oil	47	1.2	2.7	73	57	0.18 (1.5)	380
Similac Special Care	20	1.8	Nonfat cow's milk, milk whey	11	7.2	Lactose and hydrolyzed corn starch	42	3.7	MCT, 50%; coconut and soy oil	47	1.3	2.2	122	61	0.25	250
Similac Special Care 24	24	2.1	Nonfat cow's milk and whey	11	8.4	Lactose and hydrolyzed corn starch	42	4.4	MCT, 50%; coconut and soy oil	47	1.5	2.7	146	73	1.5	300
Similac PM 60/40	20	1.6	Whey sodium caseinate	9	6.9	Lactose	41	3.8	Coconut and soy oil	50	0.7	1.5	38	19	0.15	280
SMA 20 (with Fe)	20	1.5	Nonfat cow's milk, demineralized whey	8.8	7.2	Lactose	42	3.6	Oleo, oleic, coconut, and soy oil	48	0.6	1.4	42	28	0.15 (1.2)	300
SMA Preemie	24	2.0	Nonfat cow's milk, 60%; whey, 40%; casein	10	8.6	Lactose and glucose polymers	42	4.4	MCT, soy and coconut oils	48	1.4	1.9	75	40	0.3	300
Soyalac	20	2.1	Soy protein solids	12	6.8	Corn syrup, sucrose, soy bean, CHO	39	3.7	Soy oil	49	1.3	2.0	64	37	1.3	215
I-Soyalac	20	2.0	Soy protein	12	6.8	Sucrose, tapioca	40	3.6	Soy oil	48	1.4	2.0	70	50	1.2	140

D. Enteral Feeding Formula Analysis per Liter

Formula	kcal per oz	Protein % cal	Protein gm	Protein Type	Carbohydrate % cal	Carbohydrate gm	Carbohydrate Type	Fat % cal	Fat gm	Fat Type	Na (mEq)	K (mEq)	Ca (mg)	P (mg)	Fe (mg)	GI Solute Load (mOsm/kg)
Carnation Instant Breakfast	30	21.8	63.4	Casein, eggwhite, whey protein	51.5	149.	Lactose, sucrose	26.	34.	Milk fat	46	78.	2047.5	1701.4	19.2	723
Ensure with fiber	32	14.5	39.7	Na and Ca caseinate, soy protein isolate	55	162	Hydrolyzed corn starch, sucrose soy fiber	30	37	Corn oil	36.	42	708	708	12.8	480
Ensure	31	14	37.2	Na and Ca caseinate, soy protein isolate	55	145	Corn syrup, sucrose	31.	37	Corn oil	36	39.	521	521	9.4	470
Ensure Plus	44	14.7	54.9	Na and Ca caseinate, soy protein isolate	53	200	Corn syrup, sucrose	32	53	Corn oil	45.	49.	696	696	12.5	690
Glucerna	30	16.7	41.8	Na and Ca caseinate	33.3	93.7	Hydrolyzed corn starch, fiber, 53%; soy fiber, 25%; fructose, 21%	50	56	Safflower oil, 85%; soy oil, 15%	40.	40	704	704	12.7	375
Isocal	32	13	34	Na and Ca caseinate, soy protein	50	133	Maltodextrins	37	44	Soy oil, MCT oil	23	34	630	530	0.5	300

Jevity	31	44	Na and Ca caseinate	17	151	Hydrolyzed corn starch, soy fiber	53	36	MCT, 50%; corn oil; soy oil	30	40	39.	896	746	13.4	310
Nepro	60	70	Ca, Na, and Mg caseinate	14	215	Hydrolyzed corn starch, sucrose	43	96	Safflower oil, 90%; soy oil, 10%	43	36	27	1372	686	19	356.5
Osmolite	31	37	Casein soy protein isolate	14	145	Hydrolyzed corn starch	55	38	MCT, 50%; corn oil; soy oil	31	27	25.	521	521	9.4	300
Pediasure	30	29.6	Na caseinate, whey protein contentrate	12	110	Hydrolyzed corn starch, sucrose	44	50	High oleic safflower oil, 50% soy oil, 30%, MCT, 20%	44	16	34	970	800	14	<310
Peptamen	30	40	Whey protein hydrolysate	16	127	Maltodextrin, starch	51	39	MCT, 70%; sunflower, lecithin	33	22	32	600	500	9	260
Pulmocare	45	63	Na and Ca caseinate	17	106	Hydrolyzed corn starch, sucrose	28	92	Corn oil	55	56	44	1042	1042	19	490
Suplena	60	30	Na caseinate; Ca caseinate	6	255	Hydrolyzed cornstarch; sucrose	51	96	Safflower oil, 90%; soy oil, 10%	43	34	28.	1386	728	19	195
Sustacal	30	61	Na and Ca caseinate; soy protein isolate	24	140	Sucrose; corn syrup solids	55	23	Partially hydrolyzed soy oil	21	41	54	1010	930	16.9	620

(Continued.)

Formula	kcal per oz	Protein gm	Protein % cal	Protein Type	Carbohydrate gm	Carbohydrate % cal	Carbohydrate Type	Fat gm	Fat % cal	Fat Type	Na (mEq)	K (mEq)	Ca (mg)	P (mg)	Fe (mg)	GI Solute Load (mOsm/kg)
Sustacal HC	44	61	16	Na and Ca caseinate	190	50	Corn syrup solids; sucrose	58	50	Corn oil	36	38	850	850	15	650
Sustacal with fiber	30	46	17	Na and Ca caseinate; soy protein isolate	140	53	Maltodextrin; sucrose	35	53	Corn oil	31	36	840	700	12.7	480
Tolerex	30	21	8.2	Free amino acids	226	90.5	Glucose; oligosaccharide	1.4	90.5	Safflower oil	20	30	556	550	10	550
Travasorb MCT	30	49	20	Lactalbumin; K caseinate	123	50	Corn syrup solids	33	50	Sunflower oil, 20%; MCT, 80%	15	45	500	500	9	250
Vital HN	30	42	17	Partially hydrolyzed whey, meat, soy amino acids	185	74	Hydrolyzed corn starch; sucrose	11	74	Safflower oil; MCT, 45%	20	34	120	667	667	500
Vivonex TEN	30	38	15	Free amino acids	206	82	Maltodextrins	3	82	Safflower oil	20	20	500	500	9	630

IV. ENTERAL NUTRITION
A. Formula Selection in Infants (less than 12 months)

Formula Type	Indications	Examples
Human milk	First choice in enteral feeding; cellular and acellular immunoprotective elements (IgA, lactoferrin, lymphocytes, active enzymes)	
Cow's-milk based	Normal GI tract, lactose tolerant	Similac, Enfamil
Cow's-milk based, premature	Increased whey protein, calcium, and phosphorus requirements	Premature Enfamil, Premie SMA
Soy protein, lactose free	Cow's milk protein intolerance (8% of infants), lactose intolerance	Isomil, Prosobee, Nursoy
Casein hyrolysate, lactose free	Cow's milk protein intolerance, soy protein intolerance (30% of infants with cow's milk intolerance)	Nutramigen
Hypoallergenic, casein hydrolysate, lactose-free, MCT oil	Cow's milk protein intolerance, soy protein intolerance, abnormal nutrient absorption or digestion	Pregestimil, Portagen, Alimentum

B. Formula Selection in Children (older than 12 months)

Formula Type	Indication	Route	Examples
Nutritionally balanced lactose containing	Normal GI tract, lactose tolerant	Oral	Carnation Instant Breakfast
Lactose free	Normal GI tract, lactose intolerant	Oral, NG/GT	Pediasure, Ensure
		NG/GT	Osmolite, Isocal
Nutritionally complete plus fiber	Chronic diarrhea, chronic constipation	Oral, NG/GT	Ensure with fiber, Sustacal with fiber
High protein, high calorie	Increased caloric requirements, illness	NG/GT	Sustacal, Ensure plus, Sustacal HC

(Continued.)

Formula Type	Indication	Route	Examples
High fat	Pulmonary disease, decreased gastric emptying	NG/GT	Pulmocare, Glucerna
Elemental/semi-elemental	Abnormal digestion, abnormal nutrient absorption	NG/GT/JT	Tolerex, Vivonex, Travasorb MCT
Carbohydrate free	Severe carbohydrate malabsorption	NG/GT	MJ 3232A (contains tapioca starch), RCF
Low renal solute load	Renal dysfunction	NG/GT	Nepro, Suplena

Adapted from: Hendricks, K. Walker, A. Manual of Pediatric Nutrition. B.C. Decker Inc., Philadelphia, 1990.

C. Single Component Enteral Nutrition Supplements

Component	Source	Content	Calories
Protein			
Casec	Calcium caseinate	88 gm/100 gm powder	3.7 kcal/gm
Promod	Whey protein	75 gm/100 gm powder	4.2 kcal/gm
Propac	Whey protein	75 gm/100 gm powder	3.95 kcal/gm
Carbohydrate			
Moducal	Corn starch hydrolysate	95 gm/100 gm powder	3.8 kcal/gm
Polycose	Corn starch hydrolysate	50 gm/100 cc liquid	2.0 kcal/cc
		94 gm/ 100 gm powder	3.8 kcal/gm
Fat			
MCT oil	Fractionated coconut oil, 90%; C8 and C10 TGs	93 gm/100 cc	7.7 kcal/cc
Micro lipid	Safflower oil, 50% emulsion	50 gm/100 cc	4.5 kcal/cc

V. PARENTERAL NUTRITION

Ref: Committee on Nutrition of the AAP, Commentary on Parenteral Nutrition, Pediatrics, 71(4):547–552, April 1983. Kerner JA, Parenteral Nutrition, Walker A, Pediatric Gastrointestinal Disease, vol II., B.C. Decker Inc., Philadelphia, 1991;p. 1645–1675. Hendricks, K, Walker, A, Manual of Pediatric Nutrition, B.C. Decker Inc., Philadelphia, 1990; p.110–133. The Johns Hopkins Hospital Nutrition Support Service.

A. Composition

Component	Initial Dose	Advance	Maximum
Protein*	Neonates (<1000 g): 0.5 g/kg/day	0.5–1.0 g/kg/day	10–12% of calories
	Children: 1.0 g/kg/day	1.0 g/kg/day	12–16% of calories
Fat†	Neonates (<1000 g): 0.5 g/kg/day	0.5–1.0 g/kg/day	40% of calories
	Children: 1.0 g/kg/day	0.5–1.0 g/kg/day	
Carbohydrate	Neonates: 4–6 mg/kg/min	Peripheral: 12.5% dextrose	
	Children: 7–8 mg/kg/min	Central: 25 to 30% dextrose	
Electrolytes	See section IV.E.		
Heparin	0.25–1.0 units/cc		

*Restrict protein in patients who cannot tolerate nitrogen load (renal/metabolic disease).
†Rate not to exceed 0.15 g/kg/hr

B. **Peripheral Parenteral Alimentation (PPN):** The solution is restricted to a maximum of 12% dextrose, 2% amino acids and 900 mOsm. Estimate osmolality using the following formula:

$$OSM = (\%dextrose \times 50) + (\% \text{ amino acids}) \times 100) + 2(Na \text{ mEq/L} + K \text{ mEq/L} + Ca \text{ mEq/L} + Mg \text{ mEq/L})$$

C. Total Parenteral Nutrition Requirements

Component	Neonate	6 m–10 yr	>10 yr
Calories (kcal/kg/day)	90–120	60–105	40–75
Fluid (cc/kg/day)	120–180	60–150	50–75
Dextrose (mg/kg/min)	4–6	7–8	7–8 (may need to increase to supply adequate calories)
Protein (gm/kg/day)	2–3	1.5–3.0	0.8–2
Fat (gm/kg/day)	0.5–4.0	1.0–4.0	1.0–4
Sodium (mEq/kg/day)	3–4	3–4	3–4
Potassium (mEq/kg/day)	2–3	2–3	1–2

(Continued.)

Component	Neonate	6 m – 10 yr	>10 yr
Calcium (mg/kg/day)	60 – 90	40 – 80	20 – 60
Phosphate (mg/kg/day)	45 – 70	25 – 40	25 – 40
Magnesium (mEq/kg/day)	0.25 – 1.0	0.5	0.5
Zinc (μg/kg/day)	400	200	50
Copper (μg/kg/day)	20	20	20
Chromium (μg/kg/day)	0.2	0.2	0.2
Manganese (μg/kg/day)	1	1	0.3
Selenium (μg/kg/day)	3	3	3

D. Metabolic Monitoring

Variables to Be Monitored	Initial Period*	Late Period†
Growth		
Weight	Daily	2×/wk
Height	Monthly	Monthly
Head circumference (infants)	Weekly	Weekly (<3 mo)
		Monthly (3 mo – 1 yr)
Arm Circumference	Monthly	Monthly
Skin-fold thickness	Monthly	Monthly
Laboratory Studies		
Electrolytes (Na,K,Cl,HCO$_3$)	2×/wk	Weekly
BUN, creatinine	2×/wk	Weekly
Protein, albumin	Weekly	Weekly
Ca, Mg, Phos	2×/wk	Weekly
ALT, AST, Alk Phos	Weekly	Weekly
Total and direct bilirubin	Weekly	Weekly
Transferrin	Weekly	Weekly
Complete CBC	Weekly	Weekly
Serum Folate, Vitamin B$_{12}$,	Monthly	Monthly
Vitamin E	Monthly	Monthly
Copper, zinc, selenium	Monthly	Monthly
Triglycerides, cholesterol‡	With changes in lipid rate	Weekly

*The period before carbohydrate, fat, or amino acid content maximized, or any period of metabolic instability.
†When fluid composition is stable.
‡Any time in which the patient is receiving intravenous lipid emulsion.

PULMONOLOGY **23**

I. NORMAL RESPIRATORY RATES

Age (yr)	Boys	Girls
0–1	31 ± 8	30 ± 6
1–2	26 ± 4	27 ± 4
2–3	25 ± 4	25 ± 3
3–4	24 ± 3	24 ± 3
4–5	23 ± 2	22 ± 2
5–6	22 ± 2	21 ± 2
6–7	21 ± 3	21 ± 3
7–8	20 ± 3	20 ± 2
8–9	20 ± 2	20 ± 2
9–10	19 ± 2	19 ± 2
10–11	19 ± 2	19 ± 2
11–12	19 ± 3	19 ± 3
12–13	19 ± 3	19 ± 2
13–14	19 ± 2	18 ± 2
14–15	18 ± 2	18 ± 3
15–16	17 ± 3	18 ± 3
16–17	17 ± 2	17 ± 3
17–18	16 ± 3	17 ± 3

Ref: Illif A, Lee V: Child Development
1952; 23:240.

II. PULMONARY FUNCTION TESTS (PFTs)
A. Airway Function

1. **Wright Peak Flow Meter:** Hand-held instrument used to measure peak flow rate (PFR). Effort dependent; insensitive to small airway function. Provides an objective assessment of dynamic pulmonary function and clinical response to therapy.

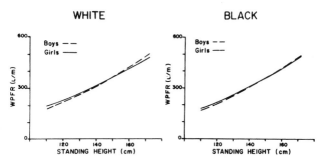

FIG 23.1.
Wright's Peak Flow Rate (WPFR)

2. **Spirometry (with and without bronchodilators):** Laboratory assessment of forced vital capacity (FVC), forced expiratory volume in one second (FEV_1), and average flow between 25 and 75% of expired vital capacity ($FEF_{25-75\%}$).

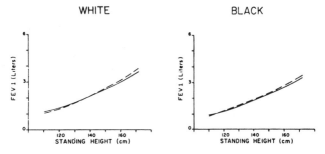

FIG 23.2.
Forced Expiratory Volume in 1 Second

3. **Flow-Volume Curves:** Two-dimensional presentation of air flow plotted against lung volume. Useful in characterizing different patterns of airway obstruction.

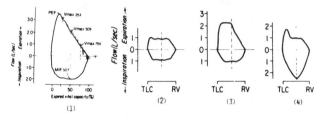

FIG 23.3.
Flow-Volume Loops

   a. Normal flow/volume loop.
   b. Fixed upper airway obstruction (tracheal stenosis): flattening of both inspiratory and expiratory phases.
   c. Variable extrathoracic obstruction (obstructive apnea): flattened **inspiratory** portion as transmural pressure gradient favors extrathoracic airway collapse on inspiration.
   d. Variable intrathoracic obstruction (tumor): Flattened **expiratory** phase as transmural pressure gradient favors intrathoracic airway collapse on inspiration.
B. **Lung Volumes:** Static parameters: total lung capacity (TLC), functional residual capacity (FRC), residual volume (RV) can be determined by helium dilution, nitrogen washout, or body plethysmography. Dynamic parameters: FEV_1, FVC are measured by spirometry.

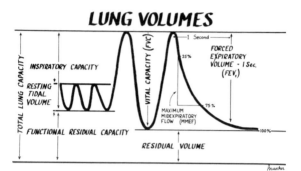

FIG 23.4.
Lung Volumes

C. Interpretation

	Obstructive (Asthma, Cystic Fibrosis§)	Restrictive (Interstitial Disease, Scoliosis)
Spirometry		
Forced vital capicity (FVC)*	Normal or reduced	Reduced
Forced expiratory volume in 1 sec (FEV₁)*	Reduced	Reduced
FEV₁/FVC(%)†	Reduced	Normal
Forced expiratory flow (FEF ₂₅₋₇₅)	Reduced	Reduced
Wright peak flow rate (WPFR)	Normal or reduced	Reduced
Lung volumes		
Total lung capacity (TLC)*	Normal or increased	Reduced
Residual volume (RV)*	Increased	Reduced
RV/TLC‡	Increased	Unchanged
Functional residual capacity (FRC)	Increased	Reduced

*Predicted normal range: ±20%.
†Predicted normal range: >85%.
‡Predicted normal range: 20±/−10.
§Cannot diagnose restrictive component by spirometry alone when obstruction is present. In this case, measure lung volumes by other methods (see Section II.B.)

III. PULMONARY GAS EXCHANGE
A. Arterial Blood Gas (ABG)

1. Henderson-Hasselbach Equation:

$$pH = pK + \log ([HCO_3]/a[PaCO_2])$$

where $pK = 6.10$ and $a = 0.0301$

2. Normal ABG Values

	pH	PaCO$_2$	HCO$_3$(mEq/L)	CO$_2$
Child	7.35–7.45	35–45	24–26	25–28
Term infant				
Birth	7.26–7.29	54.5		
1 hr	7.30	38.8		20.6
3 hr	7.34	38.3		21.9
1–3 days	7.28–7.41	34–35		21.4
Premature				
>1250 g : 1–3 days	7.38–7.39	38–39		
<1250 g : 1–3 days	7.35–7.36	37–44		

3. Abnormal ABG analysis
   a. Quick reference to pH changes in acid/base distur-
      bances
      1) Pure respiratory acidosis or alkalosis: 10 mm Hg rise
         (fall) in PaCO$_2$ accompanies a 0.08 fall (rise) in pH.
      2) Pure metabolic acidosis or alkalosis: 0.15 fall (rise)
         in pH accompanies a 10mEq/L fall (rise) in HCO$_3$.
   b. Abnormal ABG values: detailed analysis

Metabolic acidosis	PaCO$_2$ falls by 1–1.5 × fall in HCO$_3$
Metabolic alkalosis	PaCO$_2$ rises by 0.25–1 × rise in HCO$_3$
Acute respiratory acidosis	HCO$_3$ rises 1 mEq/L for each 10 mm Hg rise in pCO$_2$
Chronic respiratory acidosis	HCO$_3$ rises 4 mEq/L for each 10 mm Hg rise in PaCO$_2$
Acute respiratory alkalosis	HCO$_3$ falls 1–3 mEq/L for each 10 mm Hg fall in PaCO$_2$
Chronic respiratory alkalosis	HCO$_3$ falls 2–5 mEq/L for each 10 mm Hg fall in PaCO$_2$ (usually not < 14 mEq/L)

Ref: Adapted from Schrier RW, Renal and Electrolyte Disorders, 3rd Edition. Boston:
Little Brown,1986:146.

B. **Capillary Blood Gas (CBG)**
   1. Can be obtained from pre-warmed heel or finger sites.
   2. Correlation with arterial sampling is generally better for pH and $PaCO_2$ than for PaO_2 values.
      Ref: Sherry E. AJDC 1990; 144:168–172.

C. **Venous Blood Gas (VBG)**
   1. Requires sampling from centrally placed venous catheters. Peripheral venous samples are strongly affected by the local circulatory or metabolic environment and have limited usefulness.
   2. Although there can be a significant discrepancy between arterial and venous values, the correlation is generally best when the venous measurements are found to be within the normal physiologic range. Basing management decisions on abnormal venous measurements is not advised.
      Ref: Phillips B. Ann Intern Med 1969; 70:745–749.

D. **Pulse Oximetry**
   1. Non-invasive method of measuring beat-to-beat arterial oxygen saturation in the tissue. Related to PaO_2 through the oxyhemoglobin dissociation curve (see Figure 23.5).
   2. Technique limitations
      a. Measures **saturation** (SaO_2) and **not O_2 delivery** to tissues. A marginal saturation may be clinically significant in an anemic patient.
      b. Unreliable if not sensing peripheral pulses adequately, either due to physiologic conditions (hypothermia, hypovolemia, shock) or movement artifact.
      c. Unable to measure instantaneous changes in SaO_2.
      d. Not sensitive to hyperoxia (PaO_2 >100 mm Hg) because of the sigmoid shape of the oxyhemoglobin curve, or to extreme hypoxia (PaO_2 <70 mm Hg) as equipment has not been well validated in this range.
      e. SaO_2 **increased** by carboxyhemoglobin levels >1–2% (chronic smokers, smoke inhalation).
      f. SaO_2 **artificially decreased** by intravenous dyes, like methylene blue or indocyanine green, and opaque nail polish.
      g. SaO_2 **artificially increased or decreased** by methemoglobin levels >1–2% (nitroglycerin ingestion), patient

motion, electrosurgical interference, or xenon arc surgical lamps.

Ref: Fanconi S, et al. J Pediatr 1985; 107:362–66. Alexander CM, et al. Anesth Analg 1989: 68:368–76.

E. Transcutaneous CO_2 Monitoring (tcPCO_2)

1. Best results obtained when surface skin is vasodilated by heating probe to 42–44° C.
2. Especially useful when more invasive sampling techniques would bias results (serial samplings during a sleep study).
3. Equilibration with arterial values may be significantly slower with tcPCO_2 measurements (up to 2 minutes), than with pulse oximetry (8–10 seconds).

Ref: Herrell, N et al. J Pediatr 1980; 97:114–117. Hansen,T et al. Pediatrics 1979;64:942–945.

IV. OXYGEN DELIVERY SYSTEMS

A. Low Flow Oxygen Systems

1. Oxygen is mixed with ambient air during inspiration.
2. As tidal volume increases for a given O_2 flow rate, more air will be entrained, decreasing the net FIO_2 delivery.

Mode	O_2 Flow Supplied (LPM)	% FIO_2 Delivered
Nasal cannula	1/8–2 (infants) 1–6 (children)	24–44
Vented O_2 mask	5–8*	24–44
Mask with reservoir	6–10*	60–99

*Air flows >5LPM required to wash out expired air from mask space.

B. High Flow Oxygen Systems

1. Provide sufficient gas flow rate and reservoir capacity to supply the entire inspired atmosphere to the patient.
2. Gas temperature and humidity can be controlled.

Mode	O_2 Flow Supplied (LPM)	% FIO_2 Delivered
Venturi mask	As per flow valve	24–50
Nebulizer	8–10 L	30–100
Oxygen tent	15 L	24–100*
Oxygen hood	10–14 L	24–40

*O_2 concentration may vary by as much as 20% from the top to the bottom of the hood.

Ref: Rogers, M. Textbook of Pediatric Intensive Care, 2nd Edition. Baltimore: Williams and Wilkins, 1992:150–153.

V. MECHANICAL VENTILATION

A. Indications

1. Secure airway against possible obstruction (croup, epiglottitis) or if safety in question (altered mental status).
2. Poor oxygenation cyanosis or a measured PaO_2 <70 on FIO_2 of 60% or greater.
3. Poor ventilation manifested by a $PaCO_2$ >50–55 or rising (in the absence of chronic CO_2 retention).
4. Managed ventilation (increased intracranial pressure).
5. Decreasing metabolic cost of breathing in circumstances of shock or chronic respiratory failure.

B. Modes of Ventilatory Support

1. **Volume limited**
   a. Delivers a pre-set volume (tidal volume usually = 10–20cc/kg) of gas flow to a patient regardless of the pressure required.
   b. Risk of barotrauma reduced by pressure sensor alarms and pressure pop-off valves that limit peak pressure delivery.
   c. Changes in ventilator pressures may indicate changes in pulmonary compliance.
2. **Pressure limited**
   a. Gas flow is delivered to the patient until a pre-set pressure is administered.
   b. Useful in neonatal and infant ventilatory support (<10–15 kg) where the volume of gas being delivered to relatively small, noncompliant lungs is so small in relation to the volume of compressible air in the ventilator circuit, that reliable estimation of actual volume delivered is impossible.
   c. Reduces the risk of barotrauma to developing pulmonary parenchyma.
   d. Volume delivery may vary with changes in lung compliance.
   e. No way to assess changes in lung compliance.

C. Ventilatory Parameters

1. Peak inspiratory pressure **(PIP):** Maximum inspiratory pressure attained during the respiratory cycle.
2. Positive end-expiratory pressure **(PEEP):** Airway pressure maintained between inspiratory and expiratory phases.

Maintains open alveolar spaces, permitting continued gas exchange and decreased work of re-inflation.
3. Rate **(IMV):** The number of respiratory cycles per minute.
4. Inspired oxygen concentration (FIO_2): The percentage of FIO_2 present in inspired gas.
5. Inspiratory time **(Ti):** Length of time spent in the inspiratory phase of the respiratory cycle.
6. Tidal volume **(TV):** Volume of gas delivered by the ventilator during the inspiratory phase.

D. Initiating Ventilatory Support
1. **Volume limited**
   a. Rate: Use normal range for age.
   b. Tidal volume: Approximately 10–15 cc/kg.
   c. Inspiratory time: Generally use I:E ratio of 1:2. More prolonged expiratory times for obstructive diseases to avoid air trapping.
   d. FIO_2: Selected to maintain targeted saturations and PaO_2.
2. **Pressure limited**
   a. Rate: Use normal range for age.
   b. PEEP: Start with 3 cm H_2O and increase as clinically indicated. (Monitor for decreases in cardiac output with increasing PEEP).
   c. PIP: Ventilate patient by hand with manometer to assess necessary pressures required to inflate chest.
   d. FIO_2: Selected to maintain targeted saturations and PaO_2.
3. Blood gas measurements should be obtained immediately after initiating mechanical ventilation and periodically thereafter to assess the need for ventilator adjustments (see table below).

Ventilator Setting Changes	Effects on Blood Gases	
	$PaCO_2$	PaO_2
↑ PIP	↓	↑
↑ PEEP	↑	↑
↑ Frequency	↓	Min ↑
↑ I:E ratio	No change	↑
↑ FIO_2	No change	↑
↑ Flow	Min ↓	Min ↑

Ref: Carlo WA, Chatburn RL: Neonatal Respiratory Care, 2nd Edition. Chicago: Mosby-Year Book, 1988:331.

E. Weaning Ventilatory Support
1. Decrease ventilatory support as indicated by serial blood gas measurements.
2. Parameters predictive of successful extubation:
   a. PIP generally $<14-16$ cm H_2O.
   b. PEEP $<2-3$ cm H_2O (infants) or <5 cm H_2O (children)
   c. IMV $<2-4$ (infants); children may wean to CPAP.
   d. FIO_2 $<40\%$ (maintaining $PaO_2 > 70$).
   e. Maximum negative inspiratory pressure >45 cm H_2O (infants) or $>20-30$ cm H_2O (children).

VI. REFERENCE DATA
A. Minute Ventilation (VE)
VE = respiratory rate × tidal volume (TV)
VE × $PaCO_2$ = constant; TV = $10-15$ml/kg
B. Alveolar Gas Equation:

$$PAO_2 = PIO_2 - (PACO_2/R); PIO_2 = FIO_2 \times (PB - 47 \text{ mm Hg})$$

1. PIO_2 = partial pressure of inspired O_2: 150 mm Hg at sea level in room air.
2. R = respiratory exchange quotient (CO_2 produced/O_2 consumed) = 0.8.
3. PB = 760 mm Hg.
4. PAO_2 and $PACO_2$ are partial pressures of these gases in the alveoli.

Ref: Kendig EL, Chernick V. Disorders of the Respiratory Tract in Children. Philadelphia: WB Saunders, 1983:27.

C. Oxygen Content:

O_2 content (g/cc) = O_2 capacity × O_2 saturation + dissolved O_2

1. O_2 capacity = hemoglobin × 1.36.
2. Dissolved O_2 = PaO_2 × 0.003
D. O_2 Extraction:

O_2 extraction = (AV DO_2/CaO_2) × 100 (normal range = $28-33\%$)

1. AV DO$_2$ = CaO$_2$ − CmvO$_2$).
2. CaO$_2$ = arterial oxygen content.
3. CmvO$_2$ = mixed venous O$_2$ content (best measured from the pulmonary artery).
4. Extraction ratios are indicative of the adequacy of O$_2$ delivery to tissues, with increasing extraction ratios suggesting that metabolic needs may be outpacing the oxygen content being delivered.

Ref: Rogers M., Textbook of Pediatric Intensive Care, 2nd ed. Baltimore, Williams & Wilkins, 1992:412.

E. Oxyhemoglobin Dissociation Curve

1. Increased hemoglobin affinity for oxygen **(shift to the left)** occurs with alkalemia, hypothermia, hypocarbia, decreased 2,3-diphosphoglycerate, increased fetal hemoglobin, and anemia.
2. Decreased hemoglobin affinity for oxygen **(shift to the right)** occurs with acidemia, hyperthermia, hypercarbia, and increased 2,3-diphosphoglycerate.

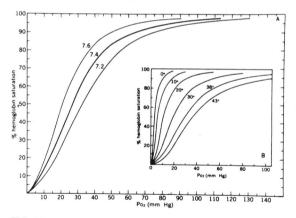

FIG 23.5.

Oxyhemoglobin Dissociation Curve

Ref: from Lanbertsten CJ. Transport of Oxygen, CO$_2$, and Inert Gases by the Blood. in Mountcastle VB (ed). Medical Physiology, 14th ed. St. Louis: Mosby-Year Book, 1980:1725.

RADIOLOGY   24

To avoid inadvertent irradiation of a fetus or embryo, elective
diagnostic radiographs of the abdomen, pelvis, hips, and upper thighs of postmenarchal women should only be performed
in the first 10 days of the menstrual cycle. If dates of menses
cannot be established, a rapid sensitive urine pregnancy test
should be performed. Gonadal shields should be used in all instances unless attempting to visualize the bony pelvis.

I. **IMAGING MODALITIES**
A. **Plain Films:** X-rays are produced when high-speed electrons
    decelerate rapidly. Structures which absorb the x-rays, such
    as bone, appear white on plain films. X-rays magnify the im-
    aged object to some extent, because of beam divergence and
    the distance between the object and the film. As this distance
    increases, so does the degree of magnification. Anterior-
    posterior (AP) films of the chest, for example, magnify ante-
    rior structures such as the heart more than posterior-anterior
    (PA) films.
    1. **Chest:** Chest films are usually obtained to look for evi-
        dence of intrathoracic pathology of pulmonary, cardiac, or
        mediastinal origin. Also commonly obtained to check
        placement of endotracheal tubes and central venous cath-
        eters.
        a. **Interlobar fissures:** Visible only when tangential to the
            x-ray beam. Minor fissure is normally located at the
            level of the 6th rib at the right lateral chest wall. The
            major fissure is usually not visible on frontal views, but
            runs at a 45° angle down from T_4-T_5 on lateral view.
        b. **Silhouette sign:** A term used to describe the blurring
            of the normally sharp borders between air-containing
            lung and other intrathoracic structures. Upper, lingu-
            lar, and middle lobe processes silhouette anterior struc-
            tures, particularly the heart border. Lower lobe pro-
            cesses silhouette posterior structures, such as the dia-
            phragm and descending aorta.

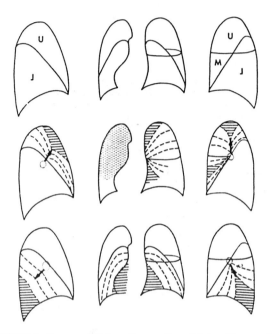

FIG 24.1. Patterns of Volume Loss or Consolidation. **Top panel:** Diagrammatic depiction of the three lobes of the right lung and the two lobes of the left lung. The lateral perspectives are shown for each lung from the side: right lung (left side), left lung (right side). **Middle panel:** Diagrammatic representation of typical patterns of atelectasis of the five major lobes. The upper and middle lobe patterns of atelectasis are shown separately from the lower lobes (bottom panel). The patterns of atelectasis reflect the manner in which the remaining aerated lung can hyperexpand to fill the space left by the atelectatic lung. The hilar structures shift accordingly. Ref: Reginald E, Greene RE. Anatomical and Functional Basis of Imaging the Respiratory System, in Radiology: Diagnosis—Imaging—Intervention. Tavaras JM and Ferrucci JT, (eds); Philadelphia, J.B. Lippincott Co, 1990.

ple epiphyseal and metaphyseal injuries of various ages. In addition, suspicions should be raised by fracture at unusual sites, or solitary spiral and transverse fractures of the long bones with a history of inadequate trauma.

B. Conventional Gray Scale Ultrasound: Images are created by echos returned from structures in the body. Measurements are based on the rate of sound wave travel and the interval between transmitted and returned signal.

1. **Applications:**
   a. Pyloric stenosis
   b. Abdominal masses in young children
   c. Acute intracranial hemorrhage in newborns
   d. Definition of renal anatomy
   e. Congenital hip dislocation
   f. Hip effusions
   g. UTI in children without reflux

2. **Advantages:** No radiation exposure, painless, no sedation required, portable.

3. **Disadvantages:** Ca^{++}, gas and fat may degrade image, operator-dependent.

C. Color Doppler Flow Imaging: Ultrasound frequency shifts caused by moving red blood cells are assigned color; usually, red is used for flow toward the transducer and blue is used for flow away from it. This modality (in conjunction with duplex Doppler) is used to evaluate deep vein thrombosis, vascular patency, intracranial blood flow, cardiac shunt flow, transplant vascularity, and scrotal perfusion.

D. CT Scan

1. **Applications**
   a. Modality of choice for evaluation of acute intracranial trauma, hydrocephalus, pulmonary parenchymal disease, calcifying processes, abdominal and chest trauma, and complicated inflammatory bowel disease. In children with blunt abdominal trauma, a CT of the abdomen, including the lower portion of the chest, should be done. In a recent study, 12% of cases with blunt abdominal trauma had thoracic injuries, 38% of which were missed or underestimated on plain films.

Ref: Sivit, CS, et al. Radiology 1989; 171:815–818.

b. Three-dimensional CT reconstruction is useful for evaluating complex craniofacial anomalies and injuries and other complex skeletal deformities.

2. **Advantages:** Cheaper than MRI, sensitive to Ca^{++}, standardized interpretation, wide field of view.

3. **Disadvantages:** Ionizing radiation exposure, not sensitive to diffuse white matter or cutaneous abnormalities, limited scanning planes.

E. **Ultrafast CT:** This technique permits cine imaging, reduced radiation dosing, and CT scanning without sedation. Each scan takes only 50–100 milliseconds. Disadvantages include high cost and somewhat decreased image quality compared to conventional CT.

F. **MRI:** MRI does not use ionizing radiation. Images are created by re-emission of absorbed energy in the form of radio signals by atomic nuclei stimulated by radio waves in a magnetic field. Four parameters (proton density within a tissue, T_1 relaxation, T_2 relaxation, chemical shift) can be weighted to best evaluate dynamic physiology and tissue composition.

1. **Applications**

   a. CNS: Better than CT for evaluating posterior fossa, brain stem, and spinal cord including defects such as meningomyelocele. Excellent for evaluating demyelinating disorders because it differentiates between areas of normal and abnormal myelin content. Useful in the workup of focal seizures, where a structural lesion may be involved. However, MRI may not reveal calcifications that characterize some neoplastic lesions.

   b. Mediastinal lymphadenopathy.

   c. Cardiac: MRI provides excellent contrast between flowing blood and myocardium, without the use of IV contrast agents.

   d. Abdomen: More sensitive than CT for evaluating extent of hepatic tumors prior to surgical resection.

   e. Skeletal: Useful in detecting early signs of osteomyelitis and avascular necrosis of the femoral head. Can detect extension of bone tumors and marrow replacement by leukemic infiltrates.

2. **Advantages:** No ionizing radiation, multiple imaging planes, sensitive to the presence of abnormal tissues.

3. **Disadvantages:** Difficult to accommodate critical care equipment, patients with implanted ferromagnetic devices cannot be scanned, sensitive to motion degradation; frequently requires sedation, poor signal from Ca^{++} and gas.

G. **Radionuclide Imaging:** Allows observation of dynamic function with a fixed amount of radiation.

1. **Bone scan:** Useful in evaluating unexplained skeletal pain. Generally positive long before plain films for both benign conditions and malignancies such as metastatic neuroblastoma and leukemia. A flow study should be ordered if infection is suspected. Bone scanning is most commonly performed with technetium (^{99m}Tc) methylene diphosphonate (MDP).

2. **Gallium-67 imaging:** Gallium-67 binds to transferrin, lactoferrin, and intracellular lysosomes, and is useful in detecting occult abscesses and some types of tumors. Because gallium-67 is partially excreted by the colon, a standard barium enema prep (See Section V.B.) with a tapwater enema should be given just prior to sending the patient to nuclear medicine. It is not necessary to keep children NPO. Images are typically obtained at 24, 48, and 72 or 96 hours after gallium-67 injection.

   Note: Gallium interferes with the detection of technetium for up to 2 weeks. Thus, when both technetium and gallium scans are indicated, the technetium scan should be done first. Injections for both scans can be made on the same day.

3. **Radionuclide cystography:** Useful in the workup of urinary tract infections in children. Allows quantitative measurements and sensitive detection of vesicoureteral reflux, with approximately 1/100th the gonadal radiation dose of VCUG. The urethra is not evaluated by this technique, so it should not be used as the initial study in males who may have obstructions such as posterior urethral valves. **Tc-DTPA** (^{99m}Tc diethylenetriamine pentaacetic acid) is eliminated by glomerular filtration, and is used for evaluation of renal function, GFR, vesicoureteral reflux, and renovascular hypertension. **Tc-DMSA** (^{99m}Tc dimercaptosuccinic acid), which selectively binds renal tubular cells, is used for evaluating renal structure and relative cortical function. Focal defects occur with pyelonephritis and scarring.

H. Gastrointestinal imaging

1. **Hepatobiliary scan:** Functional evaluation, often useful in distinguishing biliary atresia from neonatal jaundice. Requires 5 days of preparation using phenobarbital (5 mg/kg/day, po) to increase biliary excretion of the ^{99m}Tc-IDA compounds. May be useful in children with sickle cell disease, for identifying biliary causes for abdominal crises.

2. **"Meckel's scan":** ^{99m}Tc-pertechnetate is trapped and secreted in the mucus-producing cells. The scan is therefore useful for detecting ectopic gastric mucosa.

3. **Gastroesophageal reflux studies:** More informative than pH probe, and much less radiation exposure than with UGI. Allows continuous imaging for a prolonged period with visual documentation of reflux frequency and timing, esophageal clearance of refluxed material, gastric emptying, and tracheal aspiration. Esophageal and gastric outlet anatomy is not well evaluated, so patients presenting with vomiting also require a limited UGI.

4. **Cerebral imaging:** Cerebral flow imaging may be helpful in assessing presence or absence of cerebral perfusion when brain death is at issue. Also useful in cases of early encephalitis such as herpes simplex.

5. **Nuclear cardiology:** Gated blood pool (MUGA) scanning is used to evaluate ventricular function in patients with congenital or acquired heart disease, and oncology patients receiving cardiotoxic chemotherapeutic agents. Lung scanning can be used to evaluate pulmonary perfusion, and patency of surgically created systemic-to-pulmonary shunts.

   Ref: Kirchner PT (ed.). In Nuclear Medicine in Review Syllabus. Society of Nuclear Medicine, New York, 1980. Majd, Massoud. Radionuclide Imaging in Pediatrics, in *Pediatr Clin North Am* 1985;32(6):1559.

III. SEDATION: Patient motion commonly degrades the quality of pediatric imaging examinations. Gentle handling and occasional physical restraints are often all that are needed for successful studies. However, sedation is often required, particularly for children under 4 years of age undergoing CT or MRI examination. Several drug combinations for pediatric sedation appear in Pain and Sedation, Section IV. Infants should be kept NPO for 3–4 hours, if possible. The meal before the examination should be withheld for all children.

IV. **CONTRAST:** Plain film contrast agents are based on solutions with components of high atomic number which absorb x-rays well. Oral contrast agents and gadolinium (an MRI contrast agent) do not require consent for administration. IV contrast agents can rarely cause adverse reactions, including anaphylaxis, upon administration. Examinations usually will not be done if there is a previous history of allergy to iodine or severe reaction to a contrast agent. Most hospitals require that a parent or legal guardian read and sign a special consent form for administration of IV contrast agents.

V. **PREPARATORY PROCEDURES**
A. **Bisacodyl (Dulcolax)**
   1. **Contraindications:** Acute surgical abdomen, acute ulcerative colitis.
   2. **Tablets:** Bisacodyl acts directly on the colonic mucosa to produce peristalsis in the colon. Enteric-coated tablets must be swallowed whole; they must not be chewed or crushed. Use suppositories unless assured that child can swallow tablets whole. They should not be taken within 1 hour of antacids or milk. Dose: <40 kg: 1 tablet at bedtime; >40 kg: 2 tablets at bedtime:
   3. **Suppositories:** May be used at any age; for infants and children under 10 kg use a half suppository. If first suppository does not produce a good bowel movement within 45 minutes, administer a second suppository.
B. **Specific Examination Requirements**
   1. **Upper Gastrointestinal Series**
      a. Patient <18 mo: NPO for 3 hr before the study.
      b. Patient >18 mo: Clear liquids after supper. No carbonated beverages on day of study. Bisacodyl pills or suppositories (see Section V.A. above) the evening before the examination, NPO for 4 hr before procedure.
   2. **Contrast Enema**
      a. Infants <18 mo: Liquid diet starting evening before study. No carbonated beverages.
      b. Patients >18 mo: Liquid diet for 24 hr before study. No carbonated beverages. Bisacodyl pills or suppositories evening before. Bisacodyl suppository the morning of the study. If >10 years, give lukewarm tapwa-

ter enemas until clear the morning of study. Omit bisacodyl and enema when evaluation is for active colitis, acute surgical abdomen, or possible Hirschsprung disease.

   c. Air contrast barium enema (≥ 18 mo): Clear liquid diet 24 hr before study. No carbonated beverages. Bisacodyl pills or suppositories the evening before. Lukewarm tapwater enemas until clear; i.e., no stool in the water. This usually takes 2 enemas. Bisacodyl enema (Fleet Bisacodyl Prep) will be given in radiology 1 hr before the examination.

3. **Intravenous Pyelogram (IVP):** (An ultrasound exam of the kidneys frequently can substitute for an IVP.) All patients should be normally hydrated but have an empty stomach. Notation must be made on requisition of previous drug reactions and allergies.

   a. Infants <18 mo: NPO before examination for same length of time as the usual interval between feedings.

   b. Patients >18 mo: Bisacodyl pills or suppositories the night before the examination. NPO 4 hr before examination.

4. **Voiding Cystourethrogram (VCUG):** No preparation is required.

5. **Head and Body Computed Tomography (CT):** Oral and/or intravenous contrast agents may be necessary, depending upon the specific examination and the information required. IV contrast precautions and procedures apply as per Section IV above.

6. **Ultrasound Examinations:** Because sound waves do not penetrate bone, gas, or barium, sonograms should be obtained prior to barium contrast studies.

   a. Pelvic and lower abdomen: Patients should be well hydrated with oral or IV fluids and if possible, should not void for 1–3 hr before the examination. A bladder catheter may be necessary to fill the bladder.

   b. Liver, gallbladder, and biliary tree

      1) Infants: NPO 3–4 hr before examination, if possible.

      2) Children: NPO 6–12 hr before examination.

7. **Nuclear Medicine Examinations:** The general rules regarding protection from radiation as previously outlined apply for all nuclear studies. Most procedures do not require special patient preparation. Consultation with the nuclear medicine physician is encouraged before a study is performed.

PART III

Formulary

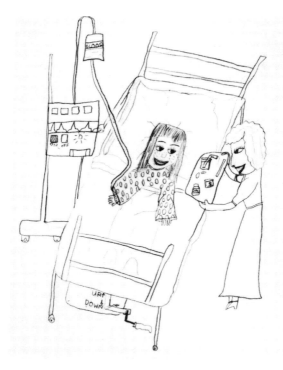

DRUG DOSES   **25**

I.   DRUG INDEX

Trade Name	Generic Name
25-Dihydroxy-cholecalciferol	Calcitriol
5-Fluorocytosine	Flucytosine
5-FU	Fluorouracil
8-Lysine Vasopressin Diapid	Lypressin
A-200 Pyrinate	Pyrethrins
A-Cillin	Amoxicillin
Abbokinase Open Cath	Urokinase
Accutane	Isotretinoin
Achromycin	Tetracycline HCl
Aclovate	Aclomethasone dipropionate
Acthar	ACTH
Actinomycin D	Dactinomycin
Adalat	Nifedipine
Adenine Arabinoside	Vidarabine
Adenocard	Adenosine
Adrenalin	Epinephrine HCl
Adriamycin	Doxorubicin
Advil	Ibuprofen
Aerobid	Flunisolide
Aftate	Tolnaftate
Akarpine	Pilocarpine HCl
Albuminar	Human albumin
Albutein	Human albumin
Aldactone	Spironolactone
Aldomet	Methyldopa
Alkeran	Melphalan
Alu-Tab	Aluminum hydroxide
Alupent	Metaproterenol
Amicar and others	Aminocaproic acid
Amikin	Amikacin sulfate
Amoxil	Amoxicillin
Amphojel	Aluminum hydroxide
Amplin	Ampicillin
Anacin	Aspirin

(Continued.)

Trade Name	Generic Name
Anacin-3	Acetaminophen
Anaprox	Naproxen
Ancef	Cefazolin
Ancill	Ampicillin
Ancobon	Flucytosine
Anectine	Succinylcholine
Aneurine HCl	Thiamine
Anspor	Cephradine
Antepar	Piperazine
Antilirium	Physostigmine salicylate
Antiminth	Pyrantel Pamoate
Apresoline	Hydralazine
Aqua-Mephyton	Vitamin K_1
Aquachloral	Chloral hydrate
Ara-A	Vidarabine
Ara-C	Cytarabine HCl
Aristocort	Triamcinolone
ASA	Aspirin
Asthmanefrin	Epinephrine HCl
Atabrine	Quinacrine
Atarax	Hydroxyzine
Ativan	Lorazepam
Atrovent	Ipratropium bromide
Augmentin	Amoxicillin—Clavulanic Acid
Auralgan	Antipyrine and benzocaine
Azactam	Aztreonam
Azidothymidine	Zidovudine
Azmacort	Triamcinolone
AZT	Zidovudine
Azulfidine	Sulfasalazine
B.A.L.	Dimercaprol
Bactocil	Oxacillin
Bactrim	Cotrimoxazole
Bactroban	Mupirocin
BCNU	Carmustine
Beclovent	Beclomethasone
Beconase	Beclomethasone
Benadryl	Diphenhydramine
Benemid	Probenecid
Beractant	Surfactant, pulmonary
Betalin S	Thiamine
Biamine	Thiamine
Biaxin FilmTabs	Clarithromycin

(Continued.)

Trade Name	Generic Name
Bicillin C-R	Penicillin G preparations: penicillin G benzathine and penicillin G procaine
Biltricide	Praziquantel
Blenoxane	Bleomycin
Breokinase	Urokinase
Brethine	Terbutaline
Bretylol	Bretylium
Bronkometer	Isoetharine
Bronkosol	Isoetharine
Bryrel	Piperazine citrate
Bufferin	Aspirin
Bumex	Bumetanide
Buminate	Human albumin
C-Lexin	Cephalexin
Cafergot	Ergotamine
Calan	Verapamil
Calciferol	Ergocalciferol
Calcijex	Calcitriol
Camphorated Opium Tincture	Paregoric
Capoten	Captopril
Carafate	Sucralfate
Catapres	Clonidine
Catapres-TTS	Clonidine
CDDP	Cisplatin
Ceclor	Cefaclor
Cefanex	Cephalexin
Cefizox	Ceftizoxime
Cefobid	Cefoperazone
Cefotan	Cefotetan
Ceftin	Cefuroxime axetil
Celontin Kapseals	Methsuximide
Cephulac and others	Lactulose
Ceptaz [arginine	Ceftazidime
Chemet	Streptomycin sulfate
Chlortrimeton and others	Chlorpheniramine maleate
Chloromycetin and others	Chloramphenicol
Choledyl	Oxtriphylline
Cholybar	Cholestyramine
Cibalith-S	Lithium
Cipro	Ciprofloxacin
Claforan	Cefotaxime
Cleocin	Clindamycin
Cleocin-T	Clindamycin

(Continued.)

Trade Name	Generic Name
Clopra	Metoclopramide
Cloxapen	Cloxacillin
Codoxy	Oxycodone and aspirin
Colace	Docusate sodium
Colfosceril palmitate	Surfactant, pulmonary
CoLyte	Polyethylene glycol electrolyte solution
Compazine	Prochlorperazine
Cordarone	Amiodarone HCl
Cordron	Flurandrenolide
Corticotropin	ACTH
Cortisporin	Polymyxin B
Cotazym	Pancreatic enzyme replacement
Coumadin	Warfarin
Creon	Pancreatic enzyme replacement
Cuprimine	Penicillamine
Cyclogyl	Cyclopentolate
Cyclomydril	Cyclopentolate
Cylert	Pemoline
Cysticillin A.S.	Penicillin G preparations: procaine
Cytovene	Ganciclovir
Cytoxan	Cyclophosphamide
Dantrium	Dantrolene
DDAVP	Desmopressin acetate
Decadron	Dexamethasone
Delta-Cortef	Prednisolone
Demerol and others	Meperidine HCl
Depakene	Valproic acid
Depakote	Divalproex sodium
Depo-Medrol	Methylprednisolone
Desferal	Deferoxamine
Dexedrine	Dextroamphetamine
DHT	Dihydrotachysterol USP
DHT Intensol	Dihydrotachysterol USP
Diamox	Acetazolamide
Dideoxyinosine	Didanosine-ddI
Diflucan	Flucanazole
Digibind	Digoxin immune Fab
Dilantin	Phenytoin
Dilautid	Hydromorphone HCl
Dipalmitoyl-phosphatidylcholine	Surfactant, pulmonary
Diprosone	Betamethasone dipropionate
Ditropan	Oxybutynin chloride
Diulo	Metolazone

(Continued.)

Trade Name	Generic Name
Diurigen	Chlorothiazide
Diuril	Chlorothiazide
Dobutrex	Dobutamine
Dolophine	Methadone HCl
Dopastat	Dopamine
DPPC	Surfactant, pulmonary
Dramamine	Dimenhydrinate
Dridase	Oxybutynin chloride
Drisdol	Ergocalciferol
Droncit	Praziquantel
Dulcolax	Bisacodyl
Duracillin A.S.	Penicillin G preparations: procaine
Duragesic	Fentanyl
Duricef	Cefadroxil
Dynapen	Dicloxacillin Sodium
E-Mycin	Erythromycin
Elimite	Permethrin
Elspar	Asparaginase
Entolase	Pancreatic enzyme replacement
Epitrol	Carbamazepine
Epogen	Epoeitin alfa
Epsom salts	Magnesium sulfate
Ery-Ped	Erythromycin
Erythrocin	Erythromycin
Esidrix	Hydrochlorothiazide USP
Eskalith	Lithium
Exosurf	Surfactant, pulmonary
Fansidar	Pyrimethamine with sulfadoxine
Festal II	Pancreatic enzyme replacement
Feverall	Acetaminophen
Flagyl	Metronidazole
Florinef acetate	Fludrocortisone acetate
Fluonide	Fluocinolone acetonide
Fluoritab	Flouride
Folvite	Folic acid
Fortaz	Ceftazidime
Fulvicin	Griseofulvin microcrystaline
Fungizone	Amphotericin B
Furadantin	Nitrofurantoin
Furomide	Furosemide
G-CSF	Filgrastim
Gamastin	Immune globulin

(Continued.)

Trade Name	Generic Name
Gamimune	Immune globulin
Gamma Benzene Hexachloride	Lindane
Gammagard	Immune globulin
Gantrisin	Sulfisoxazole
Garamycin and others	Gentamicin
Gastrocrom	Cromolyn
Geocillin	Carbenicillin
Geopn	Carbenicillin
Glucagon	Glucagon HCl
GoLYTELY	Polyethylene glycolelectrolyte solution
Grifulvin V	Griseofulvin microcrystalline
Grisactin	Griseofulvin microcrystalline
Haldol and others	Haloperidol
Halog	Halcinomide
Hexadrol	Dexamethasone
Hismanal	Astemizole
Hydro-T	Hydrochlorothiazide USP
Hydrodiuril and others	Hydrochlorothiazide USP
Hyoscine	Scopolamine hydrobromide
Hyperstat	Diazoxide
Hytakerol	Dihydrotachysterol USP
Ifex	Ifosfamide
Ilozyme	Pancreatic enzyme replacement
Imodium	Loperamide
Imodium AD	Loperamide
Imuran	Azathioprine
Inderal	Propranolol
Indocin	Indomethacin
InFeD	Iron dextran
INH	Isoniazid
Intal	Cromolyn
Intropin	Dopamine
Iosat	Potassium iodide
Isoptin	Verapamil
Isopto	Scopolamine hydrobromide
Isopto Carpine	Pilocarpine HCl
Isuprel	Isoproterenol
Janimine	Imipramine
Kabikinase	Streptokinase
Kantrex	Kanamycin
Kayexalate	Sodium polystyrene sulfonate
Keflex	Cephalexin
Keflin	Cephalothin

(Continued.)

Trade Name	Generic Name
Kefurox	Cefuroxime
Kefzol	Cefazolin
Kenacort	Triamcinolone
Kenalog	Triamcinolone
Kenalog	Triamcinolone acetonide
Ketalar	Ketamine
Klonopin	Clonazepam
Konakion	Vitamin K_1
Ku-Zyme	Pancreatic enzyme replacement
Kwell	Lindane
L-carnitine	Levocarnitine
Laniazid	Isoniazid
Larotid	Amoxicillin
Lasix	Furosemide
Levothroid	Levothyroxine
Lidex	Fluocinonide
Lioresal	Baclofen
Lithane	Lithium
Lithobid	Lithium
Lithonate	Lithium
Lithotabs	Lithium
Lopurin	Allopurinol
Lotrimin	Clotrimazole
Luminal	Phenobarbital
Luride	Flouride
Maalox	Aluminum hydroxide/magnesium hydroxide
Macrodantin	Nitrofurantoin
Magonate	Magnesium sulfate
Maloxon	Metoclopramide
Mandol	Cefamandole
Many brand names	Prednisone
Mazicon	Flumazenil
Medipren	Ibuprofen
Medrol	Methylprednisolone
Mefoxin	Cefoxitin
Mellaril	Thioridazine
Mephyton	Vitamin K_1
Mestinon	Pyridostigmine bromide
Mesylate	Deferoxamine
Metamucil	Psyllium
Metaprel	Metaproterenol

(Continued.)

Trade Name	Generic Name
Metric	Metronidazole
Mezlin	Mezlocillin
Micronefrin	Epinephrine HCl
Microsulfon	Sulfadiazine
Milk of Magnesia	Magnesium hydroxide
Minipress	Prazosin HCl
Minocin and others	Minocycline
Mithracin	Mithramycin
Monistat	Miconazole
Motrin	Ibuprofen
Mucomyst	Acetylcysteine
Myambutol	Ethambutol HCl
Mycelex	Clotrimazole
Mycifradin	Neomycin sulfate
Mycostatin	Nystatin
Mykrox	Metolazone
Mylanta	Aluminum hydroxide/magnesium hydroxide
Myleran	Busulfan
Mysoline	Primidone
Nafcil	Nafcillin
Nallpen	Nafcillin
Naprosyn	Naproxen
Narcan	Naloxone
Nasalcrom	Cromolyn
Nasalide	Flunisolide
Nebcin	Tobramycin
NebuPent	Pentamidine isethionate
Nembutal	Pentobarbital
Neo-Synephrine and others	Phenylephrine HCl
Neocalglucon	Calcium glubionate
Neomycin Sulfate	Neosporin
Nephrox	Aluminum hydroxide
Neupogen	Filgrastim
Neurosyn	Primidone
NeutraPhos	Phosphorus supplements
Nipride and others	Nitroprusside
Nitro-Bid	Nitroglycerin
Nitrostat	Nitroglycerin
Nix	Permethrin
Nizoral	Ketoconazole
Noctec	Chloral hydrate

(Continued.)

Trade Name	Generic Name
Norcuron	Vecuronium bromide
Noroxin	Norfloxacin
Norpace	Disopyramide phosphate
Nuprin	Ibuprofen
Nydrazid	Isoniazid
Ocumycin	Gentamicin sulfate
Omnipen	Ampicillin
Oncovin	Vincristine
Os-Cal	Calcium carbonate
Osmitrol	Mannitol
Oticort	Polymyxin B
Panadol	Acetaminophen
Pancrease	Pancreatic enzyme replacement
Pancreatin	Pancreatic enzyme replacement
Panmycin	Tetracycline HCL
Panwarfin	Warfarin
Pavulon	Pancuronium bromide
Pediamycin	Erythromycin
Pediapred	Prednisolone
Pediaprofen	Ibuprofen
Pediazole	Erythromycin ethylsuccinate/ sulfisoxazole
Pen Vee K	Penicillin V potassium
Penamp	Ampicillin
Pentam 300	Pentamidine isethionate
Pentothal	Thiopental sodium
Pepcid	Famotidine
Percodan	Oxycodone and aspirin
Periactin	Cyproheptadine
Permapen	Penicillin G preparations: benzathine
Pfizerpen-AS	Penicillin G preparations: procaine
PGE1	Prostaglandin E_1
Phenacetin	Acetophenetidin
Phenergan	Promethazine
Phytonadione	Vitamin K_1
Piligan	Pilocarpine HCl
Pima	Potassium iodide
Pipracil	Piperacillin
Pitressin	Vasopressin
Plasbumin-5	Human albumin
Plicamycin	Mithramycin
Polycillin	Ampicillin

(Continued.)

Trade Name	Generic Name
Polymox	Amoxicillin
Potassium Iodide Enseals	Potassium iodide
Prelone	Prednisolone
Primaxin	Imipenem-cilastatin
Principen	Ampicillin
Priscoline	Tolazoline
Procan SR	Procainamide
Procardia	Nifedipine
Procardia XL	Nifedipine
Procrit	Epoeitin alfa
Proglycem	Diazoxide
Pronestyl	Procainamide
Pronto	Pyrethrins
Prostigmin	Neostigmine
Prostin VR	Prostaglandin E_1
Protilase	Pancreatic enzyme replacement
Protostat	Metronidazole
Proventil	Albuterol
Provigan	Promethazine
Pyopen	Carbenicillin
Pyridium	Phenazopyridine
Questran	Cholestyramine
Reglan	Metoclopramide
Resectisol	Mannitol
Retrovir	Zidovudine
RID	Pyrethrins
Rimactane	Rifampin
Ritalin	Methylphenidate HCl
Ritalin SR	Methylphenidate HCl
Robinul	Glycopyrrolate
Rocaltrol	Calcitriol
Rocephin	Ceftriaxone
Roxicodone	Oxycodone
Roxilox	Oxycodone
Roxiprin	Oxycodone and aspirin
Salicylazosulfapyridine	Sulfasalazine
Sandimmune	Cyclosporine
Sandoglobulin	Immune globulin
Sandostatin	Octreotide acetate
Scabene	Lindane
Seconal	Secobarbital
Seldane	Terfenadine

(Continued.)

Trade Name	Generic Name
Selsun	Selenium sulfide
Senokot	Senna
Septra	Co-trimoxazole
Seruton	Psyllium
Slow-mag	Magnesium sulfate
Sofarin	Warfarin
Solu-cortef	Hydrocortisone
Solu-Medrol	Methylprednisolone
Somnos	Chloral Hydrate
Somophyllin	Aminophylline
Staphcillin	Methicillin
Stimate	Desmopressin acetate
Streptase	Streptokinase
Sublimaze	Fentanyl
Sudafed	Protamine sulfate
Sulamyd	Sulfacetamide sodium
Sulfatrim	Co-trimoxazole
Sumycin	Tetracycline HCl
Suprax	Cefixime
Survanta	Surfactant, pulmonary
Symadine	Amantadine hydrochloride
Symmetrel	Amantadine hydrochloride
Synalar	Fluocinolone acetonide
T$_4$ Synthroid	Levothyroxine
Tagamet	Cimetidine
Tambocor	Flecainide acetate
Tapazole	Methimazole
Tazicef	Ceftazidime
Tazidime	Ceftazidime
Tegopen	Cloxacillin
Tegretol	Carbamazepine
Tempra	Acetaminophen
Tensilon	Edrophonium
Terramycin	Tetracycline HCl
Thiaminium Chloride HCl	Thiamine
Thiuretic	Hydrochlorothiazide USP
Thorazine	Chlorpromazine
Thyro-Block	Potassium Iodide
Ticar	Ticarcillin
Tigan	Trimethobenzamide HCL
Timentin	Ticarcillin/clavulanate
Tinactin	Tolnaftate

(Continued.)

Trade Name	Generic Name
TMP-SMX	Co-trimoxazole
Tobrex	Tobramycin
Tofranil	Imipramine
Tolectin	Tolmetin Sodium
Topicort	Desoximetasone
Toradol	Ketorolac
Totacillin	Ampicillin
Totacillin	Ampicillin
Tridesilon	Desonide
Tridil	Nitroglycerin
Trimethoprim-sulfamethoxazole	Co-trimoxazole
Trimox	Amoxicillin
Trobicin	Spectinomycin
Tums	Calcium carbonate
Tylenol	Acetaminophen
Tylox	Oxycodone
Ultracef	Cefadroxil
Ultrase	Pancreatic enzyme replacement
Unipen	Nafcillin
Urecholine	Bethanechol
Utimox	Amoxicillin
V-Cillin K	Penicillin V potassium
Valisone	Betamethasone valerate
Valium	Diazepam
Vancenase	Beclomethasone
Vanceril	Beclomethasone
Vancocin and others	Vancomycin
Vaponefrin	Epinephrine HCl
Various brand names	Morphine sulfate
Vasotec	Enalapril maleate
Velban	Vinblastine
Velosef	Cephradine
Vermox	Mebendazole
Versed	Midazolam
Vibramycin	Doxycycline
Videx	Didanosine ddl
Viokase	Pancreatic enzyme replacement
Vira-A	Vidarabine
Vistaril	Hydroxyzine
Vitamin D_2	Ergocalciferol
VitaCarn	Levocarnitine
Vitamin B_1	Thiamine

(Continued.)

Trade Name	Generic Name
Vitamin B_6	Pyridoxine
Vitamin C	Ascorbic acid
VM-26	Teniposide
VP-16	Etoposide
VZIG	Varicella-zoster immune globulin
Westcort	Hydrocortisone valerate
Wycillin	Penicillin G preparations: procaine
Wymox	Amoxicillin
Xylocaine	Lidocaine
Zantac	Ranitidine HCl
Zarontin	Ethosuximide
Zaroxolyn	Metolazone
Zinacef	Cefuroxime
Zithromax	Azithromycin
Zofran	Odansetron
Zolicef	Cefazolin
Zovirax	Acyclovir
Zymase	Pancreatic enzyme replacement

II. **DRUG DOSES:** The following formulary contains both generic and trade names, how drugs are supplied, and their usual dose and routes of administration. Brief remarks about the side effects, drug interactions, precautions, and other relevant factors are included. For many generic drugs, we have provided a list of trade names. We have **not** attempted to make this list of trade names exhaustive: please consult a more complete drug information handbook (i.e., the *American Pharmaceutical Association Pediatric Dosage Handbook*) for more detailed information than is provided here.

Note: Please note in the "How Supplied" category: the unit quantity in which a drug is supplied is noted in parentheses following the drug concentration. For example, amoxicillin suspension, 125 mg/5 ml, is available in 80-, 100-, 150-, and 200-ml bottles. Also, suspension formulations marked by an asterisk are not commercially available and need to be extemporaneously compounded by a pharmacist. References for these formulations and for the contents of the Formulary are provided at the end of this chapter.

Drug	How Supplied	Dose and Route	Remarks
Acetaminophen (Tylenol, Tempra, Panadol, Feverall, Anacin-3, and others)	Tabs: 160, 325, 500, 650 mg Chewable tabs: 80 mg Drops: 80 mg/0.8 ml Oral solution: 160 mg/5 ml Elixir: 120, 130, 160, 325 mg/5 ml Caplet: 160, 325, 500 mg Suppositories: 120, 125, 300, 325, 650 mg (Combination product with Codeine, see Codeine)	*Pediatric:* 10–15 mg/kg/dose Q4–6hr; dosing by age: 0–3 mo: 40 mg/dose 4–11 mo: 80 mg/dose 12–24 mo: 120 mg/dose 2–3 yr: 160 mg/dose 4–5 yr: 240 mg/dose 6–8 yr: 320 mg/dose 9–10 yr: 400 mg/dose 11–12 yr: 480 mg/dose *Adult:* 325–650 mg/dose **Max Dose:** 4 g q 24 hr, 5 doses/24 hr	$T_{1/2}$: 1–3 hr; metabolized in the liver; some preparations contain alcohol and/or phenylalanine; see Poisonings chapter for management of overdosage; **contraindicated** in patients with known G6PD deficiency.

Acetazolamide (Diamox)	Tabs: 125, 250 mg Suspension*: 30, 50 mg/ml Capsules (sustained release): 500 mg Injection (sodium): 500 mg/5 ml	*Diuretic (PO, IV):* Child: 5 mg/kg/dose QD-QOD Adult: 250–375 mg/dose QD-QOD *Glaucoma* Child: 20–40 mg/kg/24 hr ÷ Q6 hr IM/IV; 8–30 mg/kg/24 hr ÷ Q6–8 hr PO Adult: 1000 mg/24 hr ÷ Q6 hr PO; for rapid decrease in intraocular pressure, administer 500 mg/dose IV. *Seizures:* 8–30 mg/kg/24 hr ÷ Q6–12 hr PO. **Max dose:** 1 gm/24 hr. *Urine alkalinization:* 5 mg/kg/dose repeated BID-TID *Management of hydrocephalus:* see Neurology, Chapter 21.	$T_{1/2}$: 4–10 hr; possible side effects (more likely with long-term therapy) include GI irritation, paresthesias, sedation, hypokalemia, acidosis, reduced urate secretion, aplastic anemia, polyuria, and development of renal calculi; IM injection may be painful; bicarbonate replacement therapy may be required during long-term use (see Citrate or Sodium Bicarbonate); **contraindicated** in patients with hepatic failure.
Acetylcysteine (Mucomyst)	Solution: 100 mg/ml (10%) or 200 mg/ml (20%) (4, 10, 30 ml)	For Acetaminophen Poisoning, see Chapter 3. *Meconium ileus:* 5–30 ml of 10% solution given 3–6×/24 hr PO or PR; usual dose: 10 ml QID	May induce bronchospasm, stomatitis, drowsiness, rhinorrhea, nausea, vomiting and hemoptysis.

*Indicates suspensions not commercially available; need to be extemporaneously compounded by a pharmacist. See references 6 and 7 for specific formulations.

(Continued.)

Drug	How Supplied	Dose and Route	Remarks
Acetylcysteine *(continued)*.		*Nebulizer:* 3–5 ml of 20% solution (diluted with equal volume of H_2O, or sterile saline to equal 10%), or 6–10 ml of 10% solution; administer TID-QID.	
ACTH (Corticotropin, Acthar)	Aqueous (inj): 25, 40 U/vial Gel: 40.80 U/ml (1.5 ml); 1 unit = 1 mg	*Anti-inflammatory:* Aqueous: 1.6 U/kg/24h IV, IM, or SC ÷ Q6–8 hr Gel: 0.8 U/kg/24 hr ÷ Q12–24 hr IM *Infantile spasms:* many regimens exist. Gel: 20–40 U/24 hr IM QD or 80U IM QOD: taper dose gradually.	**Contraindicated** in acute psychoses, CHF, Cushing's disease, TB, peptic ulcer, ocular herpes, fungal infections, recent surgery, sensitivity to porcine products; IV administration for diagnostic purposes only.
Acyclovir (Zovirax)	Capsules: 200 mg Tabs: 800 mg Suspension: 200 mg/5 ml Ointment: 5% (15 gm) Inj (with sodium): 500 mg/10 ml	*Herpes simplex virus:* Newborn: 30 mg/kg/24 hr ÷ Q8 hr IV Children (<12 yr): 250 mg/m²/dose IV Q8 hr Adults: 5 mg/kg/dose Q8 hr IV *Genital HSV:* 200 mg PO 5x/24 hr. Treat for 7–10 days for first infection, 5 days for recurrences.	Can cause renal impairment; adequate hydration and slow (1 hr) IV administration is essential to prevent crystallization in renal tubules; dose alteration necessary in patients with impaired renal function; has been infrequently associated with headache, vertigo, insomnia,

		encephalopathy, GI tract irritation, rash, urticaria, arthralgia, fever and adverse hematologic effects; PO dosing not well established and is not generally recommended (see Red Book, 1991).
	Chronic prophylaxis of genital HSV: 200 mg PO 2–5×/24 hr, for **max** of 12 mo. *Varicella zoster:* Children < 1yr: 30 mg/kg/24 hr ÷ Q8 hr IV; ≥1yr: 1500 mg/m²/24 hr ÷ Q8 hr IV Adults: 30 mg/kg/24 hr ÷ Q8 hr IV	
Adenosine (Adenocard)	Inj: 3 mg/ml (2 ml)	*Supraventricular tachycardia:* Children: 0.1 mg/kg rapid IV push; may increase dose by 0.05 mg/kg increments every 2 min to max of 0.25 mg/kg (up to 12 mg), or until termination of SVT. **Max dose:** 12 mg	$T_{1/2}$: <10 sec; may precipitate bronchoconstriction. Side effects include facial flushing, headache, shortness of breath, dyspnea, nausea, chest pain, lightheadedness. **Contraindicated** in 2nd and 3rd degree AV block or sick-sinus syndrome unless pacemaker placed.
Albumin, human (Albuminar, Albutein, Buminate, Plasbumin-5, Human Albumin)	Inj: 5% (50 mg/ml); 25% (250 mg/ml); each contains 130–160 mEq Na/L	*Hypoproteinemia:* Children 1 gm/kg/dose IV over 30–120 min. Adult: 25 gm/dose IV over 30–120 min; repeat Q1–2 days PRN	**Contraindicated** in cases of CHF or severe anemia; rapid infusion may cause fluid overload; hypersensitivity reactions may occur; may cause rapid increase in serum

(Continued.)

Drug	How Supplied	Dose and Route	Remarks
Albumin, human *(continued.).*		*Hypovolemia:* Children: 1gm/kg/dose IV rapid infusion. Adult 25 gm/dose IV rapid infusion; may repeat PRN. **Max dose:** 6 gm/kg/24 hr	sodium levels: **caution: 25% concentration contraindicated in preterm infants** due to risk of IVH.
Albuterol (Proventil, Ventolin)	Tabs: 2, 4 mg Sustained release tabs: 4 mg Oral solution: 2 mg/5 ml (473 ml) Aerosol inhaler: 90 μg/dose (200 doses/inhaler) Rotacaps for inhalation: 200 μg/capsule Nebulization solution: 0.5% (5 mg/ml) Prediluted nebulized solution: 2.5 mg in 3 ml NS (0.083%)	*Oral:* Children <6 yr: 0.3 mg/kg/24h PO ÷ Q8 hr; **max dose:** 12 mg/24 hr 6–11 yr: 6 mg/24 hr PO ÷ TID; **max dose:** 24 mg/24 hr ≥12 yr and adults: 2–4 mg/dose PO TID-QID; **max dose:** 32 mg/24 hr *Inhalations:* Aerosol: 1–2 puff (90–180 μg) Q4–6 hr PRN Rotacaps: 200 μg Q4–6 hr *Nebulization:* Neonate/infant: 0.05–0.15 mg/kg/dose Q4–6 hr Children: 1.25–2.5 mg/dose Q4–6 hr Adult 2.5 mg/dose Q6 hr	Possible side effects include tachycardia, palpitations, tremor, insomnia, hyperactivity, nervousness, nausea, and headache. Nebulization may be given more frequently than indicated. **Please verify concentration of solution used for nebulization.** The use of tube spacers may enhance efficacy of administering doses via metered dose inhaler.

Allopurinol (Lopurin, Zyloprim, and others)	Tabs: 100, 300 mg Suspension:* 10, 20 mg/ml	Child: 10 mg/kg/24h PO ÷ TID-QID; **max dose:** 600 mg/24 hr Adult: 200–300 mg PO ÷ BID-TID	Dose must be adjusted in cases of renal insufficiency. Must maintain adequate urine output and alkaline urine. Side effects may include rash, neuritis, hepatotoxicity, GI disturbance, bone marrow suppression, and drowsiness. Must follow liver and renal function during course of therapy.
Aluminum hydroxide (Amphojel, Dialume, Nephrox, Alu-Tab, and others)	Tabs: 300, 600 mg Caps: 475, 500 mg Suspension: 320 mg/5 ml, 600 mg/5ml, 675 mg/5 ml (150, 360 ml); each 15 ml contains <0.3 mEq Na.	*Peptic ulcer:* Child: 5–15 ml PO Q3–6 hr or 1 and 3 hr PC and HS Adult: 15–45 ml PO Q3–6 hr or 1 and 3 hr PC and HS; titrate to maintain gastric pH >5 *Prophylaxis against GI bleeding:* Infant: 2–5 ml PO Q1–2 hr Child: 5–12 ml PO Q1–2 hr Adults: 30–60 ml PO Q1–2 hr *Hyperphosphatemia* 50–150 mg/kg/24hr ÷ Q4– 6hr PO	May cause constipation, decreased bowel motility, and phosphorus depletion. Interferes with the absorption of several orally administered medications, including digoxin, indomethicin, isoniazid, tetracycline, and iron.

*Indicates suspensions not commercially available; need to be extemporaneously compounded by a pharmacist. See references 6 and 7 for specific formulations.

(Continued.)

Drug	How Supplied	Dose and Route	Remarks
Aluminum hydroxide with magnesium hydroxide (Maalox, Mylanta, and others)	Chewable tabs: (Al (OH)₃: Mg (OH)₂) 200 mg: 200 mg (Maalox, Mylanta) Susp: 200 mg: 200mg + Simethicone 20 mg (Mylanta) 225 mg: 200 mg/5 ml (Maalox); many other combinations (contain 0.04–0.1 mEq Na/5 ml)	Same as for aluminum hydroxide preparations.	May have laxative effect. May cause hypokalemia. Use with caution in patients with renal insufficiency, gastric outlet obstruction.
Amantadine hydrochloride (Symadine, Symmetrel, and others)	Capsule:100 mg Syrup: 50 mg/5 ml	Influenza A prophylaxis/ treatment: 1–9 yr: 4.4–8.8 mg/kg/24 hr PO ÷ QD-BID: **max dose:** 150 mg/24 hr >9 yr: 200 mg/24 hr ÷ QD-BID *Prophylaxis:* Single exposure: at least 10 days Repeated/uncontrolled exposure: up to 90 days. Use with influenza A vaccine when possible.	Dose must be adjusted in patients with renal insufficiency. May cause dizziness, anxiety, depression, mental status change, rash (livedo reticularis), nausea, orthostatic hypotension, edema, CHF and urinary retention. Use with **caution** in patients with liver disease, seizures, renal disease, and in those receiving CNS stimulants.

		Symptomatic treatment: Continue for 24–48 hr after disappearance of symptoms.
Amikacin sulfate (Amikin)	Injection: 50, 250 mg/ml	**Neonates:** 7.5 mg/kg/dose IV/IM Dosing Interval Postnatal Age Gestational Age / <7 days / ≥7 days <28 wk / Q24 hr / Q18 hr 28–34 wk / Q18 hr / Q12 hr >34 wk / Q12 hr / Q8 hr *Children and Adults:* 15–22.5 mg/kg/24hr ÷ Q8–12 hr IV/IM; **max dose:** 1.5 gm/24 hr	Must monitor levels. T$_{1/2}$: 2–3 hr. Dose must be adjusted in patients with renal insufficiency. May cause ototoxicity, nephrotoxicity, neuromuscular blockade, bone marrow suppression, eosinophilia, headache, and tremor. Possible synergistic ototoxic effect when used with furosemide or other diuretics. **Therapeutic levels:** peak, 20–30 mg/L: trough, 5–10 mg/L. *Infusion Rate:* Infant: 1–2 hr Children and adults: 30–60 min.
Aminocaproic acid (Amicar and others)	Tabs: 500 mg Syrup: 250 mg/ml (480 ml) Injection: 250 mg/ml	*Children:* Loading dose: 100–200 mg/kg IV, PO	Hypercoagulation may be produced when given in conjunction with oral

(Continued.)

Drug	How Supplied	Dose and Route	Remarks
Aminocaproic acid (*continued.*).		Maintenance: 100 mg/kg/dose Q4–6 hr **Max dose:** 30 gm/24 hr	contraceptives. May cause nausea, diarrhea, malaise, weakness. **Contraindications:** DIC, hematuria. May cause elevation of serum potassium, especially in patients with renal impairment.
Aminophylline (Somophylin and various other brand names)	Tabs: 100, 200, 500 mg (79% theophylline) Liquid (oral): 105 mg/5 ml (240 ml) (86% theophylline) Inj: 25 mg/ml (79% theophylline) Supp: 250, 500 mg (79% theophylline) Tablet (sustained release): 225, 300 mg (79% theophylline)	*IV loading:* 6 mg/kg IV over 20 min (each 1 mg/kg dose raises the serum theophylline concentration 2 mg/L) *IV maintenance:* Continuous IV drip: Neonates: 0.2 mg/kg/hr 6 wk–6 mo: 0.5mg/kg/hr 6 mo–1 yr: 0.6–0.7 mg/kg/hr 1–9 yr: 1–1.2 mg/kg/hr 9–12 yr and young adult smokers: 0.9 mg/kg/hr Adults, nonsmokers: 0.5 mg/kg/hr The above total daily doses may also be administered IV Q4–6 hr.	Monitoring serum levels is essential especially in infants and young children. Infants and children 1–5 yr may require Q4 hr dosing regimen due to enhanced metabolism. Side effects: restlessness, GI upset, arrhythmias, seizures (may occur in absence of other side effects with toxic levels). **Therapeutic level:** for asthma, 10–20 mg/L; for neonatal apnea, 6–13 mg/L. *Guidelines for obtaining levels:* IV Bolus: 30 min after infusion. IV continuous: 12–14 hr after initiation of infusion.

PO liquid, immediate-release tab:
Peak: 1 hr post dose.
Trough: just before dose.
PO sustained-release:
Peak: 4 hr post dose.
Trough: just before dose.
Ideally, obtain levels after steady state has been achieved.

PO: Infants (see Theophylline)
1–9 yr: 20 mg/kg/24 hr ÷ Q4–6 hr
9–16 yr: 16 mg/kg/24 hr ÷ Q6 hr
Adults: 12 mg/kg/24 hr ÷ Q6 hr
Neonatal apnea:
Loading dose: 5–6 mg/kg IV or PO
Maintenance dose: 1–2 mg/kg/dose Q6–8 hr, IV or PO

Amiodarone HCl (Cordarone)	Tabs: 200 mg	*Children:* <1 yr: 600–800 mg/1.73 m²/24 hr, then reduce to 200–400 mg/1.73 m²/24 hr ≥1 yr: 10–15 mg/kg/24 hr ÷ Q12–24 hr PO × 7–14 days, then reduce to 5 mg/kg/24 hr ÷ Q12 hr if effective. *Adults:* Loading dose: 800–1600 mg QD for 1–3 wk.	Long elimination half-life (40–55 days). Major metabolite is active. Asymptomatic corneal microdeposits. Alters liver enzymes, thyroid function. Pulmonary fibrosis reported in adults. May cause worsening of pre-existing arrhythmias with bradycardia and AV block. May cause anorexia, nausea, vomiting, dizziness, paresthesias, ataxia, and

(Continued.)

Drug	How Supplied	Dose and Route	Remarks
Amiodarone HCl *(continued).*		Maintenance: 600–800 mg QD × 1 mo, then 200–400 mg QD.	tremor. Increases digoxin, dilantin, warfarin, and quinidine levels. Safety and efficacy in children has not been established. **Therapeutic level:** 0.5–2.5 mg/L
Ammonium chloride	Tabs (enteric-coated): 500 mg Injection: 5 mEq/ml (26.75%); 1 mEq = 53 mg.	*Urinary acidification:* Child: 75 mg/kg/24 hr ÷ Q6 hr PO or IV. **Max dose:** 6 gm/24 hr Adult: 1.5 gm/dose IV Q6 hr. **Max dose:** 6 gm/24 hr IV or 8–12 gm/24 hr PO ÷ Q6 hr. Injection: Dilute to concentration not >0.4 mEq/ml. **Infusion not to exceed 50 mg/kg/hr or 1 mEq/kg/hr**	May produce acidosis, hyperammonemia. **Contraindicated** in hepatic or renal insufficiency; **use with caution in infants.** May cause GI irritation. Monitor serum chloride level, acid/base status.

Amoxicillin (Amoxil, Larotid, Trimox, Wymox, Utimox, Polymox, A-Cillin, and others)	Drops: 50 mg/ml (15, 30 ml) Susp: 125, 250 mg/5ml (80, 100, 150, 200 ml) Caps: 250, 500 mg Chewable tabs: 125, 250 mg	*Child:* 20–50 mg/kg/24 hr ÷ Q8 hr PO *Adult:* 250–500 mg/dose Q8 hr PO *Gonorrhea* (acute uncomplicated): >2 yr, ≤45 kg: 50 mg/kg single PO dose with 25 mg/kg probenicid (**max dose:** 1 gm probenicid.) >45 kg: 3 gm as single PO dose with 1 gm probenicid. See Chapter 17, for details. *SBE prophylaxis:* See Chapter 6.	Renal elimination. Serum levels about twice those achieved with equal dose of ampicillin. Less GI effects, but otherwise similar to ampicillin. Side effects: rash and diarrhea.
Amoxicillin-clavulanic acid (Augmentin)	Tabs: 250, 500 mg amoxicillin (both with 125 mg clavulanate) Chewable Tabs: 125, 250 mg Susp: 125 and 250 mg/5 ml (31.25 and 62.5 mg clavulanate) (75, 150 ml)	*Child:* <40 kg: 20–40 mg/kg/24 hr ÷ Q8 hr PO *Adult:* 250–500 mg/dose Q8 hr PO **Max dose:** 2 gm/24 hr	Clavulinic acid extends the activity of amoxicillin to include beta-lactamase producing strains of *H. influenzae, B. catarrhalis,* some *S. aureus.* Incidence of diarrhea is higher than with use of amoxicillin alone.
Amphotericin B (Fungizone)	Inj: 50-mg vials Cream: 3% Lotion: 3%	*Topical:* apply BID-QID *IV* (mix with D5W to concentration 0.1 mg/ml, pH >4.2): Infuse over 4–6 hr.	Fever, chills, nausea, vomiting are common side effects; may premedicate with acetaminophen and

(Continued.)

Drug	How Supplied	Dose and Route	Remarks
Amphotericin B (*continued*.).		*Test dose:* 0.1 mg/kg/dose IV up to max 1 mg. (Followed by remaining initial dose.) *Initial dose:* 0.25 mg/kg/24 hr *Increment:* Increase as tolerated by 0.125–0.25 mg/kg/24 hr QD OR QOD *Maintenance:* QD: 1 mg/kg/24 hr OR QOD: 1.5 mg/kg/dose **Max dose:** 1.5 mg/kg/24 hr	diphenhydramine 30 min before and 4 hr after infusion. Demerol useful for chills. Hydrocortisone, 1 mg/mg ampho (max, 25 mg) added to bottle may help prevent immediate adverse reactions. Monitor renal, hepatic, electrolyte, and hematologic status closely. Hypercalciuria, hypokalemia, RTA, renal failure, acute hepatic failure, and phlebitis may occur.
Ampicillin (Omnipen, Polycillin, Principen, Totacillin, Ancill, Amplin, Penamp)	Drops: 100 mg/ml (20 ml) Susp: 125, 250 mg/5 ml (80, 100, 150, 200 ml); 500 mg/5 ml (100 ml) Caps: 250, 500 mg Injection: 125, 250, 500 mg: 1, 2, 10 gm	*Neonate* <7 days: <2000 gm: 50–100 mg/kg/24 hr IM/IV ÷ Q12 hr ≥2000 gm: 75–150 mg/kg/24 hr IM/IV ÷ Q8 hr ≥7 days: <2000 gm: 75–150 mg/kg/24 hr ÷ Q8 hr IM/IV ≥2000 gm: 100–200 mg/kg/24 hr IM/IV ÷ Q6 hr	Use higher doses to treat CNS disease. Produces the same side effects as penicillin, with cross-reactivity. Rash commonly seen at 5–10 days. May cause interstitial nephritis. See Chapter 17.

	Child: Mild-moderate infections: 50–100 mg/kg/24 hr ÷ Q6 hr PO, IM or IV (**max PO dose:** 2–4 gm/24 hr) Severe infections: 200–400 mg/kg/24 hr ÷ Q4–6 hr IM or IV **Max IV dose:** 12 gm/24 hr	
Antipyrine and benzocaine (Auralgan)	Otic solution: Antipyrine 5.4%, Bencocain 1.4% (10, 15 ml)	Fill external ear canal Q1–2 hr prn for ear pain	Benzocaine sensitivity may develop. **Contraindicated** if tympanic membrane perforated.
Ascorbic acid (vitamin C, others)	Tabs: 25, 50, 100, 250, 500 mg, 1 gm. Chewable tabs: 100, 250, 500 mg Caps (timed release) 0.5, 1, 1.5 gm Inj: 250, 500 mg/ml Syrup: 100 mg/ml (5, 10, 120, 480 ml)	*Scurvy* Children: 100–300 mg/day ÷ QD-BID for at least 2 wk. Adults: 500–1000 mg/day ÷ QD-BID for at least 2 wk.	Adverse reactions: nausea, vomiting, heartburn, flushing, headache, faintness, dizziness, hyperoxaluria.
Aspirin (ASA, Anacin, Bufferin and various trade names) **check dose**	Tabs: 65, 75, 81, 325, 500 mg Tabs, enteric-coated: 325, 500, 650, 975 mg	*Analgesic/antipyretic:* 10–15 mg/kg/dose Q4 hr up to total 60–80 mg/kg/24 hr **max dose:** 4 gm/24 hr	Do not use in children <16 yr for treatment of chicken pox or flu-like symptoms. **Use**

(Continued.)

Drug	How Supplied	Dose and Route	Remarks
Aspirin *(continued.)*.	Tabs, time-release: 650, 800 mg Tabs, buffered: 325 mg Tabs, caffeinated: 400 mg ASA + 32 mg caffeine Tabs, chewable: 81 mg Caps: 325 mg Supp: 60, 120, 125, 130, 195, 200, 300, 325, 600, 650 mg and 1.2 gm	*Anti-inflammatory:* 60–100 mg/kg/24 hr PO ÷ Q6–8 hr *Kawasaki disease:* 100 mg/kg/24 hr PO ÷ QID during febrile phase until defervesces × 36 hr then decrease to 3–5 mg/kg/24 hr PO Q AM.	with caution in bleeding disorders. May cause GI upset, allergic reactions, liver toxicity and decreased platelet aggregation. See Chapter 3 for management of overdose. **Therapeutic levels:** antipyretic/analgesic: 150–300 mg/L. Tinnitus has been reported at levels of 200–400 mg/L.
Astemizole (Hismanal)	Tabs: 10 mg	6–12 yr: 5 mg/24 hr PO >12 yr: 10 mg/24 hr PO *To achieve therapeutic level faster:* >12 yr: day 1, 30 mg; day 2, 20 mg; day 3, 10 mg/24 hr	Long elimination half-life. Lower incidence of CNS side effects (like terfenadine). Serious cardiovascular complications have occurred rarely with higher than recommended doses. **Use with caution in patients with hepatic disease.**
Atropine sulfate	Tabs: 0.4, 0.6 mg Injection: 0.1, 0.3, 0.4, 0.5, 0.8, 1.0 mg/ml Nebulization: 0.2%, 0.5% (0.5 ml)	*Pre-anesthesia dose:* Child: 0.01 mg/kg/dose SC, IV; **max dose:** 0.4 mg/dose; **min dose:** 0.1 mg/dose; may repeat Q4–6 hr	In case of bradycardia, may give via endotracheal tube (dilute with NS to volume of 1–2 ml). Side effects include: dry mouth, blurred vision, fever,

(Continued.)

Ointment (ophthalmic): 0.5%, 1% (3.5 gm)
Solution (ophthalmic): 0.5, 1.0, 2.0, 3.0% (1, 2, 5 ml)

Adult: 0.5 mg/dose
Cardiopulmonary Resuscitation:
Child: 0.01–0.03 mg/kg/dose IV Q5 min × 2–3 PRN; **min dose:** 0.1 mg; **max dose:** 2 mg
Adult: 0.5–1mg/dose IV Q 5 min; **max dose:** 2 mg
Bronchospasm: 0.05 mg/kg/dose in 2.5 ml NS; **min dose:** 0.25 mg; **max dose:** 1 mg, Q6–8 hr
Ophthalmic:
Child: (0.5% solution) 1–2 drops in each eye TID-QD 1–3 days prior to operation.
Adult: (1% solution) 1–2 drops in each eye TID-QD 1–3 days prior to operation.

tachycardia, constipation, urinary retention, CNS signs (dizziness, hallucinations, restlessness).
Contraindicated in glaucoma, obstructive uropathy, tachycardia, thyrotoxicosis. Caution in patients sensitive to sulfites.

Aztreonam
(Azactam)

Inj: 0.5, 1, 2 gm

Neonate:
30 mg/kg/dose:
  <1.2 kg and 0–4 wk age:
  Q12 hr IV/IM
  1.2–2 kg and 0–7 days:
  Q12 hr IV/IM

Well-absorbed IM. Low cross-allergenicity between aztreonam and other beta-lactams. Adverse reactions: thrombophlebitis, eosinophilia, leukopenia,

Drug	How Supplied	Dose and Route	Remarks
Aztreonam (continued.).	Susp.* 2 or 50 mg/ml Tabs: 50 mg Injection: 5 mg/ml	1.2–2 kg and >7 days: Q8 hr IV/IM >2 kg and 0–7 days: Q8 hr IV/IM >2 kg and >7 days: Q6 hr I/IM *Children:* 90–120 mg/kg/24 hr ÷ Q6–8 hr IV/IM *Cystic fibrosis:* 150–200 mg/kg/24 hr ÷ Q6–8 hr IV/IM; **max dose: 8 gm/24 hr**	neutropenia, thrombocytopenia, elevation of liver enzymes, hypotension, seizures, confusion.
Azathioprine (Imuran)	Susp.* 2 or 50 mg/ml Tabs: 50 mg Injection: 5 mg/ml	*Immunosuppression:* Initial: 3–5 mg/kg/24 hr IV/PO QD Maintenance: 1–3 mg/kg/24 hr IV/PO QD	Toxicity: bone marrow suppression, rash, stomatitis, alopecia, arthralgias and GI disturbances. Use ¹/₄–¹/₃ dose when given with allopurinol. Monitor CBC, platelets, total bilirubin, alkaline phosphatase, BUN, creatinine.
Azithromycin (Zithromax)	Capsules: 250 mg	*Respiratory and skin infections:* Adults: 500 mg PO day 1, 250 mg QD × 4 doses. *Chlamydia:* 1 gm PO × 1	Drug should be taken at least 1 hr before or 2 hr after meals. Side effects: nausea, vomiting, diarrhea. **Caution:** do not take aluminum- or

			magnesium-containing antacids. **Contraindications:** hypersensitivity to erythromycin.
Baclofen (Lioresal)	Tabs: 10, 20 mg	*Children:* 2–7 yr: 10–15 mg/24 hr ÷ Q8 hr; titrate to **max dose:** 40 mg/24 hr ≥8 yr: **max dose:** 60 mg/day ÷ Q8 hr *Adults:* 5 mg TID; **max dose:** 80 mg/24 hr	Avoid abrupt withdrawal of drug. Use with **caution** in patients with seizure disorder, impaired renal function. Adverse effects: drowsiness, fatigue, nausea, vertigo, psychiatric disturbances, rash, urinary frequency, hypotonia.
Beclomethasone dipropionate (Vanceril, Vancenase, Beclovent, Beconase)	Inhalation, oral: 42 μg/inhalation (16.8 g) Inhalation, nasal: 42 μg/inhalation (16.8 g) Spray, aqueous nasal: 42 μg/dose 200 metered doses (25 g)	*Inhalant (oral):* 6–12 yr: 1–2 inhalations Q6–8 hr; **max:** 10 inhalations/24 hr >12 yr: 2 inhalations Q6–8 hr; **max:** 20 inhalations/24 hr (1 inhalation = 42 μg) *Inhalant (nasal):* 6–12 yr: 1 spray each nostril TID Adult: 1 spray each nostril BID-QID *Nasal spray:* 1–2 sprays each nostril BID	Rinse mouth and gargle with water after inhalation; may cause thrush. Avoid using higher-than-recommended doses, since hypothalamic, pituitary, or adrenal suppression may occur. Wean cautiously off steroids once inhalant is started to avoid rebound bronchospasm. **Not recommended** for children <6 yr. Consider using with tube spaces for oral inhalation.

*Indicates suspensions not commercially available; need to be extemporaneously compounded by a pharmacist. See references 6 and 7 for specific formulations.
(Continued.)

Drug	How Supplied	Dose and Route	Remarks
Bethanechol (Urecholine and other brand names)	Tabs: 5, 10, 25, 50 mg Susp*: 1 mg/ml Inj: 5 mg/ml	*Abdominal distention/urinary retention* PO: 0.6 mg/kg/24 hr ÷ Q6–8 hr SC: 0.15–0.2 mg/kg/24 hr ÷ Q6–8 hr *Gastroesophageal reflux:* 0.4 mg/kg/24 hr ÷ QID (AC and HS) Adults: 10–50 mg PO Q6–12 hr	**Contraindicated** in asthma, mechanical GI or GU obstruction, peptic ulcer disease, hyperthyroidism, seizure disorder. May cause hypotension, nausea, bronchospasm, salivation, flushing, abdominal cramps. **Warning:** severe hypotension may occur when given with ganglionic blockers (trimethaphan). **Do not give IV or IM.** Atropine is the antidote.
Bisacodyl (Dulcolax and various other names)	Tabs (enteric-coated): 5 mg Suppository: 5, 10 mg Enema: 10 mg/30 ml (37.5 ml)	*Oral:* Child: 0.3 mg/kg/24 hr or 5–10 mg to be given 6 hr before desired effect. Adult (>12 yr): 5–15 mg QD *Rectal:* <2 yr: 5 mg 2–11 yr: 5–10 mg >11 yr: 10 mg	Do not chew or crush tablets; do not give within 1 hr of antacids or milk. Do not use in newborn period. May cause abdominal cramps, nausea, vomiting, rectal irritation. Oral usually effective within 6–10 hr; rectal usually effective within 15–60 min.

Bretylium tosylate (Bretylol)	Inj: 50 mg/ml (10ml)	IV: 5 mg/kg/dose; may repeat Q10–20 min for total dose of 30 mg/kg. IM: 2–5 mg/kg × 1.	For specific indications, see Chapter 2. May cause initial hypertension followed by hypotension. May cause PVCs and increased sensitivity to digitalis and catecholamines. Safety and efficacy in children <12 yr.
Bumetanide (Bumex)	Tabs: 0.5, 1, 2 mg Inj: 0.25 mg/ml	<6 mo: Dose not established. ≥6 mo: 0.015–0.1 mg/kg/dose PO QD-QOD Adult PO: 0.5–2 mg/dose. QD-BID; **usual max dose: 5 mg/24 hr** IV/IM: 0.5–1 mg over 1–2 min. May give additional doses Q2–3 hr PRN; **max dose: 10 mg/24 hr.**	Side effects include cramps, dizziness, hypotension, headache, electrolyte losses (hypokalemia, hypocalcemia, hyponatremia, hypochloremia), and encephalopathy. May also lead to metabolic alkalosis. Cross-allergenicity may occur in patients allergic to sulfonamides.
Caffeine (caffeine base, caffeine citrate)	Injectable and oral liquid: *20 mg/ml (citrate salt), *10 mg/ml (caffeine base) (also available as powder for compounding)	*Neonatal apnea (caffeine base):* Loading dose: 10 mg/kg IV/ PO × 1	**Therapeutic levels 5–25 mg/L.** Cardiovascular, neurologic or GI toxicity reported at serum levels >50 mg/L. **Caffeine** *(Continued.)*

*Indicates suspensions not commercially available; need to be extemporaneously compounded by a pharmacist. See references 6 and 7 for specific formulations.

Drug	How Supplied	Dose and Route	Remarks
Caffeine *(continued.)*.		Maintenance dose: 2.5 mg/kg/dose PO/IV; QD, to begin 24 hr after loading dose. **Note: Doses for caffeine citrate are twice the doses above.**	benzoate formulation has been associated with causation of kernicterus in neonates.
Calcitriol (1,25-dihydroxy-cholecalciferol) (Rocaltrol, Calcijex)	Caps: 0.25, 0.50 µg Inj (Calcijex): 1, 2 µg/ml (1 ml)	*Renal Failure:* *Children:* Suggested dose range 0.01–0.05 µg/kg 24 hr. Titrate in 0.005–0.01 µg/kg/24 hr increments Q4–8 wk based on clinical response. *Adults:* Initial: 0.25 µg/24 hr PO. Increment: 0.25 µg/24 hr PO Q2–4 wk. IV: 0.01–0.05 µg/kg 3 ×/wk (usual 0.5–3 µg ×/wk).	Most potent vitamin D metabolite available. Monitor serum calcium and phosphorus. Avoid concomitant use of Mg^{++}-containing antacids. Side effects include: weakness, headache, vomiting, constipation, hypotonia, polydipsia, polyuria, metastatic calcification, etc. **Contraindicated** in patients with hypercalcemia, vitamin D toxicity.

Calcium carbonate (Tums, Os-Cal) (40% Ca)	Tab, chewable: 350, 420, 500, 650, 750, 850 mg Susp: 1250 mg/5ml; each gram of salt contains 20 mEq (400 mg) Ca	*Hypocalcemia:* Neonates: 50–150 mg/kg/24 hr ÷ Q4–6 hr PO: **max dose:** 1 gm/24 hr. Children: 20–65 mg/kg/24 hr PO ÷ QID. Adults: 1–2 gm or more/24 hr PO	Side effects: constipation, hypercalcemia, hypophosphatemia, nausea, vomiting, headache, confusion. May reduce absorption of tetracycline. May potentiate effects of digoxin. Some products may contain trace amounts of Na.
Calcium chloride (27% Ca)	Inj: 100 mg/ml (10%) (1.36 mEq Ca⁺⁺/ml); each gram of salt contains 13.6 mEq (270 mg) Ca.	*Cardiac Arrest:* Infant/child: 20 mg/kg/dose (0.2 ml/kg/dose) IV Q10 min. Adult: 250–500 mg/dose (2.5–5 ml/dose) IV Q10 min. **Do not exceed 1 ml/min with IV infusion.**	Use IV with extreme caution. Extravasation may lead to necrosis. Use local infiltration of hyaluronidase for calcium extravasation. Rapid IV infusion associated with bradycardia, hypotension, and peripheral vasodilation. May cause hyperchloremic acidosis.
Calcium glubionate (Neocalglucon) (6.4% Ca)	Syrup: 1.8 gm/5 ml (480 ml); each gram of salt contains 3.2 mEq (64 mg) Ca.	*Neonatal hypocalcemia:* 1200 mg/kg/24 hr PO ÷ Q4–6 hr *Maintenance:* Infant/child: 600–2000 mg/kg/24 hr PO ÷ QID; **max dose:** 9 gm/24 hr Adult: 6–18 gm/24 hr ÷ QID	Side effects include GI irritation, dizziness, and headache. Best absorbed when given before meals. Absorption inhibited by high phosphate load. High osmotic load of syrup (20% sucrose) may cause diarrhea.

(Continued.)

Drug	How Supplied	Dose and Route	Remarks
Calcium gluconate (9% Ca)	Tabs: 500, 650, 1000 mg Inj: 100 mg/ml (10%); each gram of salt contains 4.8 mEq (90 mg) Ca.	*Maintenance/hypocalcemia:* Infants: IV: 200–500 mg/kg/24 hr ÷ Q6 hr PO: 400–800 mg/kg/24 hr ÷ Q6 hr Child: 200–500 mg/kg/24 hr IV or PO ÷ Q6 hr Adult: 5–15 gm/24 hr IV or PO ÷ Q6 hr *For cardiac arrest:* Infants and children: 100 mg/kg/dose (1 ml/kg/dose) IV Q10 min. Adults: 500–800 mg/dose (5–8 ml/dose) IV Q10 min.	Avoid peripheral infusion. Extravasation may cause tissue necrosis. IV infusion associated with hypotension and bradycardia. Also associated with arrhythmias in digitalized patients. May precipatate when used with bicarbonate. **Do not use scalp veins!** Do not administer IM or SC.
Calcium lactate (13% Ca)	Tabs: 325, 650 mg; each gram of salt contains 6.5 mEq (130 mg) Ca.	*Infants:* 400–500 mg/kg/24 hr PO ÷ Q4–8 hr *Children:* 500 mg/kg/24 hr PO ÷ Q4–8 hr *Adult:* 1.5–3 gm PO Q8 hr; (**max dose** = 9 gm/24 hr)	Give with meals. Do not dissolve tablets in milk.

Captopril (Capoten)	Tabs: 12.5, 25, 50, 100 mg (smaller doses may be made by crushing tabs into powder and diluting with lactose).	Onset within 15–30 min of administration. Peak effect within 1–2 hr. Adjust with renal failure. May cause rash, proteinuria, neutropenia, cough, hypotension, or diminution of taste perception. Known to decrease aldosterone and increase renin production. Should be administered 1 hr prior to meals.
	Neonates: 0.1–0.4 mg/kg/24 hr PO ÷ Q6–8 hr. *Infants:* Initially 0.15–0.3 mg/kg/dose; Titrate upward to **max dose: 6 mg/kg/24 hr ÷ QD-QID** *Children:* Initially 0.5–1 mg/kg/24 hr ÷ Q8 hr; titrate to minimal effective dose; **max dose: 6 mg/kg/24 hr ÷ QD-QID** *Adolescents and adults:* Initially 12–25 mg/dose PO TID; increase **weekly** if necessary by 25 mg/dose to **max dose of 450 mg/24 hr.**	
Carbamazepine (Epitrol, Tegretol)	Tabs: 200 mg Chewable tabs: 100 mg Suspension: 100 mg/5 ml (450 ml)	Therapeutic blood levels: **4–12 mg/L. Contraindicated for patients taking MAO inhibitors.** Erythromycin, verapamil, cimetidine, and INH may increase serum levels. Carbamazepine may decrease activity of warfarin, doxycycline, oral
	<6yr: Initial: 5–10 mg/kg/24 hr PO ÷ BID Increment: Q5–7 days up to 20 mg/kg/24 hr PO *6–12 yr:* Initial 10 mg/kg/24 hr PO ÷ BID up to **max dose of 100 mg/dose BID**	

(Continued.)

Drug	How Supplied	Dose and Route	Remarks
Carbamazepine *(continued).*		Increment: 100 mg/24 hr at 1-day intervals (÷ TID-QID) until desired response is obtained. Maintenance: 20–30 mg/kg/24 hr PO ÷ BID-QID; **max dose:** 1000 mg/24 hr. **>12 yr:** Intial: 200 mg PO BID Increment: 200 mg/24 hr at 1-day intervals (÷ BID-QID) until desired response is obtained. Maintenance: 600–1200mg/24hr PO ÷ BID-QID; **max dose, 12–15 yr:** 1000 mg/24 hr; **max adult dose:** 1200 mg/24 hr.	contraceptives, theophylline, phenytoin, benzodiazepines, ethosuximide, and valproic acid. Side effects include sedation, dizziness, diplopia, aplastic anemia, neutropenia, urinary retention, nausea, SIADH, and Stevens-Johnson syndrome. Pretreatment CBC is suggested. Patient should be monitored for hematologic and hepatic toxicity.
Carbenicillin (Geocillin, Geopen, Pyopen)	Inj (as disodium): 1, 2, 5, 10 gm Tabs (as Indanyl sodium): 382 mg	*Mild infection:* Children: 30–50 mg/kg/ 24 hr PO ÷ Q6 hr; **max dose:** 2–3 g/24 hr; 50–200 mg/kg/24 hr ÷ Q4–6 hr IM/IV.	May cause anaphylaxis, platelet destruction. Unpredictable interaction with gentamicin. Give through separate IV tubing. May cause hypernatremia, hypokalemia,

		Adult: 382–764 mg Q6 hr PO: 200 mg/kg/24 hr ÷ Q6 hr IV/IM. *Severe infection (soft tissue):* Children: 400–500 mg/kg/24 hr IM/IV ÷ Q4–6 hr Adults: 250–500 mg/kg/24 hr ÷ Q6 hr IV/IM; **max dose: 40 g/24 hr.**	metabolic alkalosis, rash, and elevated AST. Adjust dose with renal failure. Use with **caution** in penicillin-allergic patients.
Cefaclor (Ceclor) (2nd generation)	Caps: 250, 500 mg Susp: 125, 187, 250, 375 mg/5 ml (75, 150 ml)	*Infant and child:* 40 mg/kg/24 hr PO ÷ Q8 hr; **max dose:** 2 gm/24 hr. *Adult:* 250–500 mg/dose PO Q8 hr; **max dose:** 4 gm/24 hr.	Use with **caution** in patients with penicillin allergy or renal impairment. May cause positive Coombs or false-positive test for urinary glucose. Serum sickness reactions have been reported in patients receiving multiple courses of cefaclor. Safety and efficacy in infants <1 mo has not been established.
Cefadroxil (Duricef, Ultracef) (1st generation)	Susp: 125, 250, 500 mg/5 ml (50, 100 ml) Tabs: 1 gm Caps: 500 mg	*Infant and child:* 30 mg/kg/24 hr PO ÷ Q12 hr *Adult:* 1–2 gm/24 hr PO ÷ Q12 hr; **max dose:** 2 gm/24 hr	See cephalexin. Side effects include nausea, vomiting, pseudomembranous colitis, pruritus, neutropenia, vaginitis, and candidiasis.

(Continued.)

Drug	How Supplied	Dose and Route	Remarks
Cefamandole (Mandol) (2nd generation)	Inj: 0.5, 1, 2, 10 gm (3.3 mEq Na/gm)	*Child:* 50–150 mg/kg/24 hr IM/IV ÷ Q4–6 hr. *Adult:* 4–12 mg/24 hr IM/IV ÷ Q4–8 hr; **max dose:** 12 gm/24 hr, 2 gm/dose.	See cefaclor. May cause elevated liver enzymes, coagulopathy, transient neutropenia and disulfiram-like reaction with ethanol.
Cefazolin (Ancef, Kefzol, Zolicef, others) (1st generation)	Inj: 0.25, 0.5, 1, 5, 10 gm (2 mEq Na/gm)	*Neonate:* Age <7 days: 40 mg/kg/24 hr IV/IM ÷ Q12 hr. Weight <2000 gm, age ≥7 days: 40 mg/kg/24 hr IV/IM ÷ Q12 hr Weight ≥2000 gm, age ≥7 days: 60 mg/kg/24 hr ÷ Q8–12 hr IV/IM *Infant >1 mo/children:* 50–100 mg/kg/24 hr ÷ Q6–8 hr IV/IM *Adult:* 2–6 gm/24 hr ÷ Q6–8 hr IV/IM; **max dose:** 6 gm/24 hr	See cephalexin. Use with **caution** in renal impairment or in penicillin-allergic patients. May cause phlebitis, leukopenia, thrombocytopenia, elevated liver enzymes, false-positive urine reducing substance.
Cefixime (Suprax) (3rd generation)	Tabs: 200, 400 mg Susp: 100 mg/5 ml (50, 100 ml)	*Infant and child:* 8 mg/kg/24 hr ÷ Q12–24 hr PO; **max dose:** 400 mg/24 hr. *Adult:* 400 mg/24 hr ÷ Q12–24 hr PO. *N. gonorrhoeae infection:* 400 mg × 1 PO may be as effective as ceftriaxone.	Use with **caution** in patients with penicillin allergy or renal failure. Adverse reactions include diarrhea, abdominal pain, nausea, headaches.

Cefoperazone (Cefobid) (3rd generation)	Inj: 1, 2 gm (1.5 mEq Na/gm)	*Infant and child:* 100–200 mg/kg/24 hr ÷ Q12 hr IM/IV. *Adult:* 2–4 gm/24 hr ÷ Q12 hr IM/IV; **max dose:** 12 gm/24 hr	Use with **caution** in penicillin-allergic patients or in patients with renal failure. May cause disulfiram-like reaction with ethanol.
Cefotaxime (Claforan) (3rd generation)	Inj: 1, 2, 10 gm (2.2 mEq Na/gm)	*Neonate:* *<1.2 kg:* 0–4 wk: 100 mg/kg/24 hr ÷ Q12 hr IV/IM. *≥1.2 kg* 0–7 days: 100 mg/kg/24 hr ÷ Q12 hr IV/IM. >7 days: 150 mg/kg/24 hr ÷ Q8 hr IV/IM. *Infant and child:* (<50 kg): 100–200 mg/kg/24 hr ÷ Q6–8 hr IV/IM. Meningitis: 200 mg/kg/24 hr ÷ Q6 hr IV/IM. *Adult:* (≥50 kg): 2–12 gm/24 hr ÷ Q4–8 hr IV/IM; **max dose:** 12 gm/24 hr.	Use with **caution** in penicillin-allergic patients or in presence of renal impairment. Toxicities similar to other cephalosporins: allergy, neutropenia, thrombocytopenia, eosinophilia, positive Coombs, elevated BUN, creatinine, and liver enzymes.

(Continued.)

Drug	How Supplied	Dose and Route	Remarks
Cefotetan (Cefotan) (2nd generation)	Inj: 1, 2 gm (3.5 mEq Na/gm)	*Infant and child:* 40–80 mg/kg/24 hr ÷ Q12 hr IV/IM. *Adult:* 2–6 gm/24 hr ÷ Q12 hr IV/IM; **max dose:** 6 gm/24 hr.	Use with **caution** in penicillin-allergic patients or in presence of renal impairment.
Cefoxitin (Mefoxin) (2nd generation)	Inj: 1, 2 gm (2.3 mEq Na/gm)	*Infant and child:* 80–160 mg/kg/24 hr ÷ Q4–6 hr IM/IV. *Adult:* 4–12 gm/24 hr ÷ Q6–8 hr IM/IV; **max dose:** 12 gm/24 hr.	Use with **caution** in penicillin-allergic patients or in presence of renal impairment.
Ceftazidime (Fortaz, Tazidime, Tazicef, Ceptaz [arginine salt]) (3rd generation)	Inj: 0.5, 1, 2, 6 gm (2.3 mEq Na/gm)	*Neonate:* <1.2 kg: 0–4 wk: 100 mg/kg/24 hr ÷ Q12 hr IV/IM. ≥1.2 kg: 0–7 days: 100 mg/kg/24 hr ÷ Q12 hr IV/IM. >7 days: 150 mg/kg/24 hr ÷ Q8 hr IV/IM.	Use with **caution** in penicillin-allergic patients or in presence of renal impairment.

	Infant and child: 90–150 mg/kg/24 hr ÷ Q8 hr IV/IM. *Cystic fibrosis:* 150 mg/kg/24 hr ÷ Q8 hr IV/IM. *Adult:* 2–6 gm/24 hr ÷ Q8–12 hr IV/IM; **max dose:** 6 gm/24 hr.	
Ceftizoxime (Cefizox) (3rd generation)	Inj: 1, 2 gm (2.6 mEq Na/gm)	*Infant and child:* 150–200 mg/kg/24 hr ÷ Q6–8 hr IV/IM. *Adult:* 2–12 gm/24 hr ÷ Q8–12 hr IV; **max dose:** 12 gm/24 hr.	Use with **caution** in penicillin-allergic patients or in presence of renal impairment.
Ceftriaxone (Rocephin) (3rd generation)	Inj: 0.25, 0.5, 1, 2, 10 gm (3.6 mEq Na/gm)	*Infant and child:* 50–75 mg/kg/24 hr ÷ Q12–24 hr IM/IV. *Meningitis:* loading dose 50–75 mg/kg IM/IV. Maintenance: 100mg/kg/24 hr ÷ Q12 hr IV/IM. *Adult:* 1–4 gm/24 hr ÷ Q12–24 hr IV/IM; **max dose:** 4 gm/24 hr. *Gonococcal prophylaxis:* see Chapter 17.	Use with **caution** in penicillin-allergic patients or in presence of renal impairment. May cause reversible cholelithiasis, sludging in gallbladder, and jaundice. Use with **caution** in neonates at risk for hyperbilirubinemia.

(Continued.)

Drug	How Supplied	Dose and Route	Remarks
Cefuroxime (Zinacef, Kefurox) (2nd generation)	Inj: 0.75, 1.5, 7.5 gm (2.4 mEq Na/gm)	*Neonates:* 20–50 mg/kg/24 hr ÷ Q12 hr IM/IV. *Infant and child:* 75–150 mg/kg/24 hr ÷ Q8 hr IV/IM; **max dose: 6** gm/24 hr. *Adults:* 750 mg–1.5 gm/dose Q8 hr IM/IV; **max dose: 9** gm/24 hr.	Use with **caution** in penicillin-allergic patients or in presence of renal impairment. May cause thrombophlebitis at infusion site. Other toxicities are those of other cephalosporins. **Not recommended for meningitis.**
Cefuroxime axetil (Ceftin) (2nd generation)	Tabs: 125, 250, 500 mg	*Children:* 30 mg/kg/24 hr PO ÷ BID. Otitis media: 40 mg/kg/24 hr PO ÷ BID.	Same as cefuroxime.
Cephalexin (Keflex, Cefanex, C-Lexin, and others) (1st generation)	Tabs: 250, 500 mg, 1 gm Caps: 250, 500 mg Susp: 125 ml/5 ml, 250 mg/5 ml (60, 100, 200 ml) Drops: 100 mg/ml (10 ml)	*Infant and child:* 25–50 mg/kg/24 hr PO ÷ Q6–12 hr. *Adult:* 1–4 gm/24 hr PO ÷ Q6–12 hr; **max dose: 4** gm/24 hr.	Some cross-reactivity with penicillins. GI disturbance frequent. Safety and efficacy in children <1 mo of age **has not been established.** Use with **caution** in renal insufficiency.
Cephalothin (Keflin) (1st generation)	Inj: 1, 2, 4 gm (2.8 mEq Na/gm)	*Infant and child:* 80–160 mg/kg/24 hr ÷ Q4–6 hr IV or deep IM. *Adults:* 2–12 gm/24 hr ÷ Q4–6 hr IV/IM; **max dose: 12** gm/24 hr.	See cephalexin. May cause phlebitis.

Cephradine (Velosef, Anspor, and others) (1st generation)	Susp: 125, 250 mg/5 ml (100, 200 ml) Caps: 250 and 500 mg Tabs: 1 gm Injection: 0.25, 0.5, 1, 2, 4 gm	*Child:* PO: 25–50 mg/kg/24 hr ÷ Q6–12 hr; IM/IV: 50–100 mg/kg/24 hr ÷ Q6–12 hr. *Adult:* PO: 1–4 gm/24 hr ÷ Q6 hr; IV: 2–8 gm/24 hr ÷ Q6 hr; **max oral dose:** 4 gm/24 hr; **max parenteral dose:** 8 gm/24 hr.	See cephalexin. Safety of parenteral cephradine in children less than 9 mo old **has not been established.**
Charcoal, activated	See Chapter 3.		
Chloral hydrate (Noctec, Somnos, Aquachloral)	Caps: 250, 500 mg Syrup: 250, 500 mg/5 ml Supp: 324, 500, 648 mg	*Children:* Sedative: 5–15 mg/kg/dose Q8 hr PO/PR Preprocedure: see Chapter 27. Hypnotic: 50–75 mg/kg/dose PO/ PR; **max dose:** 1 gm/dose, 2 gm/24 hr. *Adult:* Sedative: 250 mg/dose TID PO/PR	Irritating to mucous membranes; (consider administering with water or ginger ale) may cause laryngospasm if aspirated. May cause GI irritation, paradoxical excitement, delirium, peripheral vasodilation, hypotension, myocardial and respiratory depression. May accumulate with repeated

(Continued.)

Drug	How Supplied	Dose and Route	Remarks
Chloral hydrate *(continued.)*		Hypnotic: 500–1000 mg/dose PO/PR; **max dose: 2 gm/24 hr.**	use; sudden withdrawal may cause delirium tremens. **Contraindicated** in hepatic or renal impairment. **Caution** when using with furosemide and anticoagulants. **Use with caution in patients with cardiac disease.**
Chloramphenicol (Chloromycetin and others)	Caps: 250, 500 mg Susp: 150 mg/5 ml (60 ml) Inj: 1 gm (100 mg/ml) Otic solution: 0.5% (7.5 ml) Ophthalmic solution: 0.5% Ophthalmic ointment: 1% (3.5 gm) Topical cream: 1%	*Loading dose (all ages):* 20 mg/kg IV or PO *Maintenance:* *Neonates:* <2 kg: 25 mg/kg/24 hr QD IV/PO. ≤7 days: 25 mg/kg/24 hr IV/PO QD. >7 days: 50 mg/kg/24 hr IV/PO ÷ Q12 hr. *Infants/children/adults:* 50–100 mg/kg/day IV/PO ÷ Q6 hr; **max dose: 4 gm/24 hr.** *Ophthalmic:* 1–2 drops or ribbon of ointment in each eye Q3–6 hr.	Dose recommendations are just guidelines for therapy; monitoring of blood levels is essential in neonates and infants. Follow hematologic status for dose related or idiosyncratic marrow suppression. "Gray baby" syndrome may be seen with levels >50 mg/L. Concomitant use of phenobarbital and rifampin may lower its serum levels. Chloramphenicol may increase phenytoin levels. **Therapeutic levels:** 15–25 mg/L for meningitis; 10–20

	Topical: apply to affected area TID-QID	mg/L for other infections. Trough: 5–15 mg/L for meningitis; 5–10 mg/L for other infections. **Note: higher serum levels may be achieved using the oral, rather than the IV route.**
Chlorothiazide (Diuril, Diurigen)	Tabs: 250, 500 mg Susp: 250 mg/5 ml (237 ml) Inj: 40 mg/ml (500 mg)	*<6 mo:* 20–40 mg/kg/24 hr ÷ Q 12 hr PO/IV *≥6 mo:* 20 mg/kg/24 hr ÷ Q12 hr PO/IV *Adults:* 250–1000 mg/dose QD-QID PO/IV; **max dose:** 2gm/24 hr.	Use with **caution** in liver and severe renal disease. May cause hypercalcemia, hyperbilirubinemia, hypokalemia, alkalosis, hyperglycemia, hyperuricemia, hypomagnesemia, blood dyscrasias, pancreatitis. **Avoid IM administration.**
Chlorpheniramine maleate (Chlor-Trimeton and others)	Tabs: 4, 8, 12 mg Sustained-release caps and tabs: 8, 12 mg Syrup: 2 mg/5 ml (120, 473 ml) Inj: 10, 100 mg/ml Tab (chewable): 2 mg	*Children 2–6 yr:* 1 mg/dose PO Q4–6 hr PRN; **max dose:** 4 mg/24 hr. *6–12 yr:* 2 mg/dose PO Q4–6 hr; **max dose:** 12 mg/24 hr. Sustained release: 8–12 mg/dose PO BID PRN. *≥12 yrs/adults:* 4 mg/dose Q4–6 hr PO PRN; **max dose:** 24 mg/24 hr.	May cause drowsiness, dry mouth, polyuria, sedation, or disturbed coordination. Young children may be paradoxically excited.

(Continued.)

Drug	Dose and Route	How Supplied	Remarks
Chlorpromazine (Thorazine)	*Children >6 mo:* IM or IV: 2.5–6 mg/kg/24 hr ÷ Q6–8 hr PO: 2.5–6 mg/kg/24 hr ÷ Q4–6 hr PR: 1 mg/kg/dose Q6–8 hr; **max IV/IM dose:** <5 yrs: 40 mg/24 hr; **max IV/IM dose:** 5–12 yr: 75 mg/24 hr. *Adult:* Initial: 25 mg IM/IV; increase by 25–50 mg/dose Q1–4 hr up to **max** of 400 mg/dose Q4–6h. PO: 10–25 mg/dose Q4–6 hr; may be increased up to 1200 mg/24 hr; **max dose:** 2 gm/24 hr.	Tabs: 10, 25, 50, 100, 200 mg Extended-release caps: 30, 75, 150, 200, 300 mg Syrup: 10 mg/5 ml (120 ml) Supp: 25, 100 mg Oral conc: 30 mg/ml (120 ml), 100 mg/ml (60, 240 ml) Inj: 25 mg/ml	Adverse effects include drowsiness, jaundice, lowered seizure threshold, extrapyramidal/anticholinergic symptoms, hypotension, arrhythmias, agranulocytosis. May potentiate effects of narcotics, sedatives, other drugs. Monitor BP closely. ECG changes include prolonged PR interval, flattened T waves and ST depression.
Cholestyramine (Questran, Cholybar)	*Children:* 240 mg/kg/24 hr cholestyramine ÷ TID. Give PO as slurry in water, juice or	Powder: 5, 9 gm packets, each containing 4 gm of anhydrous resin	May cause constipation, diarrhea, vomiting, vitamin deficiencies (A, D, E, K), and

	Cans: 378 gm powder, containing 168 gm of anhydrous resin (each 9 gm of powder contains 4 gm of resin) Chewable bars: 4 gm	milk before meals. *Adult:* 3–4 gm of cholestyramine TID; **max dose: 32 gm/24 hr**	rash. Give other oral medications 4–6 hr after cholestyramine or 1 hr. before dose to avoid decreased absorption. Hyperchloremic acidosis may occur with prolonged use.
Cimetidine (Tagamet)	Tabs: 200, 300, 400, 800 mg Inj: 150 mg/ml Syrup: 300 mg/5 ml (237 ml)	*Infants:* 10–20 mg/kg/24 hr PO/IV ÷ Q6 hr *Children:* 20–40 mg/kg/24hr PO/IV ÷ Q6 hr *Adults* (PO/IM/IV): 300 mg/dose QID, 400 mg/dose BID or 800 mg/dose QHS; Ulcer Prophylaxis: 400–800 mg PO QHS; **max dose: 2400 mg/24 hr**	Use with caution in all patients. Diarrhea, rash, myalgia, confusion, neutropenia, gynecomastia, elevated liver function tests or dizziness may occur. IV/IM dosing should be titrated to maintain gastric pH > 5. Inhibits cytochrome P-450 oxidase system.
Ciprofloxacin (Cipro)	Tabs: 250, 500, 750 mg Inj: 200 mg/20 ml Opthalmic solution: 3.5 mg/ml (2.5, 5.0 ml)	*Children:* 20–30 mg/kg/24 hr IV/PO ÷ Q12 hr *Adults:* Oral: 250–750 mg/dose PO Q12 hr **max dose: 2 gm/24 hr.** IV: 200–400 mg/dose Q12 hr;	Side effects: nausea, vomiting, renal failure, GI bleeding, restlessness. Like other quinolones, ciprofloxacin causes cartilage arthropathy in experimental animals. **Not recommended for children <16–18 yr.**

(Continued.)

Drug	How Supplied	Dose and Route	Remarks
Citrate mixtures, (oral)	Each ml contains (mEq): Na K Citrate Polycitra 1 1 2 Polycitra-K 0 2 2 Bicitra 1 0 1 Oracit 1 0 1	*Children:* 5–15 ml/dose Q6–8 hr PO or 2–3 mEq/kg/24 hr ÷ Q6–8 hr *Adult:* 15–30 ml/dose Q6–8 hr PO or 100–200 mEq/24 hr ÷ Q6–8 hr; dilute dose in 30–90 ml of water; chilling may enhance palatibility.	Adjust dose to maintain desired urine pH. 1 mEq of citrate is equivalent to 1 mEq HCO₃. Use with **caution** in patients already receiving potassium supplements. May have laxative effect.
Clarithromycin (Biaxin FilmTabs)	Tabs: 250, 500 mg	*Children:* 15 mg/kg/24 hr PO ÷ Q12 hr *Adult:* 250–500 mg/dose Q12 hr	Side effects: diarrhea, nausea, abnormal taste, dyspepsia, abdominal discomfort, headache. May increase carbamazepine, theophylline concentration. **Contraindicated** in patients sensitive to erythromycin.
Clindamycin (Cleocin-T, Cleocin, and others)	Caps: 75, 150, 300 mg Oral liquid: 75 mg/5 ml (100 ml) Inj: 150 mg/ml (contains 9.45 mg/ml benzyl alcohol) Solution, topical: 1% (3960 ml) Gel: 1% (7.5, 3 gm)	*Neonates:* Preterm: 15 mg/kg/24 hr ÷ Q8 hr IV/IM Term: 20–40 mg/kg/24 hr ÷ Q6 hr IV/IM *Children:* 20–30 mg/kg/24 hr ÷ Q6 hr PO; 25–40 mg/kg/24 hr ÷ Q6–8 hr IM/IV	Not indicated in meningitis. Pseudomembraneous colitis may occur up to several weeks after cessation of therapy, but generally is uncommon in pediatric patients. May cause diarrhea, rash, Stevens-Johnson

		Adults: 150–450 mg/dose Q6–8 hr PO; 600–3600 mg/24 hr IM/IV ÷ Q6–12 hr; **max dose:** 4.8 gm/24 hr IV/IM; 1.8 gm/24 hr PO. Topical: apply to affected area BID	patients. May cause diarrhea, rash, Stevens-Johnson syndrome, granulocytopenia, thrombocytopenia or sterile abscess at injection site.
Clonazepam (Klonopin)	Tabs*: 0.5, 1.0, 2.0 mg Susp*: 100 μg/ml	*Children:* ≤10 yr or 30 kg: Initial: 0.01–0.03 mg/kg/24 hr ÷ Q8 hr PO Increment: 0.25–0.5 mg/kg/24 hr Q3 days, up to **max maintenance dose** of 0.1–0.2 mg/kg/24 hr ÷ Q8 hr. *Adult:* Initial: 1.5 mg/24 hr PO ÷ TID. Increment: 0.5–1 mg/24 hr Q3 days; **max dose:** 20 mg/24 hr	CNS depression, drowsiness, and ataxia common. May cause behavioral changes, and other CNS symptoms; increased bronchial secretions. GI, CV, GU and hematopoietic toxicity (thrombocytopenia, leukopenia) may occur. Use with **caution** in renal impairment. **Therapeutic levels:** 20–80 ng/ml.
Clonidine (Catapres, Catapres-TTS)	Tabs: 0.1, 0.2. 0.3 mg Transdermal patch: 0.1, 0.2, 0.3 mg/24 hr (7 day)	*Children:* 5–7 μg/kg/24 hr ÷ Q6 hr. If needed, increase gradually at 5–7 day intervals to 5–25 μg/kg/day ÷ Q6 hr.	T₁/₂: 6–20 hr. Applying >2 of the 0.3 mg/24 hr patches does not provide additional benefit. Side effects: dry *(Continued.)*

*Indicates suspensions not commercially available; need to be extemporaneously compounded by a pharmacist. See references 6 and 7 for specific formulations.

Drug	How Supplied	Dose and Route	Remarks
Clonidine *(continued).*		*Adult:* 0.1 mg BID initially; increase in 0.1 mg/24 hr increments until desired response is achieved: **max dose:** 2.4 mg/day. Transdermal patch: 0.1 mg/24 hr patch 1st week; increase weekly, if necessary up to 0.3 mg/24 hr patch.	mouth, dizziness, drowsiness, fatigue, constipation, anorexia, arrhythmias, local skin reactions with patch. Do not abruptly discontinue—signs of sympathetic overactivity may occur; taper gradually over >1wk.
Clotrimazole (Lotrimin, Mycelex)	Cream: 1% (15, 30, 45, 90 gm) Solution: 1% (10, 30 ml) Vaginal tabs: 100, 500 mg Vaginal cream: 1% (45, 90 gm) Oral troche: 10 mg	*Topical:* apply to skin BID × 4–8 wks *Vaginal candidiasis:* 1 tab or applicator dose (5 g) /24 hr × 7–14 days *Alternative plans:* Two 100 mg tabs 1 dose × 3 days or one 500 mg tab 1 dose × 1 *Thrush:* Dissolve slowly one troche in the mouth 5 times/24 hr × 14 days	May cause erythema, blistering, or urticaria where applied. Safety and efficacy in children <3 yrs **has not been established.**
Cloxacillin (Tegopen, Cloxapen)	Caps: 250, 500 mg Oral solution: 125 mg/5 ml (100, 200 ml)	*Infant/child:* 50–100 mg/kg/24 hr ÷ Q6 hr PO. *Adult:* 250–1000 mg/dose Q6 hr PO; **max dose:** 4 gm/24 hr.	Same side effects as other penicillins. Give on an empty stomach.

Codeine (various brands)	Tabs: 15, 30, 60 mg Inj: 30, 60 mg/ml Syrup: 10, 60 mg/5 ml Oral solution: 15 mg/5 ml Elixir: Acetaminophen 120 mg and codeine 12 mg/5 ml Caps: Acetaminophen 325 + 15 mg codeine Acetaminophen 325 + 30 mg codeine Acetaminophen 325 + 60 mg codeine Tabs: (all contain 300 mg acetaminophen per tab) Tylenol #1: 7.5 mg codeine. Tylenol #2: 15 mg codeine Tylenol #3: 30 mg codeine. Tylenol #4: 60 mg codeine.	*Analgesic:* Children: 0.5–1.0 mg/kg/dose Q4–6 hr IM, SC, or PO; **max dose:** 60 mg/dose. Adults: 30–60 mg/dose Q4–6 hr IM, SC, or PO *Antitussive:* (all doses PRN) Children (2–6 yr): 2.5–5 mg/dose Q4–6 hr; **max dose:** 30 mg/24 hr. Children (6–12 yr): 5–10 mg/dose Q4–6 hr; **max dose:** 60 mg/24 hr. Adults: 15–30 mg/dose Q4–6 hr; **max dose:** 120 mg/24 hr	Side effects: CNS and respiratory depression, constipation, cramping. May be habit forming. For analgesia, use with acetaminophen orally. **Do not use in children <2 yr old as antitussive.** Not intended for IV use, due to large histamine release and cardiovascular effects. See Chapter 27 for equianalgesic dosing.
Cortisone acetate (Cortone acetate)	Tabs: 5, 10, 25 mg Inj: 25, 50 mg/ml	*Physiologic replacement:* 0.5–0.75 mg/kg/24 hr ÷ Q8 hr PO or 0.25–0.35 mg/kg/24 hr QD IM *Stress/preoperative:* 31.5–50 mg/m²/24 hr IM QD for days −2, −1, 0, 1, 2, 3, and 4 of perioperative period	IM slowly absorbed over several days. See steroid section of Chapter 26. May produce glucose intolerance, Cushing's syndrome, pituitary-adrenal suppression, edema, hypertension, cataracts, hypokalemia, and skin atrophy.

(Continued.)

Drug	How Supplied	Dose and Route	Remarks
Cortisone acetate (continued.).		*Anti-inflammatory/ immunosuppressive:* 2.5–10 mg/kg/24 hr ÷ Q6–8 hr PO or 1–5 mg/kg/24 hr ÷ Q12–24 hr IM	
Co-trimoxazole (Trimethoprim-Sulfamethoxazole) (Bactrim, Septra, TMP-SMX, Sulfatrim, others)	Tabs (reg strength): 80 mg TMP/400 mg SMX Tabs (double strength): 160 mg TMP/800 mg SMX Susp: 40 mg TMP/200 mg SMX per 5 ml (20, 100, 150, 200, 480 ml) Inj: 16 mg TMP/ml and 80 mg SMX/ml	Doses based on TMP component. *Minor infections (PO or IV):* Child: 8–10 mg/kg/24 hr ÷ Q12 hr Adult (>40 kg): 160 mg/dose Q12 hr *UTI prophylaxis:* 2 mg/kg/24 hr QD *Severe infections and Pneumocystis carinii pneumonitis (PO or IV):* 20 mg/kg/24 hr ÷ Q6–8 hr *Pneumocystis prophylaxis:* 5–10 mg/kg/24 hr ÷ Q12 hr or 150 mg/m²/24 hr ÷ Q12 hr 3 consecutive days/wk; **max dose:** 320 mg/24 hr.	Not recommended for use with infants <2 mo. May cause kernicterus in newborns; may cause blood dyscrasias, crystalluria, glossitis, renal or hepatic injury, GI irritation, allergy, hemolysis in G6PD. Reduce dose in renal impairment. See Infectious Disease chapter for guidelines.

| Cromolyn (Intal, Nasalcrom, Opticrom, Gastrocrom) | Caps: 20 mg (for inhalation via "spinhaler") Nebulized solution: 10 mg/ml (2 ml) Nasal solution: 4% (13 ml) Aerosol inhaler: 800 µg/spray (8.1, 14.2 gm) Capsule: 100 mg | *Inhalant:* 20 mg Q6 hr (for adults and children >5 yr) *Nebulization:* 20 mg Q6–8 hr (adults and children >2 yr old) *Nasal:* 1 spray each nostril TID-QID *Aerosol inhaler:* 2 puffs QID *Food allergy/inflammatory bowel disease:* 100 mg PO QID 15–20 min before each meal; **max dose:** 40 mg/kg/day. *Systemic mastocytosis:* <2 yr: 20 mg/kg/24 hr ÷ QID PO; **max dose:** 30 mg/kg/24 hr 2–12 yr: 100 mg PO QID; **max dose:** 40 mg/kg/24 hr. Adults: 200 mg PO QID. | Not for treatment of acute asthmatic attack. Allow 2–4 weeks of use for adequate trial. May cause rash, cough, bronchospasm, nasal congestion. May cause headache, diarrhea with oral use. Use with caution in patients with renal or hepatic dysfunction. Give dose <1 hr before anticipated exercise or exposure. Bronchospasm and pharyngeal irritation may occur when using spinhaler product. |
| **Cyclopentolate** (Cyclogyl, and others) | Solution: 0.5%, 1%, 2% (2, 5, 15 ml) | *Infant:* 1 drop of 0.5% OU 5–10 min before exam. *Children:* 1 drop of 0.5–1%, followed by repeat drop if necessary. | Do not use in narrow-angle glaucoma. May cause a burning sensation, behavioral disturbance, loss of visual accommodation. To minimize |

(Continued.)

Drug	How Supplied	Dose and Route	Remarks
			absorption, apply pressure over nasolacrimal sac for at least 2 min. Observe patient closely for at least 30 min after dose.
Cyclopentolate/ phenylephrine (Cyclomydril)	Solution: 0.2% cyclopentolate/ 1% phenylephrine	1 drop OU Q5–10 min; **max dose:** 3 drops per eye.	Used to induce mydriasis.
Cyclosporine (Sandimmune)	Injection: 50 mg/ml Oral solution: 100 mg/ml (50 ml) Cap: 25, 50, 100 mg	*Oral:* 15 mg/kg/24 hr as a single dose 4–12 hr pre-transplant. Give the same dose daily × 1–2 wk posttransplant, then reduce by 5% per wk to 5–10 mg/kg/24 hr. *IV:* 5–6 mg/kg/24 hr ÷ Q12–24 hr 4–12 hr pre-transplant. Give slowly over 2–6 hr. Continue the same dose daily posttransplant until the patient can tolerate the oral solution.	Plasma concentrations decreased with use of rifampin, phenobarbital and phenytoin. Peaks about 4 hr after PO dose; plasma half-life 5–40 hr. May cause nephrotoxicity, hepatotoxicity, hypomagnesemia, hypertension, hirsutism, acne, GI symptoms, tremor, leukopenia, sinusitis.

			Recommended Trough Levels
			RIA (monoclonal):100–200 ng/ml RIA (polyclonal):250–800 ng/ml HPLC: 100–450 ng/ml
			Note that targeted trough levels vary according to transplantation protocol.
Cyproheptadine (Periactin)	Tabs: 4 mg Syrup: 2 mg/5 ml (473 ml)	*Children:* 0.25–0.5 mg/kg/24 hr ÷ Q8–12 hr PO *Adult:* 12–32 mg/24 hr ÷ TID PO **Max. dose:** 2–6 yr: 12 mg/24 hr 7–14 yr: 16 mg/24 hr Adults: 32 mg/24 hr	**Contraindicated** in neonates, patients currently on MAO inhibitors and patients suffering from asthma, glaucoma or GI/GU obstruction. May produce anticholinergic (atropine-like) effects, sedation, appetite stimulation.
Dantrolene (Dantrium)	Cap: 25, 50, 100 mg Inj: 20 mg	*Chronic spasticity:* Children (<5 yr): Initial: 0.5 mg/kg/dose PO BID Increment: Increase frequency to TID-QID at 4–7 day intervals, **then** increase doses by 0.5 mg/kg	Contrandicated in active hepatic disease. Monitor transaminases for hepatotoxicity. May cause change in sensorium, weakness, and diarrhea. Avoid unnecessary exposure

(Continued.)

Drug	How Supplied	Dose and Route	Remarks
Dantrolene (*continued.*).		**Max dose:** 3 mg/kg/dose PO BID-QID, up to 400 mg/24 hr. Adults: Initial: 25 mg PO QD Increment: Increase frequency to TID-QID, **then** increase dose by 25 mg/dose at 4–7 day intervals. **Max dose:** 400 mg/24 hr. *Malignant hyperthermia:* Prevention: 4–8 mg/kg/24 hr PO ÷ Q6–8 hr × 2 days prior to surgery Treatment: 1 mg/kg IV, repeat PRN up to a **max cumulative dose** of 10 mg/kg, then continue at 4–8 mg/kg/24 hr PO ÷ QID for 3 days.	to sunlight. When using IV, prevent extravasation into tissues. A decrease in spasticity sufficient to allow daily function should be therapeutic goal. Discontinue if benefits are not evident in 45 days. Use with **caution** in children with cardiac or pulmonary impairment. Dose in children < 5 yr of age **has not been established.**

Deferoxamine (Desferal, Mesylate)	Injection: 500 mg	*Iron poisoning:* 15 mg/kg/hr IV or 90 mg/kg/dose IM Q8 hr; **max** **dose:** 6 gm/24 hr. *Chronic iron overload:* IV: 15 mg/kg/hr. SC: 20–40 mg/kg/24 hr infusion over 8–12 hr.	**Contraindicated** in anuria, hemochromatosis. May cause flushing, erythema, urticaria, hypotension, tachycardia, diarrhea, leg cramps, fever, cataracts, hearing loss. Iron mobilization may be poor in children <3 yr.
Desmopressin acetate (DDAVP, Stimate)	Nasal solution: 100 μg/ml (2.5, 5 ml) Inj: 4 μg/ml Spray: 10 μg/5 ml Conversion: 100 μg = 400 IU arginine vasopressin	*Diabetes insipidus:* 3 mo–12 yr: 5–30 μg/24 hr ÷ QD-BID intranasally. Adults: Intranasal, 10–40 μg/24 hr ÷ QD-TID; titrate dose to achieve control of excessive thirst and urination; **max intranasal** **dose:** 40 μg/24 hr IV/ SC: 2–4 μg/24 hr ÷ BID *Hemophilia A and von* *Willebrand's disease:* 2–4 μg/kg/dose intranasally or 0.2–0.4 μg/kg/dose IV over 15–30 min. *Nocturnal enuresis (>6 yr):* 20 μg at bedtime intranasally, range 10–40 μg.	Injection may be used SC or IV at approximately 10% of intranasal dose. Adjust fluid intake to decrease risk of water intoxication. Use with caution in hypertension and coronary artery disease. Peak of effect is 1–5 hr. May cause headache, nausea, hyponatremia, nasal congestion, abdominal cramps, and hypertension.

(Continued.)

Drug	How Supplied	Dose and Route	Remarks
Dexamethasone (Decadron and other brand names)	Tabs: 0.25, 0.5, 0.75, 1.5, 2, 4, 6 mg Inj: 4, 10, 24 mg/ml (sodium phospate); 8, 16 mg/ml (acetate) Elixir: 0.5 mg/5 ml (100 ml) Oral solution: 0.1, 1 mg/ml (30 ml) Inhalation: 84 μg/metered dose (12.6 gm)	*Cerebral edema:* Initial dose: 0.5–1.5 mg/kg IV or IM (adult dose: 10 mg). Maintenance: 0.2–0.5 mg/kg/24 hr ÷ Q6 hr IV or IM × 5 days, then taper (adult dose: 4 mgQ6 hr) *Airway edema:* 0.25–0.5 mg/kg/dose Q6 hr PRN for croup or beginning 24 hr before elective extubation, then for 4–6 doses. *Antiemetic:* 4–8 mg/m² IV loading dose, then 2–4 mg/m²/dose IV Q6 hr. *Anti-inflammatory:* Children: 0.03–0.15 mg/kg/24 hr ÷ Q6–12 hr. IV/PO/IM. Adult: 0.75–9 mg/24 hr ÷ Q6–12 hr. PO/IV/IM. *Meningitis:* 0.15 mg/kg/dose IV Q6 hr × 4 days.	See Chapter 15. Toxicity: same as for prednisone. Oral peak serum levels occur at 1–2 hr and within 8 hr following IM administration.

| **Dextroamphetamine** (Dexedrine and many other brand names) | Tabs: 5, 10 mg
Elixir: 5 mg/5 ml
Sustained-release caps: 5, 10, 15 mg | *Attention deficit hyperactivity disorder:*
3–5 yr: 2.5 mg/24 hr Q AM; increase by 2.5 mg/24 hr at weekly intervals to a **max dose** of 40 mg/24 hr.
≥6 yr: 5 mg/24 hr QAM; increase by 5 mg/24 hr at weekly intervals to a **max dose** of 40 mg/24 hr.
Narcolepsy:
6–12 yr: 5 mg/24 hr; increase by 5 mg/24 hr at weekly intervals to a maximum of 60 mg/24 hr.
>12 yr: 10 mg/24 hr; increase by 10 mg/24 hr at weekly intervals to a maximum of 60 mg/24 hr. | Use with caution in presence of hypertension or cardiovascular disease. **Not** recommended for <3 yr olds. Interrupt administration occasionally to determine need for continued therapy. Many side effects, including insomnia, restlessness, anorexia, psychosis, headache, vomiting, abdominal cramps, dry mouth, growth failure. Tolerance develops. (Same guidelines as for methylphenidate apply.) **Do not give** with MAO inhibitors, general anesthetics. |
| **Diazepam** (Valium and others) | Tabs: 2, 5, 10 mg
Oral solution: 1, 5 mg/ml
Inj: 5 mg/ml
Sustained-release cap: 15 mg | *Sedative/muscle relaxant:*
Children:
IM or IV: 0.04–0.2 mg/kg/dose Q2–4 hr (**max dose**: 0.6 mg/kg within an 8-hr period). | Hypotension and respiratory depression may occur. Use with **caution** in glaucoma, shock, and depression. Give undiluted no faster than 2 mg/min. **Do not** mix with IV |

(Continued.)

Drug	How Supplied	Dose and Route	Remarks
Diazepam *(continued.)*.		PO: 0.12–0.8 mg/kg/24 hr ÷ Q6–8 hr. Adults: IM or IV: 2–10 mg/dose Q3–4 hr PRN. PO: 2–10 mg/dose Q6–8 hr PRN. *Status epilepticus:* Neonate: 0.3–0.75 mg/kg/dose IV Q15–30 min × 2–3 doses >1 mo: 0.2–0.5 mg/kg/dose IV Q15–30 min. **Max total dose: <5 yr:** 5 mg; **≥5 yr:** 10 mg. *Rectal dose:* 0.5 mg/kg/dose. Adults: 5–10 mg/dose IV Q10–15 min (**max total dose:** 30 mg).	fluids. In status epilepticus, diazepam must be followed by long acting anticonvulsants. For management of status epilepticus see Chapter 2.
Diazoxide (Hyperstat, Proglycem)	Inj: 15 mg/ml Caps: 50 mg Susp: 50 mg/ml (30 ml)	*Hypertensive crisis:* 1–3 mg/kg IV up to 150 mg; repeat Q5–15 min PRN, then Q4–24 hr.	May cause hyponatremia, salt and water retention, GI disturbances, ketoacidosis, rash, hyperuricemia,

hypertrichosis, and
arrhythmias. Monitor BP
closely for hypotension.
Hyperglycemia occurs in
majority of patients.
Hypoglycemia should be
treated initially with IV
glucose; diazoxide should be
introduced only if refractory to
glucose infusion.

Hyperinsulinemic hypoglycemia
(due to insulin-producing
tumors):
Newborns and infants: 8–15
mg/kg/24 hr ÷ Q8–12 hr
PO
Children and adults: 3–8
mg/kg/24 hr ÷ Q8–12 hr
PO (start at lowest dose)

Children (<40 kg):
Mild/moderate: 12.5–25
mg/kg/24 hr PO ÷ Q6 hr.
Severe: 50–100 mg/kg/24 hr
PO ÷ Q6 hr.
Adults (>40 kg): 125–500
mg/dose PO Q6 hr; **max
dose:** 4 gm/24 hr.

Toxicity and side effects similar
to cloxacillin. Give 1–2 hr
before meals or 2 hr after
meals. Limited experience in
neonates and very young
infants. Higher doses
(50–100 mg/kg/24 hr) are
indicated following IV therapy
for osteomyelitis. Large
volumes of oral suspension
may be needed.

Dicloxacillin sodium
(Dynapen, and others)

Caps: 125, 250, 500 mg
Oral susp: 62.5 mg/5 ml (80,
100, 200 ml)

(Continued.)

Drug	How Supplied	Dose and Route	Remarks
Didanosine (ddI) (Dideoxyinosine) (Videx)	Tabs (buffered, chewable/dispersable): 25, 50, 100, 150 mg Oral powder, buffered (single-dose packets for solution): 100, 167, 250, 375 mg Oral pediatric powder (for solution): 2, 4 gm.	*Children:* (Based on 200 mg/m²/24 hr avg. recommended dose) |	Peds Powder BSA Tablets	Dose
---	---	---
<0.4	25mg Q12 hr	31mg Q12 hr
0.5–0.7	50mg Q12 hr	62mg Q12 hr
0.8–1	75mg Q12 hr	94mg Q12 hr
1.1–1.4	100mg Q12 hr	125mg Q12 hr | *Adult:* | Weight (kg)	Tablets	Buffered Powder
---	---	---
35–49	125mg Q12 hr	167mg Q12 hr
50–74	200mg Q12 hr	250mg Q12 hr
≥75	300mg Q12 hr	375mg Q12 hr		**Adminster all doses on empty stomach.** Reported side effects in adults (in decreasing incidence): headaches (36%), diarrhea, peripheral neuropathy, nausea, vomiting, rash/pruritus, abdominal pain (21%), CNS depression, constipation, stomatitis, myalgia, arthritis (11%), pancreatitis (9%), alopecia (8%), dizziness. Use with **caution** in patients on sodium restriction (264.5 mg Na/ buffered tablet, 1380 mg Na/ single dose packet). Impairs absorption of drugs requiring an acidic environment (i.e., ketoconazole, dapsone.) **Consult package insert for additional details.**

	Caps: 50, 100, 200 μg
Digoxin	Tabs: 125, 250, 500 μg
	Elixir: 50 μg/ml (60 ml)
	Inj: 100, 250 μg/ml

Digitalizing: Total digitalizing dose (TDD) and maintenance doses in μg/kg/24 hr:

	TDD		Maintenance	
Age	PO	IV/IM	PO	IV/IM
Premature	20	15	5	3–4
Full term	30	20	8–10	6–8
<2 yr	40–50	30–40	10–12	7.5–9
2–10 yr	30–40	20–30	8–10	6–8
>10 yr	750–1250 μg/24hr		125–250 μg/24hr	

Initial: 1/2 TDD, then 1/4 TDD Q8–18 hr × 2 doses. Obtain ECG 6 hr after dose to assess for toxicity.

Maintenance:
<10 yr: Give maintenance dose ÷ BID
≥10 yr: Give maintenance dose QD

Excreted via the kidney. Use with caution in renal failure. Contraindicated in patients with ventricular dysrhythmias. May cause AV block or dysrhythmias. In the patient treated with digoxin, cardioversion or calcium infusion may lead to ventricular fibrillation (pretreatment with lidocaine may prevent this). For signs and symptoms of toxicity, Chapter 3. **Therapeutic concentration:** 0.8–2 μg/ml. Higher doses may be required for supraventricular tachycardia. Neonates may have falsely elevated digoxin levels, due to maternal digoxin-like substances.

Digoxin immune Fab (ovine) (Digibind)	Inj: 40 mg

First, determine total body digoxin load:

TBL(mg) = serum digoxin level (ng/ml) × 5.6 × wt (kg) ÷ 1000

May cause rapidly developing severe hypokalemia. Digoxin therapy may be reinstituted in 3–7 days, when toxicity has been corrected.

(Continued.)

Drug	How Supplied	Dose and Route	Remarks
Digoxin immune Fab (ovine) *(continued.).*		*Calculate dose of digoxin immune Fab (mg):* Fab(mg) = TBL × 66.7 Infuse over 15–30 min (through 0.22 micron filter).	**Contraindicated** if hypersensitivity to sheep products, or if renal or cardiac failure.
Dihydrotachysterol USP (DHT, Hytakerol, DHT Intensol)	Solution: 0.2 mg/ml (20% alcohol) Solution (in oil): 0.25 mg/ml (15 ml) Caps: 0.125 mg Tabs: 0.125, 0.2, 0.4 mg 1 mg = 120,000 IU vitamin D_2	*Hypoparathyroidism:* Neonates: 0.05–0.1 mg/24 hr PO Infants/young children: 0.1–0.5 mg/24 hr PO Older children/adults: 0.5–1. mg/24 hr PO *Hypophosphatemic vitamin D-resistant rickets:* 0.25–1. mg/24 hr PO *Nutritional rickets:* 0.5 mg × 1 dose PO *Renal osteodystrophy:* 0.6–6 mg/24 hr PO until healing occurs; then 0.25–0.6 mg/24 hr to achieve normal Calcium levels.	Monitor serum Ca^{++} and PO_4. Toxicities include hypercalcemia or hypervitaminosis D. More potent than vitamin D_2, but more rapidly inactivated (half-life is hours vs. weeks). Titrate dose with patient response. Oral Ca^{++} supplementation may be required. Activated by 25-hydroxylation in liver; does not require 1-hydroxylation in kidney.

Dimenhydrinate (Dramamine and other brand names)	Tabs (chewable): 50 mg Solution: 12.5 mg/4 ml (90 ml) 16 mg/5 ml Inj: 50 mg/ml	*Children (<12 yr):* 5 mg/kg/24 hr ÷ Q6 hr PO or IM *Adult:* 50–100 mg/dose Q4–6 hr PRN PO, IM, IV **Max PO doses:** 2–6 yr: 75 mg/24 hr 6–12 yr: 150 mg/24 hr Adults: 400 mg/24 hr **Max IM dose: 300 mg/24 hr**	May mask vestibular symptoms. **Caution** when taken with ototoxic agents. Causes drowsiness. Use should be limited to management of prolonged vomiting of *known* etiology. **Not recommended** in children <2 yrs.
Dimercaprol (B.A.L., British anti-Lewisite)	Inj (in oil): 100 mg/ml (3 ml)	Give all injections deep **IM**. *Lead poisoning:* See Chapter 3 for management. *Arsenic or gold poisoning:* Days 1 and 2: 2.5–3 mg/kg/dose Q6 hr Day 3: 2.5–3 mg/kg/dose Q12 hr Days 4–14: 2.5–3 mg/kg/dose Q24 hr	May cause hypertension, tachycardia, GI disturbance, headache, fever (30% of children), transient neutropenia. Symptoms are usually relieved by antihistamines. **Contraindicated** in hepatic or renal insufficiency. Urine *must* be alkaline. May result in renal toxicity. Use **cautiously** in patients with G6PD deficiency. **Do not use** concomitantly with iron.

(Continued.)

Drug	How Supplied	Dose and Route	Remarks
Diphenhydramine (Benadryl and other brand names)	Elixir, syrup: 12.5 mg/5 ml (120 ml) Caps: 25, 50 mg Tabs: 25, 50 mg Injection: 10, 50 mg/ml Cream: 2% (30 gm, 60 gm) Lotion: 1% (75 ml)	*Children:* 5 mg/kg/24 hr ÷ Q6 hr PO/IM/IV (**Max dose:** 300 mg/24 hr) *Adult:* 10–50 mg/dose Q6–8 hr PO/IM/IV (**Max dose:** 400 mg/24 hr) *For anaphylaxis or phenothiazine overdose:* 1–2 mg/kg IV slowly.	Side effects common to antihistamines. CNS side effects more common than GI disturbances. **Contraindicated** in neonates, or with concurrent MAO inhibitor use or acute attacks of asthma.
Disopyramide Phosphate (Norpace and others)	Caps: 100, 150 mg Extended-release caps (CR): 100, 150 mg	*<1 yr:* 10–30 mg/kg/24 hr ÷ Q6 hr PO *1–4 yr:* 10–20 mg/kg/24 hr ÷ Q6 hr PO *4–12 yr:* 10–15 mg/kg/24 hr ÷ Q6 hr PO *12–18 yr:* 6–15 mg/kg/24 hr ÷ Q6 hr PO *Adult:* 200–300 mg/dose × 1 dose PO, then 400–800 mg/24 hr ÷ Q6 hr PO With **extended-release caps,** give same daily dose ÷ Q12 hr.	Modify dose in renal or hepatic failure. May cause decreased cardiac output. Anticholinergic effects may occur. Causes dose-related AV block, wide QRS, increased QTc, ventricular dysrhythmias. Erythromycin may increase serum levels. **Therapeutic levels:** 3–8 mg/L.
Divalproex Sodium (Depakote)	Enteric coated tabs: 125, 250, 500 mg Sprinkle caps: 125 mg	Dose: See Valproic Acid	Remarks: See Valproic Acid. Preferred over valproic acid for patients on ketogenic diet.

Dobutamine (Dobutrex)	Injection: 12.5 mg/ml (contains sulfites)	*Continuous IV infusion:* 2.5–15 µg/kg/min **Max recommended dose:** 40 kg/min. *To prepare infusion:* see inside front cover.	Monitor BP and vital signs. T½: 2 min. Peak effects in 10–20 min. **Contraindicated** in IHSS. Tachycardia, arrhythmias (PVCs) and hypertension may occasionally occur (especially at higher infusion rates). Adjust rate and duration of therapy according to patient response. **Correct hypovolemic states before use.** Increases AV conduction, may precipitate ventricular ectopic activity.
Docusate sodium (Colace and others)	Caps: 50, 240, 250, 300 mg Tabs: 50, 100 mg Syrup: 20 mg/5 ml (240 ml) Solution: 10 mg/1 ml (30 ml), 50 mg/1 ml (60 ml)	*PO:* (take with liquids) <3 yr: 10–40 mg/24 hr ÷ QD-QID 3–6 yr: 20–60 mg/24 hr ÷ QD-QID 6–12 yr: 40–120 mg/24 hr ÷ QD-QID >12 yr: 50–500 mg/24 hr ÷ QD-QID	Oral dosage effective only after 1–3 days of therapy. Incidence of side effects is exceedingly low. Oral solution is bitter; give with milk, fruit juice or formula to mask taste.

(Continued.)

Drug	How Supplied	Dose and Route	Remarks
Docusate sodium (*continued*).		*Rectal:* Older children and adults: add 50–100 mg of oral solution to enema fluid.	
Dopamine (Intropin, Dopastat, and others)	Inj: 40, 80, 160 mg/ml Prediluted in D₅W: 800, 1,600 µg/ml	*Low dose:* 2–5 µg/kg/min IV. Increases renal blood flow. Minimal effect on heart rate and cardiac output. *Intermediate dose:* 5–15 µg/kg/min IV. Increases renal blood flow, heart rate, cardiac contractility, and cardiac output. *High dose:* >20 µg/kg/min IV. Alpha adrenergic effects are prominent. **Decreases** renal perfusion. **Max dose recommended:** 20–50 µg/kg/min IV. *To prepare infusion:* See inside front cover.	Monitor vital signs and blood pressure continuously. **Correct hypovolemic states.** Tachyarrhythmias, ectopic beats, hypertension, vasoconstriction, vomiting may occur. Extravasation may cause tissue necrosis; treat with phentolamine. Use **cautiously** with phenytoin since hypotension and bradycardia may be exacerbated. **Do not use** in pheochromocytoma, tachyarrhythmias, or hypovolemia. Administration into an umbilical arterial catheter is **NOT** recommended.

Doxycycline (Vibramycin and others)	Caps: 50, 100 mg Tabs: 50, 100 mg Syrup: 50 mg/5 ml (30 ml) Susp: 25 mg/5 ml (60 ml) Inj: 100, 200 mg	*Initial:* ≤45 kg: 5 mg/kg/24 hr ÷ BID PO/IV × 1 day to **max dose** of 200 mg/24 hr >45 kg: 200 mg/24 hr ÷ BID PO/IV × 1 day *Maintenance:* ≤45 kg: 2.5–5 mg/kg/24 hr ÷ QD-BID PO or IV >45 kg: 100–200 mg/24 hr ÷ QD-BID PO/IV **Max adult dose:** 300 mg/24 hr PID: see Chapter 17.	Use with **caution** in hepatic and renal disease. May cause increased intracranial pressure. **Do not use** in children <8 yr; may result in tooth enamel hypoplasia and discoloration. May cause GI symptoms, photosensitivity, hemolytic anemia, hypersensitivity reactions. Infuse IV over 1–4 hr. Avoid direct sunlight. See Tetracycline.
Edrophonium chloride (Tensilon)	Inj: 10 mg/ml (1, 10 ml)	*Test for myasthenia gravis (IV):* Neonate: 0.1 mg single dose Infant and Child: 0.2 mg/kg/dose. Give 20% as a test dose slowly; if no re- sponse in 1 min give 1 mg increments to **max** of 10 mg.	Keep **atropine** available in syringe and have resuscitation equipment ready. May precipitate cholinergic crisis, arrhythmias, bronchospasm. Hypersensitivity to test dose (fasciculations or intestinal cramping) is indication to stop

(Continued.)

Drug	How Supplied	Dose and Route	Remarks
Edrophonium chloride (*continued.*).		Adult: 2 mg test dose IV; if no reaction give 8 mg after 45 seconds	giving drug. **Contraindicated in GI or GU obstruction, or arrhythmias.** Short duration of action (minutes). **Antidote: Atropine 0.01–0.04 mg/kg/dose.**
EDTA calcium disodium (Calcium disodium versenate)	Inj: 200 mg/ml (5 ml)	*Lead poisoning* (see Chapter 17 for risk classification; Chapter 3 for treatment regimens): Child: 1–1.5 gm/m²/24 hr IM/IV ÷ Q4–12 hr for 3–5 days depending on severity **or** 50 mg/kg/24 hr IM/IV ÷ Q6–12 hr for 5 days, then 50 mg/kg/24 hr IM/IV ÷ Q8–12 hr for 3–5 days. **Do not exceed 7 days of therapy.** Adult: 2–4 gm/24 hr IV/IM ÷ Q12–24 hr for 5 days; repeat course × 1 after 2 day break. **Max dose:** 75 mg/kg/24 hr	May cause renal tubular necrosis. **Do not use** if anuric. Follow urinalysis and renal function. Monitor ECG continuously for arrhythmia when giving IV. Rapid IV infusion may cause sudden increase in intracranial pressure in patients with cerebral edema. May cause zinc deficiency by chelation effect. Monitor Ca⁺⁺ and PO₄. IM route preferred; give IM with 0.5% procaine.

Enalapril maleate/enalapriat (Vasotec, Vasotec IV)	Tabs: 2.5, 5, 10 and 20 mg (Enalapril) Inj: 1.25 mg/ml (Enalapriat)	*Adult:* 2.5–5 mg PO QD initially up to **max dose** of 40 mg/24 hr ÷ QD-BID IV: 0.625–1.25 mg/dose IV Q6 hr.	Safety and efficacy in children has **not been** established. Use in children only when other measures have been unsuccessful. Reduce dose in renal impairment. Administer IV over 5 min. Enalapril is converted to its active form (Enalapriat) by the liver. Side effects: nausea, diarrhea, headache, dizziness, hypotension, and hypersensitivity may occur.
Epinephrine HCl (Adrenalin and others)	*1:1000 (Aqueous):* Inj: 1 mg/ml (1, 30 ml) *1:200 (Sus-phrine):* Inj: 5 mg/ml (0.3, 0.5 ml) *1:10,000 (Aqueous):* Prefilled syringes: 0.1 mg/ml (10 ml) *Epi-pen:* 0.15, 0.3mg autoinjection.	*1:1000 (Aqueous):* 0.01 ml/kg/dose SC (**max single dose:** 0.3 ml); repeat Q15 min × 3–4 doses or Q4 hr PRN. Adult: 0.3–0.5 ml/dose. *1:200 (Sus-phrine):* 0.005 ml/kg/dose SC (**max single dose:** 0.15 ml); repeat Q8–12 hr PRN. Adult: 0.1–0.3 ml/dose.	May produce arrhythmias, tachycardia, hypertension, headaches, nervousness, nausea, vomiting. Necrosis may occur at site of repeated local injection. May be given via ETT. Do not use in acute coronary disease, hyperthyroidism, hypertension, diabetes.

(Continued.)

Drug	How Supplied	Dose and Route	Remarks
Epinephrine HCl *(continued.).*	*Aerosol:* Each contains 300 metered doses equivalent to 0.16 mg/dose or 0.2 mg/dose of epinephrine (15 ml)	*Inhalation:* 1–2 puffs during attack. Repeat Q4 hr PRN. *Bradycardia/hypotension:* (1:10,000) Child: 0.1 ml/kg IV Q3–5 min Adult: 5 ml IV Q3–5 min IV drip: 0.1–1 μg/kg/min, titrated to effect. *To prepare infusion:* see inside front cover. *Nebulization* (alternative to racemic epinephrine): 0.5 ml/kg of 1:1000 (1 mg/ml) concentration diluted in 3 ml NS. **Max dose:** ≤4 yr: 2.5 ml/dose >4 yr: 5 ml/dose	
Epinephrine, racemic (Vaponefrin, Micronefrin, Asthmanefrin)	Solution: 2.25% (7.5, 15, 30 ml), 2% (15, 30 ml)	*Croup:* 0.05 ml/kg/dose diluted to 3 ml with saline. Given via nebulizer over 15 min PRN, but not more frequently than Q2 hr. **Max dose:** 0.5 ml	Tachyarrhythmias, headache, nausea, palpitations reported. Observe patient for recurrence of symptoms if indicated.

Epoetin alfa (Epogen, Procrit)	2,000, 3,000, 4,000, 10,000 U/ml	*Renal failure:* 50–100 U/kg 3× wk SC/IV *AZT-treated HIV patients:* 100U/kg/dose 3× wk SC/IV for 8 wks. *Anemia of prematurity:* 25–100 U/kg/dose SC 3× wk	Evaluate serum iron, ferritin, TIBC before therapy. Monitor Hct, BP, clotting times, platelets, BUN, serum creatinine. **Peak** effect in 2–3 wk. Reduce drugs when target Hct is reached, or when Hct increases >4 points in any 2-wk period. May cause hypertension, seizure, hypersensitivity reactions, headache, edema, dizziness.
Ergocalciferol (Drisdol, Calciferol, vitamin D_2)	Caps: 25,000 IU (0.625 mg); 50,000 IU (1.25 mg) Tabs: 50,000 IU Solution: 10,000 IU (0.25 mg/ml) Inj: 500,000 IU/ml Drops: 8,000 IU/ml (200 IU/gtt) (60ml) 1 mg = 40,000 IU	*Dietary supplementation:* *Preterm:* 400–800 IU/24 hr PO *Infants/Children:* 400 IU/24 hr PO; please refer to Chapter 22 for details. *Renal osteodystrophy:* 25,000–250,000 IU/24 hr PO until healing occurs, then 10,000–25,000 IU/24 hr PO	Monitor serum Ca^{++}, PO_4, and alkaline phos. Serum Ca^{++}, PO_4 product should be <70 mg/dl. Titrate dosage to patient response. Watch for symptoms of hypercalcemia: weakness, diarrhea, polyuria, metastatic calcification, nephrocalcinosis. Vitamin D_2 is activated by

(Continued.)

Drug	How Supplied	Dose and Route	Remarks
Ergocalciferol (continued.).		*Rickets:* Vitamin D-dependent: 5,000–60,000 IU/24 hr PO Vitamin D-resistant: 25,000–1,000,000 IU/24 hr PO Nutritional: 10,000 IU/24 hr × 30 days **or** 100,000 IU/dose × 1 PO.	25-hydroxylation in liver and 1-hydroxylation in kidney. May use IM route in cases of fat malabsorption.
Ergotamine (Cafergot and others)	Tabs: 1 mg and caffeine (100 mg) Sublingual tabs: 2 mg Supp: 2 mg and caffeine (100 mg)	*Older children and adolescents:* 1 tab at onset of attack then 1 tab Q30 min PRN up to **max 3 tabs** *Adults:* 2 tablets at onset of attack; then one tablet Q 30 min. up to 6 per attack. Suppository: 1 at first sign of attack; follow with second dose after 1 hour. Max. dose 2 per attack, not to exceed 5/week.	Caution in renal or hepatic disease. May cause paresthesias, or disturbance, muscle cramps, nausea, vomiting.
Erythromycin preparations (Erythrocin, Pediamycin, E-Mycin, Ery-Ped, and others)	*Erythromycin base:* Caps: 125, 250 mg Tabs: 250, 333, 500 mg Topical solution: 1.5%, 2% (60 ml)	*Oral:* Neonates: ≤7 days or <1.2 kg (0–4 wk): 20 mg/kg/24 hr ÷ Q12 hr	Avoid IM route (pain, necrosis). GI side effects common (nausea, vomiting, abdominal cramps). Give doses after meals. Use with **caution** in

Ophthalmic oint: 0.5% (3.75 gm)

Erythromycin ethyl succinate (EES):
Susp: 200, 400 mg/5 ml (60, 100, 200 ml)
Drops: 100 mg/2.5 ml (50 ml)
Tabs: 200, 400 mg

Erythromycin lactobionate:
Inj: 500, 1000 mg

Erythromycin estolate:
Tabs: 500 mg
Chewable tabs: 125, 250 mg
Drops: 100 mg/ml (10 ml)
Caps: 125, 250 mg
Susp: 125, 250 mg/5 ml

Erythromycin stearate:
Tabs: 125, 250, 500 mg

Erythromycin gluceptate
Inj: 250, 500, 1000 mg

>7 days and ≥1.2 kg: 30 mg/kg/24 hr ÷ Q8 hr
Children: 30–50 mg/kg/24 hr ÷ Q6–8 hr. **Max dose: 2 gm/24 hr**
Adults: 1–4 gm/24 hr ÷ Q6 hr; **max dose: 4 gm/24 hr**
Parenteral:
Children: 20–50 mg/kg/24 hr ÷ Q6 hr IV or as continuous infusion.
Adults: 15–20 mg/kg/24 hr ÷ Q6 hr IV or as continuous infusion. **Max dose: 4 gm/24 hr**
Rheumatic fever prophylaxis: 500 mg/24 hr ÷ Q12 hr PO
Endocarditis prophylaxis: See Chapter 6.
Ophthalmic: Apply 0.5 in. ribbon to affected eye BID-QID
Pertussis: Use estolate salt 50 mg/kg/24 hr PO ÷ Q6 hr
Preoperative bowel prep: 20 mg/kg/dose PO erythromycin base × 3 doses, with neomycin, 1 day before surgery.

liver disease. Estolate may cause cholestatic jaundice, although hepatotoxicity is uncommon (2% of reported cases). May produce elevated digoxin, theophylline, carbamazepine, cyclosporine, methylprednisolone levels. Oral therapy should replace IV as soon as possible. Because of different absorption characteristics, higher oral doses of EES are needed to achieve therapeutic effects. May produce false positive urinary catecholamines. Formulations of IV lactobionate dosage form may contain benzyl alcohol. **Note: formulations other than the estolate have a high incidence of relapse in the treatment of pertussis.**

(Continued.)

Drug	How Supplied	Dose and Route	Remarks
Erythromycin ethylsuccinate and acetyl sulfisoxazole (Pediazole)	Susp: 200 mg erythromycin and 600 mg sulfa/5 ml (100, 150, 200 ml)	*Otitis media:* 50 mg/kg/24 hr (as erythromycin) and 150 mg/kg/24 hr (as sulfa) ÷ Q6 hr PO **or** give 1.25 ml/kg/24 hr ÷ Q6 hr PO **Max dose:** 6 gm sulfisoxazole/24 hr	See adverse effects of erythromycin and sulfisoxazole. Not recommended in infants <2 mo old.
Ethambutol HCl (Myambutol)	Tabs: 100, 400 mg	*Adolescents and adults:* 15–25 mg/kg/24 hr as single PO dose **or** 50 mg/kg/dose twice weekly up to **max dose** of 2.5 gm/day.	May cause reversible optic neuritis, especially with larger doses. Obtain baseline ophthalmologic studies before beginning therapy and then monthly. Follow visual acuity, visual fields, and (red-green) color vision. Discontinue if any visual deterioration occurs. Monitor uric acid, heme status and renal function. May cause GI disturbances. Give with food. Adjust dose with renal failure. **Not recommended for children ≤12 yr old.**

Ethosuximide (Zarontin)	Caps: 250 mg Syrup: 250 mg/5 ml	*Initial:* 3–6 yr: 250 mg/24 hr ÷ QD-BID PO >6 yr: 500 mg/24 hr ÷ QD-BID PO Adults: 750 mg/24 hr ÷ QD *Increment:* Increase by 250 mg/24 hr every 4–7 days *Maintenance:* 3–6 yr: 20–40 mg/kg/dose QD >6 yr: 20–30 mg/kg/dose QD Adults: 750–1500 mg/dose QD **Max dose:** 1500 mg/24 hr	Monitor levels. Use with **caution** in hepatic and renal disease. Ataxia, anorexia, drowsiness, sleep disturbances, rashes, and blood dyscrasias are rare idiosyncratic reactions. May cause lupus-like syndrome; may increase frequency of grand mal seizures in patients with mixed type seizures. To minimize GI distress, may administer with food or milk. **Therapeutic levels:** 40–100 mg/L.
Famotidine (Pepcid)	Inj: 10 mg/ml (multidose vials contain 0.9% benzyl alcohol) Liquid: 40 mg/5ml (contains parabens) Tabs: 20, 40 mg	*Children:* IV: Initial: 0.6–0.8 mg/kg/24 hr ÷ Q8–12 hr up to a **max** of 40 mg/24 hr. PO: Initial: 1–1.2 mg/kg/24 hr ÷ Q8–12 hr up to a **max** of 40 mg/24 hr.	**Pediatric dosage not well established.** A Q12 hr dosage interval is generally recommended; however, infants and young children may require a Q8 hr interval due to enhanced elimination.

(Continued.)

Drug	How Supplied	Dose and Route	Remarks
Famotidine *(continued.)*.		*Adult:* PO: 20 mg BID or 40 mg QHS IV: 20 mg BID	Headaches, dizziness, constipation, diarrhea, and drowsiness have occurred. Dosage adjustment is required in severe renal failure.
Fentanyl (Sublimaze, Duragesic, and others)	Injection: 50 μg/ml SR patch: 25, 50, 75, 100 μg/hr	1–2 μg/kg/dose IM or IV Q30–60 min PRN. May be used as continuous IV infusion. Start with 1 μg/kg/hr; titrate to effect. **Max dose:** 3 μg/kg/hr. See Chapter 27 for equianalgesic dosing.	Onset of action 1–2 min with a peak action about 10 min. As with other opiates, respiratory depression occurs and may persist beyond the period of analgesia. May cause chest wall rigidity in neonates. Give IV dose over 3–5 min; rapid infusion may cause respiratory depression. Safety and efficacy for transdermal patch has not been established in pediatrics.
Ferrous sulfate (See Iron Preparations)			
Filgrastim (G-CSF Neupogen)	Inj: 300 μg/ml	Initial: 5 μg/kg/dose QD SC/IV; continue for up to 14 days, or until ANC of	Pediatric dosage and efficacy have **not been** well established. May cause bone

10,000/mm^3. Dosage may be increased in 5-µg/kg increments for each chemotherapy cycle. Discontinue therapy when ANC >10,000/mm^3.

pain, fever, rash. Monitor CBC, platelets, uric acid, liver function tests. **Contraindicated** for patients sensitive to *E. coli*-derived proteins. SC routes of administration preferred because of prolonged serum levels over IV route.

Flecainide acetate (Tambocor)	Tabs: 50, 100, 150 mg	*Children:* 3–6 mg/kg/24 hr ÷ Q8–12 hr PO. *Adults:* 100 mg PO Q12 hr. May increase dose by 50 mg Q12 hr every 4 days to **max dose** of 400 mg/24 hr.	Safety and efficacy in children have not been established. Give $\frac{1}{2}$–$\frac{1}{4}$ dose when GFR <20 ml/min. May aggravate LV failure, sinus bradycardia, preexisting ventricular arrhythmias. May cause AV block, dizziness, blurred vision, dyspnea, nausea, headache, increased PR or QRS intervals. Reserve for life-threatening cases. **Trough level:** <0.7–1 mg/L.

(Continued.)

Drug	How Supplied	Dose and Route	Remarks
Flucanazole (Diflucan)	Tabs: 50, 100, 200 mg Inj: 2 mg/ml	*Children (3–13 yr):* Loading dose: 10 mg/kg IV/PO, then Maintenance: (begin 24 hr after loading dose) 3–6 mg/kg/24 hr IV/PO QD *Adults:* *Oropharyngeal and esophageal candidiasis:* Loading dose of 200 mg PO/IV followed by 100 mg QD 24 hr after. Doses up to **max dose** of 400 mg/24 hr may be used for esophageal candidiasis. *Systemic candidiasis:* Loading dose of 400 mg PO/IV, followed by 200 mg QD 24 hr later. *Cryptococcal meningitis:* Loading dose of 400 mg PO/IV, followed by 200–400 mg QD 24 hr later.	PO and IV doses are equivalent. May cause nausea, headache, rash, vomiting, abdominal pain, and diarrhea. Reduce maintenance dose in renal dysfunction (see Chapter 26). May interact with warfarin, phenytoin, cyclosporin, oral hypoglycemic agents, and rifampin.

Flucytosine (Ancobon, 5-FC, 5-Fluorocytosine)	Caps: 250, 500 mg Oral liquid*: 10 mg/ml	*Neonates:* 20–40 mg/kg/dose Q6 hr PO *Children and adults:* 50–150 mg/kg/24 hr ÷ Q6 hr PO	Common side effects: nausea, vomiting, diarrhea, rash, CNS disturbance, anemia, leukopenia, thrombocytopenia. Monitor CBC, BUN, serum creatinine, alkaline phos, AST, ALT (see Chapter 26). **Therapeutic levels:** 25–100 mg/L
Fludrocortisone acetate (Florinef acetate, 9-Fluorohydrocortisone)	Tabs: 0.1 mg	*Infants:* 0.05–0.1 mg/24 hr QD PO *Children and adults:* 0.05–0.2 mg/24 hr QD PO; titrate dose to suppress plasma renin activity to normal levels.	**Contraindicated** in CHF, systemic fungal infections. Preferably administered in conjunction with cortisone or hydrocortisone. Has primarily mineral ocorticoid activity. If BP rises, decrease dose to 0.05 mg/24 hr. 0.1 mg 9-fluorocortisol = 1mg DOCA (see Chapter 26).
Flunisolide (Nasalide, Aerobid)	Nasal solution: 25 µg/spray (200 sprays/bottle) Aerosol inhaler: 250 µg/dose (50 doses/inhaler)	*Nasal solution* (for nasal use only): *Children:* (6–14 yr): 1 spray per nostril TID or 2 sprays per nostril BID	Reduce dose to smallest maintenance dose that will control symptoms. Stop gradually after 3 wk if no clinical improvement is seen.

*Indicates suspensions not commercially available; need to be extemporaneously compounded by a pharmacist. See references 6 and 7 for specific formulations.

(Continued.)

Drug	How Supplied	Dose and Route	Remarks
Flunisolide (*continued.*).		**Max dose: 4 sprays/** nostril/24 hr *Adult:* 2 sprays/nostril BID **Max dose: 8** sprays/nostril/24 hr. *Inhaler:* *Children >6 yr:* 1 puff BID, up to 4 puffs/24 hr *Adults:* 2 puffs BID, **max dose: 8 puffs/24 hr**	Shake inhaler well before use. Rinse mouth after administering drug.
Flouride (Luride, Fluoritab and others)	Solution: 0.5, 2, 2.25, 5.5, 5.9 mg/ml Chewable tabs: 0.25, 0.5, 1.0 mg Tabs: 1 mg (expressed as fluoride ion)	Dose/24 hr Concentration of flouride in drinking water (ppm): | Age	<0.3	0.3–0.7	>0.7 | |---|---|---|---| | 2 wk–2 yr | 0.25 mg | 0 | 0 | | 2–3 yr | 0.5 mg | 0.25 mg | 0 | | 3–16 yr | 1.0 mg | 0.50 mg | 0 |	Acute overdose: GI distress, salivation, CNS irritability, tetany, seizures, hypocalcemia, hypoglycemia, cardiorespiratory failure. Chronic excess use may result in mottled teeth or bone changes.

Flumazenil
(Mazicon)

Inj: 0.1 mg/ml (5, 10 ml)

For management of suspected benzodiazepine overdose:
0.3 mg IV. If desired level of consciousness is not obtained, administer additional doses of 0.3 mg at 1 min intervals up to **max cumulative dose** of 3 mg.

For IV use only, using a freely running infusion into a large vein. Infuse over 30 sec. **Contraindicated** if patient shows signs of TCA coingestion or if using benzodiazepines for seizure management. May cause seizures in some patients. Use with **caution** in patients with hepatic impairment. Safety and efficacy in children **has not** been established. Use in reversing conscious sedation is controversial.

Folic acid
(Folvite and others)

Tabs: 0.1, 0.4, 0.8, 1.0 mg
Oral solution*: 1 mg/ml
Inj: 5, 10 mg/ml

Folic acid deficiency load:
Infants: 15 μg/kg/dose QD;
max dose: 50 μg/kg/24 hr
Children: 0.5–1. mg/24 hr QD
Adult: 1–3 mg/24 hr ÷ QD-TID

Normal levels: serum >4 ng/ml, whole blood >50 ng/ml. May mask hematologic effects of vitamin B_{12} deficiency, but will not prevent progression of neurologic abnormalities. May give PO, IM, IV, or SC.

*Indicates suspensions not commercially available; need to be extemporaneously compounded by a pharmacist. See references 6 and 7 for specific formulations. *(Continued.)*

Drug	How Supplied	Dose and Route	Remarks
Folic acid *(continued.)*.		*Maintenance:* Premature infants: 50 µg/24 hr <1 yr: 30–45 µg/24 hr 1–3 yr: 100 µg/24 hr 4–6 yr: 200 µg/24 hr 7–10 yr: 300 µg/24 hr 11 yr–adult: 400 µg/24 hr Pregnant, lactating women: 800 µg/24 hr	
Furosemide (Furomide, Lasix and others)	Tabs: 20, 40, 80 mg Inj: 10 mg/ml Oral liquid: 10 mg/ml (60 ml), 40 mg/5 ml	*Oral:* Infants and children: 2 mg/kg/dose Q6–8 hr PRN; may increase by 1–2 mg/kg/dose Adult: 20–80 mg/24 hr QD or BID; may increase 20 or 40 mg up to total of 600 mg/24 hr *Parenteral:* Infants and children: 1 mg/kg/dose Q6–12 hr IM or IV PRN; may increase by 1 mg/kg/dose Adult: 20–80 mg/dose IM/IV; **max single dose** (PO, IM, IV): 6 mg/kg	Ototoxicity may occur in presence of renal disease, especially when used with aminoglycosides. Use with caution in hepatic disease. May cause hypokalemia, alkalosis, dehydration, hyperuricemia, and increased calcium excretion. Prolonged use in premature infants may result in nephrocalcinosis. **Max rate of infusion:** 0.5mg/kg/min.

Gamma benzene hexachloride (Kwell, Lindane, Scabene)	Shampoo: 1% (60, 480 ml) Lotion: 1% (60, 480 ml) Cream: 1% (57, 450 gm)	*Shampoo:* Use ≤30 ml/application. Leave in place 4–8 min before rinsing. Repeat in 7 days if lice or mites still present. *Lotion:* Apply to skin, leave on 8–12 hr, then wash off. Change clothing and bedsheets after starting treatment. Treat family members. **Note:** Second application usually not necessary but may repeat application in 7–10 days if lice persist.	Systemically absorbed. Risk of toxic effects is greater in young children; use other agents (permethrin) in infants, young children, and during pregnancy. Avoid contact with face, urethral meatus, or mucous membranes. May cause a rash; rarely may cause seizures or aplastic anemia.
Ganciclovir (Cytovene)	Inj: 500 mg	*Cytomegalovirus infections:* Children >3 mo and adults: Induction therapy: 5 mg/kg/dose Q12 hr IV or 2–5 mg/kg/dose Q8 hr IV for 14–21 days	Limited experience with use in children <12 yr old. **Use with extreme caution.** Reduce dose in renal failure (see Chapter 26). Common side effects: neutropenia, thrombocytopenia, retinal

(Continued.)

Drug	How Supplied	Dose and Route	Remarks
Ganciclovir *(continued.)*.		Maintenance therapy: 5 mg/kg/dose QD IV or 6 mg/kg/dose QD IV for 5days/wk	detachment, confusion. Drug reactions alleviated with dose reduction or temporary interruption. Minimum dilution is 10 mg/ml and should be infused IV over ≥1 hr. IM and SC administration are **contraindicated** because of high pH (pH = 11).
Gentamicin (Garamycin and others)	Inj: 10, 40 mg/ml Ophthalmic ointment: 0.3% (3.5 gm) Drops: 0.3% (5 ml) Topical ointment: 0.1% Intrathecal inj.: 2 mg/ml	*Parenteral (IM or IV):* Neonates: 2.5 mg/kg/dose IV/IM Children: 6–7.5 mg/kg/24 hr ÷ Q8 hr Adults: 3–5 mg/kg/24 hr ÷ Q8 hr **Max dose:** 300 mg/24 hr	Monitor levels (peak and trough) after steady state is achieved. Monitor renal status: may cause proximal tubule dysfunction. Watch for ototoxicity. Intrathecal or intraventricular administration is adjunctive to parenteral administration. **Therapeutic levels:** 6–10 mg/L **(peak)**; <2 mg/L **(trough)**. Eliminated more quickly in patients with cystic fibrosis, multiple sclerosis, burn patients, or neutropenic patients.

Dosing Interval

	Postnatal Age	
Gestational Age	≤7 Days	>7 days
<28 wk	Q24 hr	Q18 hr
28–34 wk	Q18 hr	Q12 hr
>34 wk	Q12 hr	Q8 hr

Intrathecal/intraventricular:
>3 mo: 1–2 mg daily
Adult: 4–8 mg daily
Ophthalmic ointment: apply
Q6–8 hr
Ophthalmic drops: 1–2 drops
Q4 hr

Glucagon HCl (Glucagon)	Inj: 1, 10 mg/vial (1 unit = 1 mg)	*For hypoglycemia:* <10 kg: 0.1 mg/kg IM, SC, IV up to 1 mg Q30 min. ≥10 kg: 1 mg/dose IM, SC, IV Q30 min or Children: 0.03–0.1 mg/kg/dose IM, SC, IV Q5–20 min. **Max dose:** 1 mg/dose. Adults: 0.5–1 mg/dose IM, IV, SC Q5–20 min.	Also noted to have cardiostimulatory effect at high doses even in the presence of beta blockade. **Do not** delay starting glucose infusion while awaiting effect of glucagon.
Glycopyrrolate (Robinul)	Tabs: 1, 2 mg Inj: 0.2 mg/ml	*Respiratory antisecretory:* Children: 0.004–0.01 mg/kg/dose Q4–8 hr IV/IM Adults: 0.1–0.2 mg/dose Q4–8 hr IV/IM. **Max dose:** 0.2 mg/dose or 0.8 mg/24 hr	Atropine-like side effects: tachycardia, nausea, constipation, confusion, bronchospasm, blurred vision and dry mouth. Use with **caution** in hepatic and renal disease, ulcerative colitis, asthma, glaucoma, ileus, or

(Continued.)

Drug	How Supplied	Dose and Route	Remarks
Glycopyrrolate (*continued.*).		*Reverse neuromuscular block:* 0.2 mg per each mg neostigmine IV *Oral:* Adult: 1–2 mg BID-TID Children: Dose not established	urinary retention. PO dose is about 10 times the IV dose.
Griseofulvin microcrystalline (Grifulvin V, Grisactin, Fulvicin)	*Microsize:* Tabs: 250, 500 mg Caps: 125, 250 mg Susp: 125 mg/5 ml (120ml) *Ultramicrosize tabs:* 125, 165, 250, 330 mg, 250 mg ultra ~500 mg micro.	*Microsize:* Children >2 yr: 10–15 mg/kg/24 hr PO QD; give with milk, eggs, fatty foods. Adult: 500–1000 mg/24 hr QD. **Max dose:** 1 gm/24 hr *Ultramicrosize:* Children >2 yr: 7 mg/kg/24 hr PO QD. Adults: 330–750 mg/24 hr PO ÷ BID-QD.	Monitor hematologic, renal, and hepatic function. May cause leukopenia. Possible cross-reactivity in penicillin-allergic patients. **Contraindicated** in porphyria, hepatic disease. Usual treatment period is 4–6 wk (for tinea unguium, 4–6 mo). Photosensitivity reactions may occur.
Haloperidol (Haldol and others)	Inj (IM use only): 5 mg/ml; 50, 100 mg/ml (decanoate) Tabs: 0.5, 1, 2, 5, 10, 20 mg Solution: 2 mg/ml (15, 20 ml)	*Children 3–12 yr:* Agitation: 0.01–0.03 mg/kg/24 hr QD PO Psychosis: 0.05–0.15 mg/kg/24 hr ÷ BID-TID PO	Use with **caution** in patients with cardiac disease because of the risk of hypotension and in patients with epilepsy since the drug lowers the seizure

		threshold. Acutely aggravated patients may require doses as often as Q60 min. Extrapyramidal symptoms can occur. For treatment of toxicity see Chapter 3. Safety and efficacy of IM administration in children have not been established. Decanoate salt is given every 3–4 wk in doses that are 10–15 times the individual patient's stabilized oral dose.
	Tourette's syndrome: 0.05–0.075 mg/kg/24 hr ÷ BID-TID PO; may increase dose by 0.5 mg/24 hr. *>12 yr:* Acute agitation: 2–5 mg IM **or** 1–15 mg PO. Repeat in 1 hr if needed. Psychosis: 2–5 mg/dose Q4–8 hr IM PRN **or** 1–15 mg/24 hr ÷ BID-TID PO; **max dose:** 100 mg/24 hr. Tourette's 6–15 mg/24 hr ÷ BID-TID PO	
Heparin sodium (various trade names)	Inj: 10; 100; 1,000; 2,500; 5,000; 7,500; 10,000; 20,000; 40,000 U/ml Repository inj; 20,000 U/ml 120 U = ~1 mg	Adjust dose to give clotting time of 20–30 min or PTT of 1.5–2.5 times control value before dose. Toxicities: bleeding, allergy, alopecia, thrombocytopenia. Use preservative-free heparin in neonates. **Note:** heparin flush doses may alter PTT in small patients; consider using more dilute heparin in these cases.
	Infants and children: Initial: 50 U/kg IV bolus Maintenance: 10–25 U/kg/hr as constant infusion, **or** 50–100 U/kg/dose Q4 hr IV *Adults:* Initial: 5,000–10,000 U IV bolus Maintenance: 20,000–40,000 U IV/24 hr as constant infusion **or** 5,000–10,000 units Q4–6 hr IV	

(Continued.)

Drug	How Supplied	Dose and Route	Remarks
Heparin sodium (*continued.*).		*DVT prophylaxis:* 5,000 U/dose SC Q8–12 hr until ambulatory *Heparin flush:* Peripheral IV: 1–2 ml of 10 U/ml solution Q4 hr Central lines: 2–3 ml of 100 U/ml solution Q24 hr Flush dose should be less than heparinizing dose!	**Antidote:** Protamine sulfate (1 mg per 100 U heparin in previous 4 hr).
Hydralazine (Apresoline)	Tabs: 10, 25, 50, 100 mg Inj: 20 mg/ml Oral liquid*: 2 mg/ml	*Hypertensive crisis:* Children: 0.1–0.2 mg/kg/dose IM or IV Q4–6 hr PRN (Not to exceed 20mg) Adults: 10–50 mg IM or IV Q3–6 hr PRN *Chronic hypertension:* Children: 0.75–3 mg/kg/24 hr ÷ Q6–12 hr PO. **Max dose:** 200mg/24 hr or 7.5 mg/kg/24 hr Adults: 10–50 mg/dose PO QID. **Max dose:** 300 mg/24 hr.	Use with **caution** in severe renal and cardiac disease. May cause lupus-like syndrome (generally reversible). CV, neurologic, GI, hematologic, dermatologic reactions may be seen. Follow blood pressure closely. May cause reflex tachycardia. Maximum effect seen in 3–4 days.

Hydrochlorothiazide, USP (Esidrix, Hydro-T, Thiuretic, Hydrodiuril and others)	Tabs: 25, 50, 100 mg	*Infants and children:* 2–3 mg/kg/24 hr ÷ BID PO *Adult:* 25–100 mg/24 hr ÷ QD-BID PO **Max adult dose:** 200 mg/24 hr	See chlorothiazide. May cause fluid and electrolyte imbalances, hyperuricemia.
Hydrocortisone (Solu-cortef)	Tabs: 5, 10, 20 mg Susp: 10 mg/5 ml (120 ml) *Na Phosphate* Inj: 50 mg/ml *Na Succinate (Solu-Cortef):* Inj: 100, 250, 500, 1000 mg/vial *Acetate (Hydrocortone):* Inj: 25, 50 mg/ml	*Physiologic replacement/stress doses:* See Special Drugs, Chapter 26. *Status asthmaticus (loading)* (**max dose:** 4–8 mg/kg/dose (max dose: 250 mg) then 8 mg/kg/24 hr ÷ Q6 hr IV *Adult:* 100–500 mg/dose Q6 hr IV *Anti-inflammatory:* 0.8–4 mg/kg/24 hr ÷ Q6 hr IV	Na succinate used for IV dosing. Na phosphate may be given IM, SC, or IV. A corticosteroid with less mineralocorticoid activity is recommended for prolonged use (see Chapter 26).
Hydromorphone HCl (Dilaudid, and others)	Tabs: 1, 2, 3, 4 mg Inj: 1, 2, 3, 4, 10 mg/ml (contains benzyl alcohol) Suppository: 3 mg	*Analgesia:* *Older children/adults:* 1–4 mg/dose Q4–6 hr PO/IV/IM/SC. *Oral Antitussive:* *Children 6–12 yr:* 0.5 mg Q3–4 hr PRN *>12 yr:* 1 mg Q3–4 hr PRN	Refer to Chapter 27 for details of use. See morphine for side effects and warnings. Side effects may be less frequent with the use of this drug, as compared to morphine.

*Indicates suspensions not commercially available; need to be extemporaneously compounded by a pharmacist. See references 6 and 7 for specific formulations.

(Continued.)

Drug	How Supplied	Dose and Route	Remarks
Hydroxyzine (Atarax, Vistaril)	Tabs (HCl): 10, 25, 50, 100 mg Caps (pamoate): 25, 50, 100 mg Syrup (HCl): 10 mg/5 ml Susp (pamoate): 25 mg/5 ml (120 ml) Inj (HCl): 25, 50 mg/ml	*Oral:* Children: 2 mg/kg/hr ÷ Q6 hr Adult: 25–100 mg/dose TID-QID *IM:* Children: 0.5–1.0 mg/kg/dose Q4–6 hr PRN Adult: 25–100 mg/dose Q4–6 hr PRN. (**max dose: 600 mg/24 hr.)**	May potentiate barbiturates, meperidine, and other depressants. May cause dry mouth, drowsiness, tremor, convulsions, blurred vision, hypotension. May cause pain at injection site. IV administration is **not** recommended.
Ibuprofen (Motrin, Advil, Nuprin, Medipren, Children's Motrin, and others)	Suspension: 100 mg/5 ml Tabs: 200, 300, 400, 600, 800 mg	*Children:* Antipyretic: 20 mg/kg/24 hr ÷ Q8 hr PO JRA: 20—40 mg/kg/24 hr ÷ Q6–8 hr PO **Max dose:** 40 mg/kg/24 hr *Adults:* Inflammatory disease: 400–800 mg/dose Q6–8 hr Pain/fever/dysmenorrhea: 200–400 mg/dose Q4–6 hr **Max dose:** 3.2 gm/24 hr	GI distress (lessened with milk), rashes, ocular problems, granulocytopenia, anemia. Inhibits platelet aggregation. Use **caution** with aspirin hypersensitivity, or hepatic/renal insufficiency.

Imipenem-Cilastatin (Primaxin)	Inj: 250, 500, 750 mg. Each gram contains 3.2 mEq Na.	*Children >12 yr:* 50–100 mg/kg/24 hr ÷ Q6–8 hr IV *Adults:* 250–1000 mg/dose Q6–8 hr IV **Max dose:** 4 gm/24 hr or 50 mg/kg/24 hr, whichever is less	For IV use, give slowly over 30–60 minutes. Adverse effects: pruritus, urticaria, GI symptoms, seizures, dizziness, hypotension, elevated LFTs, blood dyscrasias, and penicillin allergy. Safety and efficacy in children <12 yr has **not** been established.
Imipramine (Tofranil, Janimine)	Tabs: 10, 25, 50 mg Caps: 75, 100, 125, 150 mg Inj: 12.5 mg/ml	*Anti-depressant:* Not FDA approved for age <12 yr Children: Initial: 1.5 mg/kg/24 hr ÷ TID PO Increment: increase 1–1.5 mg/kg/24 hr Q3–4 days to **max** of 5 mg/kg/24 hr. Adult: Initial: 75–100 mg/24 hr ÷ TID PO Maintenance: 50–300 mg/24 hr QHS	Minor side effects include dry mouth, drowsiness, constipation, dizziness. One evening dose may reduce sedation during first weeks of therapy. Monitor ECG, BP, CBC at start of therapy and with dose changes. Decrease dose if PR interval reaches 0.22 sec, QRS reaches 130% of baseline, HR rises above 140/min, or if BP is more than 140/90. Tricyclics may cause mania.

(Continued.)

Drug	How Supplied	Dose and Route	Remarks
Imipramine (*continued*).		**Max PO dose: 300 mg/24 hr**	**Therapeutic levels** for depression: 150–225 ng/ml. Janimine 10 and 25 mg tablets and Tofranil PM 100 and 125 mg capsules contain tartrazine, which may cause allergic reactions. PO route preferred. May be given IM.
		Max initial IM dose: 100 mg/24 hr	
		Enuresis:	
		Not recommended in children <6 yr.	
		Initial: 10–25 mg QHS PO	
		Increment: 10–25 mg/dose at 1–2 wk intervals until max dose for age or desired effect achieved. Continue × 2–3 mo, then taper slowly.	
		Max dose:	
		6–12 yr: 50 mg/24 hr	
		12–14 yr: 75 mg/24 hr	
Immune Globulin (Gamastan, Gammagard, Sandoglobulin, Gamimune-N)	Gamastan: 165 ± 5 mg/ml Gammagard, Sandoglobulin: 0.5, 1, 2.5, 3, 5, 6, 10 gm/vial Gamimune-N: 50 mg/ml	See indications and doses in Chapter 15. **Note:** Gamastan is an IM preparation; Gammagard, Sandoglobulin, and Gamimune-N are IV preparations. Infusion rates vary among manufacturers. In general, start with a low dose and increase slowly to maximum rate.	May cause tenderness, erythema, and induration at injection site, flushing, chills, fever, headache. Rare hypersensitivity reaction, especially when given rapidly. Gamimune-N contains maltose and may cause an osmotic diuresis.

Indomethacin
(Indocin)

Caps: 25, 50 mg
Sustained-release caps: 75 mg
Inj: 1 mg
Suppositories: 50 mg
Suspension: 25 mg/5ml

Anti-inflammatory:
>14 yr old: 1–3 mg/kg/24 hr
÷ TID-QID PO.
Max dose: 200 mg/24 hr.
Adults: 50–150 mg/24 hr ÷
BID-QID PO.
Closure of ductus arteriosus:
0.1–0.25 mg/kg/dose IV over
20–30 min. Repeat at
intervals of 12–24 hr up to
a total of 3 doses.

Age	Dose (mg/kg)		
	1	2	3
<48 hr	0.20	0.10	0.10
2–7 days	0.20	0.20	0.20
>7 days	0.20	0.25	0.25

In neonates, monitor renal and
hepatic function before and
during use. **Contraindicated**
in neonates with BUN ≥30
mg/dl and Cr ≥1.8 mg/dl.
Keep urine output >0.6
ml/kg/hr. IV is the preferred
route of administration for
treatment of PDA. May cause
decrease platelet aggregation
and GI distress (ulcer,
nausea, diarrhea), headache,
blood dyscrasias. Some early
evidence suggests that
duration of therapy should be
prolonged in specific
instances.

Insulin

Many preparations, at
concentrations of 40, 100
U/ml

Insulin preparations: See
Chapter 26.
Hyperkalemia: See Chapters 2
and 10.
DKA: See Chapter 2.

(Continued.)

Drug	How Supplied	Dose and Route	Remarks
Ipecac	Syrup: 70 mg/ml (15, 30, 473, 4000 ml) (contains 1.5–2% alcohol)	See Chapter 3 for indications. 6–12 mos: 5–10 ml Ipecac with 10–20 ml/kg water. 1–12 yr: 15 ml ipecac with 10–20 ml/kg water.	May cause GI irritation, cardiotoxicity.
Ipratropium bromide (Atrovent)	Aerosol: 18 μg/dose (200 inhalations/canister)	*Children <12 yr:* 1–2 puffs Q6–8 hr *Children ≥12 yr:* 2–4 puffs Q6 hr up to 12 puffs/24 hr	Safety and efficacy for use in children <12 yr has not been established. **Not** indicated for the initial treatment of acute bronchospasm. Shake inhaler well prior to use. Use with **caution** in narrow-angle glaucoma or bladder neck obstruction.
Iron dextran (InFeD)	Inj: 50mg/ml (contains 50 mg elemental Fe/ml)	*Iron deficiency anemia:* Wt (kg) × 4.5 × (desired Hgb − patient's Hgb gm%) = mg Fe needed IM or IV *Iron replacement after blood loss:* Blood loss (ml) × Hct(%) ÷ 100 = mg Fe needed (based on 1 ml RBC = 1 mg Fe) IM or IV	Oral therapy with iron salts is preferred. Numerous adverse effects including anaphylaxis, fever, hypotension, rash, myalgias, arthralgias. Use "Z-track" technique for IM administration. **Inject test dose** (0.5 ml) on first day. Give IV at **maximum** rate of 50 mg/min. For IV infusion,

Iron preparations		

| | | diluting in NS may result in lower incidence of phlebitis than diluting in dextrose. |

Max daily (IM) dose:
<5 kg: 0.5 ml (25 mg)
5–10 kg: 1.0 ml (50 mg)
10–50 kg: 2.0 ml (100 mg)
>50 kg: 2.0 ml (100 mg)
IV: Give 25 mg test dose over 5 minutes. If no reaction, give remainder of replacement ÷ over 2–3 daily doses.

| Iron preparations | *Ferrous sulfate (20% elemental Fe):*
Drops (Fer-In-Sol): 75 mg (15 mg Fe)/0.6 ml (50 ml)
Syrup (Fer-In-Sol): 90 mg (18 mg Fe)/5 ml
Elixir (Feosol): 220 mg (44 mg Fe)/5 ml (355 ml)
Capsules: 250 mg (50 mg Fe)
Tabs: 195 mg (39 mg Fe), 300 mg (60 mg Fe), 324 mg (65 mg Fe)
Ferrous gluconate (12% elemental Fe):
Elixir: 300 mg (34 mg Fe)/5 ml (7% alcohol)
Tabs: 300 mg (34 mg Fe), 320 mg (37 mg Fe), 325 mg (38 mg Fe) | *Iron deficiency anemia:*
3–6 mg elemental Fe/kg/24 hr ÷ TID PO
Prophylaxis:
Children: Give dose below PO ÷ QD-TID
Premature: 2 mg elemental Fe/kg/24 hr
Full-term: 1–2 mg elemental Fe/kg/24 hr
Max dose: 15 mg elemental Fe/24 hr
Adults: 100 mg elemental Fe/24 hr PO ÷ QD-BID | Iron preparations are variably absorbed. **Do not** use in hemolytic disorders. Less GI irritation when given with or after meals. Vitamin C, 200 mg per 30 mg iron, may enhance absorption. Liquid iron preparations may stain teeth. Give with dropper or drink through straw. May produce constipation, dark stools, nausea, and epigastric pain. Iron and tetracycline inhibit each other's absorption. Antacids may decrease iron absorption. |

(Continued.)

Drug	How Supplied	Dose and Route	Remarks
Iron preparations *(continued.)*.	Sustained-release caps: 320 mg (37 mg Fe), 435 mg (50 mg Fe) Caps: 86 mg (10 mg), 325 mg (38 mg Fe), 435 mg (50 mg)		
Isoetharine (Bronkosol, Bronkometer)	Aerosol: 20 metered doses/ml, each dose 340 µg isoetharine (10, 15 ml dispensers) Sol: 1% (10 mg/ml) (0.25, 0.5, 10, 30 ml) Also available in concentrations of 0.062, 0.08, 0.11, 0.125, 0.14, 0.167, 0.17, 0.2, 0.25, 0.5%.	*Adults:* Aerosol: 1–2 puffs Q3–4 hr PRN *Children:* 0.01 ml/kg, minimum dose 0.1 ml, **max dose** 0.5 ml Q2–4 hr PRN Metered dose inhaler: 1–2 puffs Q4–6 hr PRN Nebulization: 0.25–0.5 ml 1% Sol (= 0.1–0.2 mg/kg/dose) diluted to 2 ml in NS (1:8–1:4 dilution) Q4 hr PRN.	May cause nausea, tachycardia, hypertension, anxiety, headache. Not recommended in children.
Isoniazid (INH, Nydrazid, Laniazid)	Tabs: 50, 100, 300 mg Syrup: 50 mg/5 ml (473 ml) Inj: 100 mg/ml	See Infectious Diseases, Chapter 17, for details. *Prophylaxis:* Infants and children: 10 mg/kg/24 hr PO QD **or** 20	Should not be used alone for treatment. Peripheral neuropathy, optic neuritis, seizures, encephalopathy, psychosis, hepatic side effects

mg/kg/dose PO twice weekly (after 1 mo of daily therapy) for total of 9 mo of treatment.

Adults: 5 mg/kg/24 hr PO QD (usual dose 300 mg) for 9 mo

Treatment:

Infants and children: 10–20 mg/kg/24 hr QD PO **or** 20–40 mg/kg/dose twice weekly for 9 mo with rifampin.

Adults: 5 mg/kg/24 hr QD PO **or** 15 mg/kg/24 hr twice weekly for 9 mo with rifampin.

For INH resistant TB: Consult an ID specialist.

Max daily dose: 300 mg

Max single biweekly dose: 900 mg

may occur with higher doses. Hepatotoxicity is rare in children; follow LFTs monthly. Supplemental pyridoxine (1–2 mg/kg/24 hr) is recommended. May cause false positive urine glucose test. Inhibits hepatic microsomal enzymes; decrease dose of carbamazepine, diazepam, phenytoin, and prednisone. May be given IM when oral therapy is not possible.

| **Isoproterenol**
(Isuprel) | *Isoproterenol HCl:*
Tabs: 10, 15 mg | *Aerosol:* 1–2 puffs up to 5 ×/24 hr | Use with care in CHF, ischemia, or aortic stenosis. May |

(Continued.)

Drug	How Supplied	Dose and Route	Remarks
Isoproterenol (*continued*).	Solutions: 1:400 (2.5 mg/ml) (0.5, 15 ml); 1:200 (5 mg/ml) (0.5, 10, 60 ml); 1:100 (10 mg/ml) Aerosol: 80, 131 µg/dose, about 300 metered doses per container (15 ml) Inj: 200 µg/ml (1:5000) (1,5 ml)	*Nebulized Sol:* Children: 0.05 mg/kg/dose = 0.01 ml/kg/dose of 1:200 Sol (**min dose** 0.5 mg; **max dose:** 1.25 mg) diluted with NS to 2 ml Q4 hr PRN. Adults: 2.5–5.0 mg of 0.25–0.5 ml of 1:100 solution diluted with NS to 2 ml Q4 hr PRN. *IV:* 0.1–1.5 µg/kg/min; begin with 0.1 µg/kg/min and increase every 5–10 min by 0.1 µg/kg/min until desired effect, tachycardia >180 bpm, or arrhythmia occurs **Max dose:** 2 µg/kg/min See inside front cover for preparation of infusion.	precipitate arrhythmias when used in combination with epinephrine. Avoid "abuse" of inhaler. Patients with continuous IV infusion should be observed for evidence of arrhythmias, hypertension, and myocardial ischemia. Not for treatment of asystole or for use in cardiac arrests, unless bradycardia is due to heart block.
Isotretinoin (Accutane)	Caps: 10, 20, 40 mg	Cystic acne: 0.5–2.0 mg/kg/24 hr ÷ Q12 hr PO × 15–20 wk.	**Caution** in females during childbearing years. **Contraindicated** during pregnancy; known teratogen. May cause conjunctivitis, xerosis, pruritus, epistaxis,

		hyperlipidemia, pseudotumor cerebri, cheilitis, bone pain muscle aches, skeletal changes, lethargy, nausea, vomiting, elevated ESR. To avoid additive toxic effects, do not take vitamin A concomitantly.

Kanamycin
(Kantrex)
	Caps: 500 mg
	Inj: 37.5, 250,
	333 mg/ml
		IM or IV administration:
		Neonates *<7 days* *≥7 days*
		BW<2 kg: 15 mg/kg/24 hr 20 mg/kg/24 hr
		    ÷Q12 hr ÷Q8 hr
		BW<2 kg: 20 mg/kg/24 hr 30 mg/kg/24 hr
		    ÷Q12 hr ÷Q8 hr
		Infants and Children: 15–30
		  mg/kg/24 hr ÷ Q8–12 hr
		  IV/IM. **Max dose:** 1.5
		  gm/24 hr
		Adults: 15 mg/kg/24 hr ÷
		  Q8–12 hr IV/IM; **max
		  dose:** 1.5 gm/24 hr
		PO administration: 150–250
		  mg/kg/24 hr ÷ Q6 hr. **Max
		  dose:** 4 gm/24 hr.
			Retinal toxicity and ototoxicity.
			Give over 30 min if IV.
			Reduce dosage frequency
			with renal impairment. Poorly
			absorbed orally. PO used to
			treat GI bacterial overgrowth.
			Therapeutic levels: peak:
			15–30 mg/L; trough: **<5–10**
			mg/L.

(Continued.)

Drug	How Supplied	Dose and Route	Remarks
Ketamine (Ketalar)	Inj: 10, 50, 100 mg/ml	*Children:* IV: sedation for procedures: 0.5–1 mg/kg; induction: 1–2 mg/kg IM: 3–7 mg/kg *Adults:* 1.–4.5 mg/kg IV; 3–8 mg/kg IM	May cause hypertension, tachycardia, respiratory depression, laryngospasm. **Contraindicated** in elevated ICP, hypertension, aneurysms, thyrotoxicosis, CHF, angina, and psychotic disorders. Closely monitor cardiac function when using halothane with this medication.
Ketoconazole (Nizoral)	Tabs: 200 mg Susp*: 100 mg/5 ml (120 ml) Cream: 2% (15, 30, 60 gm)	Children ≥2 yr: 5–10 mg/kg/24 hr ÷ QD-BID PO Adult: 200–400 mg/24 hr QD PO **Max dose:** 1 gm/24 hr Topical: 1–2 applications/24 hr	Monitor liver function tests in long-term use. Drugs that decrease gastric acidity will decrease absorption. May cause nausea, vomiting, rash, headache, pruritus, and fever.
Ketorolac (Toradol)	Inj: 15 mg/ml, 30 mg/ml Tab: 10 mg	Loading: Adults: 30–60 mg × 1 IM **Max dose:** 150 mg/24 hr IM 1st day Maintenance: 15–30 mg Q6 hr IM PRN max maintenance dose: 120 mg/24 hr Oral: 10 mg PRN Q4–6 hr. **Max dose:** 40 mg/24 hr	**Parenteral form should not be used for more than 5 days.** See Chapter 27 for equianalgesic dosing. May cause nausea, dyspepsia, drowsiness. Do not use in hepatic or renal failure. Safety and efficacy in children have not been established.

Lactulose (Cephulac and others)	Syrup: 10 gm/15 ml	*Chronic constipation:* *Infants:* 2.5–10 ml/24 hr ÷ TID-QID PO *Older children and* *adolescents:* 40–90 ml/24 hr ÷ TID-QID PO *Adults:* 30–45 ml/dose TID-QID PO *Acute portal-systemic* *encephalopathy:* *Adults:* 30–45 ml Q1–2 hr until laxative effect observed. *Rectal (adults):* 300 ml diluted in 700 ml water or NS in 30–60 min retention enema; may give Q4–6 hr.	Use with **caution** in diabetes mellitus. GI discomfort, diarrhea may occur. If initial dose causes diarrhea, reduce immediately. Discontinue drug if diarrhea persists. Goal is 2–3 soft stools per day. **Contraindicated** in galactosemia. Do not use with concomitant antacids.
Levocarnitine (L-carnitine) (Carnitor, VitaCarn)	Tabs: 330 mg Caps: 250 mg Sol: 100 mg/ml	*Children:* 50–100 mg/kg/24 hr ÷ Q8–12 hr; increase slowly to **max dose** of 3 gm/24 hr *Adult:* Start at 1 gm/24 hr QD; increase cautiously to 2–3 gm/24 hr QD	May cause nausea, vomiting, abdominal cramps, diarrhea, body odor, myasthenia.

*Indicates suspensions not commercially available; need to be extemporaneously compounded by a pharmacist. See references 6 and 7 for specific formulations.

(Continued.)

Drug	How Supplied	Dose and Route	Remarks
Levothyroxine (T₄) (Synthroid, Levothroid)	Tabs: 12.5, 25, 50, 75, 100, 112, 125, 150, 175, 200, 300 μg Inj: 200, 500 μg	*Children PO dosing:* 0–6 mo: 8–10 μg/kg/24 hr 6–12 mo: 6–8 μg/kg/24 hr 1–5 yr: 5–6 μg/kg/24 hr 6–12 yr: 4–5 μg/kg/24 hr >12 yr: 2–3 μg/kg/24 hr *IM/IV dose:* 75% of oral dose *Adults:* PO: Initial: 12.5–50 μg/24 hr Increment: Increase by 25–50 μg/24 hr at intervals of Q2–4 wk Maintenance: 100–200 μg/24 hr (1.4–3 μg/kg/24 hr) IM,IV: 50% of oral dose QD *Myxedema coma or stupor:* 200–500 μg × 1, then 100–300 μg the next day if needed.	Use with **caution** in patients on anticoagulants. Total replacement dose may be used in children unless there is evidence of cardiac disease; in that case, begin with 1/4 of maintenance and increase weekly. Titrate dosage with clinical status and serum T₄ and TSH. May cause hyperthyroidism, rash, growth disturbances. 100 μg levothyroxine=65 mg thyroid USP.
Lidocaine (Xylocaine and others)	Inj: 0.5, 1.0, 1.5, 2.0, 4.0, 10.0, 20% (1% solution = 10 mg/ml) Ointment: 2.5, 5% (35 gm) Susp (viscous): 2% (20,100 ml)	*Anesthetic:* Injection: **Max dose** of 7 mg/kg/dose with epinephrine Q2 hr **or** 4–5 mg/kg/dose without	Use sparingly orally to minimize aspiration. Side effects: hypotension, seizures, asystole, respiratory arrest. Decrease dose in presence of

Jelly: 2% (30 ml)
Prefilled syringes:
10 mg/ml (1%)
100 mg/5 ml (2%)
Oral spray: 10% (0.1 ml/dose)

epinephrine Q2 hr. **Max dose: 500 mg**
Topical: **Max dose of 3 mg/kg/dose no less than Q2 hr. Max dose: 200 mg**
Anti-arrhythmic: Single bolus 1 mg/kg/dose slowly IO, ET, IV. May repeat in 10–15 min × 2. **Max dose: 3.0–4.5 mg/kg/hr**
Continuous infusion: 20–50 µg/kg/min IV
Infusion preparation: See inside front cover.

hepatic or renal failure. **Contraindicated** in Stokes-Adams attacks, SA, AV, or intraventricular block. Prolonged infusion (24 hr) may result in toxic accumulation of lidocaine. **Therapeutic levels 1.5–5.0 µg/L.** Toxicity occurs at >7 mg/L.

| **Lindane** (gamma benzene hexachloride) (Kwell, Scabene) | Shampoo: 1% (60, 480 ml) Lotion: 1% (60, 480 ml) Cream: 1% (57, 450 gm) | *Shampoo:* Use ≤30 ml per application. Leave in place 4–8 min before rinsing. Repeat in 7 days if lice or mites still present. *Lotion:* Apply to skin, leave on 8–12 hr, then wash off. Change clothing and bed sheets after starting treatment. Treat family members. **Note:** Second | Systemically absorbed. Risk of toxic effects is greater in young children; use other agents (permethrin) in infants, young children, and during pregnancy. Avoid contact with face, urethral meatus, or mucous membranes. May cause a rash; rarely may cause seizures or aplastic anemia. |

(Continued.)

Drug	How Supplied	Dose and Route	Remarks
Lindane *(continued.).*			application usually not necessary but may repeat application in 7–10 days if lice persist.
Lithium (Eskalith, Lithane, Lithonate, Lithotabs, Lithobid, Cibalith-S)	*Carbonate:* Caps: 150, 300, 600 mg Tabs: 300 mg Controlled-release tabs: 450 mg Slow-release tabs: 300 mg *Citrate:* Syrup: 8 mEq/5 ml (10, 480 ml); 5 ml is equivalent to 300 mg Li carbonate (8.12 mEq Li) Cibalith-S is citrate; All other brands are carbonate.	*Children:* Initial: 15–60 mg/kg/24 hr ÷ TID-QID PO Maintenance: Adjust as needed to achieve therapeutic levels. *Adults:* Initial: 300 mg TID PO Maintenance: Adjust as needed to achieve therapeutic levels. Usual dose is about 300 mg TID-QID. **Max dose:** 2.4 gm/24 hr	Increased sodium intake will depress lithium levels. Decreased sodium intake or increased sodium-wasting will increase lithium levels. **Therapeutic levels: 0.6–1.5 mEq/L.** May cause goiter, nephrogenic diabetes insipidus, or sedation at therapeutic doses. In either acute or chronic toxicity, confusion and somnolence may be seen at levels of 2.0–2.5 mEq/L. Seizures or death may occur at levels >2.5 mEq/L.
Loperamide (Imodium, Imodium AD, and others)	Caps: 2 mg Tabs: 2 mg Liquid: 1 mg/5 ml (60, 90, 120 ml)	*Active diarrhea* Children: (>2 yr): 0.4–0.8 mg/kg/24 hr ÷ Q6–12 hr PO until diarrhea resolves. **Max dose:** 2 mg	May cause nausea, vomiting, constipation, cramps, dry mouth, CNS depression. Avoid use in children <2 yr. Dosage has not been clearly

Adults: 4 mg/dose × 1, followed by 2 mg/dose after each stool up to **max dose** of 16 mg/24 hr

Chronic diarrhea:

Children: 0.08–0.24 mg/kg/24 hr ÷ BID-TID **Max dose:** 2 mg/dose

Adults:

Maintenance: 4–8 mg/24 hr ÷ BID-QID PO for **max dose** of 16 mg/24 hr.

established for the treatment of chronic diarrhea in children. Discontinue use if no clinical improvement is observed within 48 hr.

Lorazepam
(Ativan)

Tabs: 0.5, 1, 2 mg
Injection: 2, 4 mg/ml
Oral Sol conc: 2 mg/ml

Status epilepticus:

Neonates: 0.05–0.1 mg/kg/dose IV (over 2–3 min)

Infants and children: 0.1 mg/kg/dose IV/PR up to **max dose** of 4 mg/dose. May repeat 0.05 mg/kg × 1 in 5 min if needed.

Adults: 2.5–10.0 mg/dose IV/PR. May repeat in 15–20 min

May cause respiratory depression, especially in combination with other sedatives. May also cause sedation, dizziness, mild ataxia, mood changes, rash, and GI symptoms. Injectable product may be given rectally. Some preparations contain benzyl alcohol.

(Continued.)

Drug	How Supplied	Dose and Route	Remarks
Lorazepam *(continued.)*.		*Premedication:* 0.05 mg/kg/dose IM to **max dose** of 4 mg/dose, 2 hr before procedure. *Anxiolytic/sedation:* Infants/children: 0.05 mg/kg/dose Q4–8 hr PO/IV Adults: 1–10 mg/24 hr PO ÷ BID-TID	
Lypressin (8-lysine vasopressin) (Diapid)	Nasal spray: 185 µg/ml (8 ml); each spray delivers 7 mg or 2 pressor units.	*Diabetes insipidus:* 1–2 sprays into each nostril QID and HS. If patient requires more than 2–3 sprays per dose, increase frequency of doses rather than amounts/dose.	Titrate dose to thirst, urinary frequency. Coronary vasoconstriction may occur with large doses. May cause nasal congestion, headache, conjunctivitis, and abdominal cramps.
Magnesium citrate (16.17% Mg)	Sol: (300 ml): 5 ml = 4.0–4.7 mEq Mg	*Children:* 4 ml/kg/dose PO; repeat Q4–6 hr until liquid stool results. **Max dose:** 200 ml *Adults:* 240 ml QD PO PRN	Use with **caution** in renal insufficiency. May cause hypermagnesemia, hypotension, respiratory depression; up to about 20% of dose is absorbed.

Magnesium hydroxide (milk of magnesia) (41.69% Mg)	Susp (USP magma): 8% (120, 360 ml) 5 ml = 13.7 mEq Mg Tabs: 325 mg	*Children:* 0.5 ml/kg/dose PO PRN **or** 40 mg/kg/dose PO PRN *Adults:* 15–30 ml/dose **or** 1200 to 2400 mg/dose PO PRN	See Mg citrate.
Magnesium oxide (60.32% Mg) **or gluconate** (5.4% Mg)	Mg oxide: Tabs: 400, 420, 500 mg Caps: 140 mg (241.3 mg Mg/ 400 mg oxide) Mg gluconate: 500 mg tab (27 mg Mg)	*Children:* 3–6 mg elemental Mg^{++}/kg/24 hr ÷ TID-QID PO (**max dose** 400 mg/24 hr) *Adults:* 200–400 mg elemental Mg^{++}/24 hr ÷ TID-QID PO.	See Mg citrate.
Magnesium sulfate (Epsom salts) (Mg-plus, Slow-mag, Magonate) (20.20% Mg)	Inj: 100 mg/ml (0.8 mEq/ml), 125 mg/ml (1 mEq/ml), 250 mg/ml (2 mEq/ml), 500 mg/ml (4 mEq/ml) Oral Sol*: 50% (crystals)	*Cathartic:* Child: 0.25 gm/kg/dose PO Q4–6 hr Adult: 10–30 gm/dose PO Q4–6 hr *Hypomagnesemia or hypocalcemia:* IV/IM: 25–50 mg/kg/dose Q4–6 hr × 3–4 doses; repeat PRN. PO: 100–200 mg/kg/24 hr ÷ QID Maintenance: 0.25–0.5 mEq/kg/24 hr or 30–60 mg/kg/24 hr IV. **Max dose:** 1 gm/24 hr	When given IV, beware of hypotension, respiratory depression, hypermagnesemia. Calcium gluconate (IV) should be available as antidote. Use with **caution** in renal insufficiency, patients on digoxin.

*Indicates suspensions not commercially available; need to be extemporaneously compounded by a pharmacist. See references 6 and 7 for specific formulations.

(Continued.)

Drug	How Supplied	Dose and Route	Remarks
Mannitol (Osmitrol, Resectisol)	Injection: 50, 100, 150, 200, 250 mg/ml (5, 10, 15, 20, 25%)	*Anuria/oliguria* (test dose): 0.2 gm/kg/dose IV over 3–5 min. If there is no diuresis within 2 hr, discontinue mannitol Initial 0.5–1.0gm/kg Maintenance 0.25–0.5 gm/kg/dose Q 4–6 hr *Cerebral edema:* 0.25 gm/kg IV push, repeat Q5 min PRN. (May give furosemide 1 mg/kg concurrently or 5 min before mannitol.) May increase dose gradually to 1 gm/kg/dose if necessary for satisfactory response. *Preoperative for neurosurgery:* 1.5–2.0 gm/kg IV over 30–60 min.	May cause circulatory overload and electrolyte disturbances. For hyperosmolar therapy, keep serum osmolality at 310–320 mOsm/kg. **Caution:** may crystallize with concentration 20%; use line filter. May cause hypovolemia, headache, and polydipsia.
Mebendazole (Vermox)	Chewable tabs: 100 mg	*Pinworms:* 100 mg PO × 1, repeat in 2 wk if not cured *Hookworms, roundworms (Ascaris), and whipworm*	May cause diarrhea and abdominal cramping in cases of massive infection. Use with **caution** in children <2 yr.

	(Trichuris): 100 mg PO BID × 3 days	Family may need to be treated as a group. Therapeutic effect may be decreased if administered to patients receiving carbamazipine or phenytoin.
Meperidine HCl (Demerol and others)	Tabs: 50, 100 mg Syrup, elixir: 50 mg/5 ml Inj: 10, 25, 50, 75, and 100 mg/ml *PO, IM, IV, and SC:* Children: 1.0–1.5 mg/kg/dose Q3–4 hr PRN. **Max dose:** 100 mg. Adults: 50–150 mg/dose Q3–4 hr PRN	See Chapter 27 for details of use and equianalgesic dosing. **Contraindicated** in cardiac arrhythmias, asthma, increased ICP. Potentiated by MAO inhibitors, phenothiazines, other CNS-acting agents and isoniazid. Lower dose if IV. May cause nausea, vomiting, respiratory depression, smooth muscle spasm, constipation, and lethargy. **Caution** in renal failure; accumulated metabolite has CNS effects. Other analgesics may be preferred in patients with sickle cell disease.

(Continued.)

Drug	How Supplied	Dose and Route	Remarks
Metaproterenol (Metaprel, Alupent, and others)	Syrup: 10 mg/5 ml Tabs: 10, 20 mg Inhaler: 650 µg/metered dose, 300 doses/inhaler (15 ml) Inhalant Sol: 5% (10 ml) Single-dose inhalant Sol: 0.4%–0.6% (2.5 ml)	*Inhalation:* Aerosol: 1–3 puffs Q3–4 hr to **max dose** of 12 puffs/24 hr Nebulized solution: Dilute 0.1–0.3 ml of 5% Sol in 2.5 ml NS **or** give 2.5 ml of 0.6% Sol. Usual dose: Q4–6 hr and up to Q1 hr for severe bronchospasm. *Oral:* Children: 0.3–0.5 mg/kg/dose Q6–8 hr Adults: 20 mg/dose Q6–8 hr	Adverse reactions as with other β-adrenergic agents. Excessive use may result in cardiac arrhythmias and death. Also causes tachycardia, increased myocardial O_2 consumption, hypertension, nausea, palpitations, and tremor. The use of tube spacers may enhance efficacy of administering doses via metered dose inhaler.
Methadone HCl (Dolophine)	Tabs: 5, 10 mg Inj: 10 mg/ml Sol: 5, 10 mg/5 ml	*Children:* 0.7 mg/kg/24 hr ÷ Q4–6 hr PO, SC, IM, or IV PRN pain. **Max dose:** 10 mg/dose. *Adults:* 2.5–10.0 mg/dose Q3–4 hr PO, SC, IM, or IV PRN pain *Detoxification or maintenance:* See package insert	Respiratory depression, hypotension. $T_{1/2}$ in nontolerant patients is approximately 22–25 hr. **Not** recommended in children. SC injections may cause local irritation. Refer to Chapter 27 for equianalgesic dosing.

Methicillin (Staphcillin)	Inj: 1, 4, 6, 10 gm 2.6–3.1 mEq Na/gm.	*Neonates IV or IM:* *<2 kg:* ≤1 wk: 25–50 mg/kg/dose Q12 hr >1 wk: 25–50 mg/kg/dose Q8 hr *≥2 kg:*≤1 wk: 25–50 mg/kg/dose Q8 hr >1 wk: 25–50 mg/kg/dose Q6 hr *Infants >1 mo and children:* 100–400 mg/kg/24 hr ÷ Q4–6 hr IV/IM *Adults:* 4–12 gm/24 hr ÷ Q4–6 hr IV/IM. **Max dose:** 12 gm/24 hr	Allergic cross-reactivity with and same toxicity as penicillin. May cause hematuria, nephritis, reversible bone marrow depression, phlebitis at infusion site, eosinophilia, rash. Adjust dose in patients with renal failure (see Chapter 28).
Methimazole (Tapazole)	Tabs: 5, 10 mg	*Children:* Initial: 0.4 mg/kg/24 hr PO ÷ Q8 hr Maintenance: 0.2 mg/kg/24 hr ÷ TID **Max dose:** 30 mg/24 hr PO	Readily crosses placental membranes. Blood dyscrasis, dermatitis, hepatitis, arthralgia, CNS reactions, pruritus, nephrotic syndrome, agranulocytosis, headache,

(Continued.)

Drug	How Supplied	Dose and Route	Remarks
Methimazole *(continued.).*		*Adults:* Initial: 15–60 mg/24 hr PO ÷ TID Maintenance: 5–30 mg/24 hr PO ÷ TID PO	fever, hypothyroidism may occur. $T_{1/2} = 6$ hr.
Methsuximide (Celontin Kapseals)	Caps: 150, 300 mg	*Children:* 10–15 mg/kg/24 hr ÷ Q6–8 hr; increase weekly up to **max** 30 mg/kg/24 hr *Adults:* Initial: 300 mg/24 hr PO ÷ BID–QID for 1 wk *Increment:* Increase by 300 mg/24 hr each wk for 3 wk to **max dose** of 1.2 gm/24 hr ÷ BID–QID *Maintenance:* 10 mg/kg/24 hr PO	GI symptoms, blood dyscrasias, CNS symptoms, and behavioral changes may occur. **Caution** in presence of renal or liver disease. Follow LFTs and urinalysis. Avoid abrupt withdrawal of methsuximide.
Methyldopa (Aldomet)	Tabs: 125, 250, 500 mg Inj: 50 mg/ml Susp: 250 mg/5 ml	*Hypertension:* Children: 10 mg/kg/24 hr ÷ Q6–12 hr PO: increase PRN Q2 days. **Max dose:** 65 mg/kg or 3 gm/24 hr, whichever is less.	**Contraindicated** in pheochromocytoma and active liver disease. Positive Coombs' test, fever, hemolytic anemia, leukopenia, sedation, GI disturbances, orthostatic

		Adults: 250–750 mg PO Q8–12 hr. *Hypertensive crisis:* Children: 20–40 mg/kg/24 hr IV ÷ Q6–8 hr. Adults: 250–1000 mg IV Q6 hr	hypotension may occur. Use with **caution** if patient is receiving haloperidol, propranolol, lithium, sympathomimetics. May interfere with lab tests for creatinine, urinary catecholamines.
Methylene blue		Tabs: 55, 65 mg Inj: 10 mg/ml (1%)	*Methemoglobinemia:* 1–2 mg/kg/dose IV over 5 min. May repeat in 1 hr if needed.	Use **cautiously** in G6PD deficiency or renal insufficiency. May cause nausea, vomiting, headache, diaphoresis, and abdominal pain; causes blue-green discoloration of urine.
Methylphenidate HCl (Ritalin, Ritalin SR, others)		Tabs: 5, 10, 20 mg Slow-release tabs: 20 mg (8 hr duration)	*Attention deficit hyperactivity disorder:* ≥6 yr: Initial: 0.3 mg/kg/dose given with breakfast and lunch (or 2.5–5.0 mg/dose) Interval: If tolerated, may increase by 0.1 mg/kg/dose (or 5–10 mg/dose) weekly until maintenance dose is reached.	Insomnia, weight loss, anorexia, rash, nausea, emesis, abdominal pain, hyper- or hypotension, tachycardia, arrhythmias, hallucinations, fever, tremor. High dose may slow growth by appetite suppression. Rebound overactivity may disrupt sleep.

(Continued.)

Drug	How Supplied	Dose and Route	Remarks
Methylphenidate HCl *(continued).*		Maintenance: 1–2 mg/kg/24 hr **Max dose:** 2 mg/kg/24 hr **or** 60 mg/24 hr. Discontinue use if no improvement seen within 1 mo. Supervise closely.	**Contraindications:** glaucoma, epilepsy, hypertension, MAO inhibitor use.
Methylprednisolone (Medrol, Solu-Medrol, Depo-Medrol, and others)	Tabs: 2, 4, 8 16, 24, 32 mg Inj: Na succinate (Solu-Medrol) 40, 125, 500, 1000, 2000 mg (IV/IM use) Inj: Acetate 20, 40, 80 mg/ml (IM repository)	*Anti-inflammatory/ immunosuppressive:* 0.16–0.8 mg/kg/24 hr PO/IV/IM ÷ Q6–12 hr *Status asthmaticus:* Child: Loading: 1–2 mg/kg/dose IV × 1 Maintenance: 2. mg/kg/24 hr ÷ Q6 hr IV Adult: 10–250 mg/dose Q4–6 hr IM/IV	See Chapter 26. Other dosing regimens exist for specific disorders. Dose of methylprednisolone=1/6 dose of cortisone. Repository used mainly for local therapy. Acetate may be used for intraarticular or intralesional injection. Can be used IM as infrequently as once a week.
Metoclopramide (Clopra, Maloxon, Reglan, and others)	Tabs: 5, 10 mg Injection: 5 mg/ml Syrup (sugar-free): 5 mg/5 ml	*Gastroesophageal reflux or GI dysmotility:* Infants and children: 0.2–0.4 mg/kg/24 hr ÷ QID IV or PO	For gastroesophageal reflux, give 30 min before meals and at bedtime. May cause extrapyramidal symptoms, especially at higher doses.

	Max dose: 0.5 mg/kg/24 hr Adult: 10–15 mg/dose QAC and QHS IV/IM/PO Anti-emetic: 1–2 mg/kg/dose Q2–6 hr IV	Premedicate with diphenhydramine when using as an anti-emetic. Use with **caution** in patients with history of seizure disorder.
Metolazone (Zaroxolyn, Diulo, Mykrox)	Tabs: 2.5, 5, 10 mg Susp*: 1 mg/ml	*Child:* 0.2–0.4 mg/kg/24 hr ÷ QD-BID PO *Adults:* Hypertension: 2.5–5.0 mg QD PO; Edema: 5–20 mg QD PO	Electrolyte imbalance, GI complaints, hyperglycemia, marrow suppression, hyperuricemia, rash.
Metronidazole (Flagyl, Protostat, Metric, and others)	Tabs: 250, 500 mg Susp*: 100 mg/5 ml, or 50 mg/ml Inj: 500 mg Ready to use inj: 5 mg/ml	*Amebiasis:* Children: 35–50 mg/kg/24 hr PO ÷ TID × 10 days. Adults: 750 mg/dose PO TID × 5–10 days. *Anaerobic infection:* Loading dose: 15 mg/kg IV Maintenance: Preterm: 7.5 mg/kg/dose IV Q12 hr beginning 48 hr after load Term: 7.5 mg/kg/dose IV Q12 hr beginning 24 hr after load	Nausea, diarrhea, urticaria, dry mouth, leukopenia, vertigo, peripheral neuropathy. Candidiasis may worsen. Patients should not ingest alcohol for 24 hr after dose (disulfuram-type reaction). Potentiates anticoagulants. IV infusion must be given slowly over 1 hr. Except for amebiasis, safe use of metronidazole in children <12 yr has not been established. Avoid in first-trimester

*Indicates suspensions not commercially available; need to be extemporaneously compounded by a pharmacist. See references 6 and 7 for specific formulations.

(Continued.)

Drug	How Supplied	Dose and Route	Remarks
Metronidazole (*continued*).		Infants, children, and adults: Maintenance: 7.5 mg/kg/dose Q6 hr IV or PO. **Max dose:** 4 gm/24 hr *Gardnerella vaginalis vaginitis:* 500 mg PO BID × 7 days *Giardiasis:* Children: 15 mg/kg/24 hr PO ÷ TID × 10 days *Trichomonas vaginitis:* Children: 15 mg/kg/24 hr PO ÷ TID × 7 days Adults: 250 mg/dose PO TID × 7 days **or** 2 gm PO × 1. *Clostridium difficile* (adult): 0.75–2 gm/24 hr PO ÷ TID-QID × 7–14 days Infants/children: PO 20 mg/kg/24 hr ÷ Q6 hr *Inflammatory bowel disease* (as alternative to sulfasalazine): Adults: 400 mg BID PO Refractory perianal disease: 20 mg/kg/24 hr PO ÷ 3–5 doses.	pregnancy. Use with **caution** in patients with liver or renal disease (GFR <10 ml/min). See Chapter 26.

Mezlocillin (Mezlin)	Inj: 1, 2, 3, 4 gm (contains 1.85 mEq Na/gm)	*Neonates IV or IM:* ≤7 days: 75 mg/kg/dose Q12 hr >7 days: <2 kg: 75 mg/kg/dose Q8 hr >2 kg: 75 mg/kg/dose Q6 hr *Infants and children IV or IM:* 200–300 mg/kg/24 hr ÷ Q4–6 hr *Adults IV or IM:* 1–4 gm/dose Q4–6 hr **Max dose:** 24 gm/24 hr	May cause allergic reactions, seizure, nausea, vomiting, and hematologic abnormalities, (eosinophilia, leukopenia, neutropenia, anemia), elevated BUN, creatinine, and liver enzymes.

Miconazole (Monistat)	Cream: 2% (15, 40, 85 gm) Lotion: 2% (30, 60 ml) Vaginal cream: 2% (45 gm) Inj: 10 mg/ml Powder: 2% (45 gm) Vaginal Suppository: 100, 200 mg	*Topical:* Apply BID × 2–4 wk *Vaginal:* 1 applicator dose **or** 100 mg suppository QHS × 7 days **or** 200 mg suppository QHS × 3 days *IV:* >1 yr: 15–40 mg/kg/24 hr ÷ Q8 hr **Max dose:** 15 mg/dose Adults: 200–1200 mg/dose Q8 hr	Side effects of IV therapy: phlebitis, pruritus, rash, nausea, vomiting, fever, drowsiness, diarrhea, anorexia, and flushes. Decrease in Hct, Na, and platelets have been reported. May cause lipemia.

(Continued.)

Drug	How Supplied	Dose and Route	Remarks
Midazolam (Versed)	Inj: 1, 5 mg/ml	*Children:* Pre-op sedation: 0.08 mg/kg/dose IM or 0.3 mg/kg/dose PR *Sedation for procedures:* Begin with 0.035 mg/kg IV over 2 min; repeat PRN. **Max total dose:** 0.2 mg/kg **or** 2.5 mg *Adults:* Pre-op sedation: 0.07–0.08 mg/kg IM. See Sedation for procedures above	Causes respiratory depression, hypotension, bradycardia as with other benzodiazepines. Lower the dose by 25% when narcotics are given concurrently. May give injectable preparation rectally. **Contraindicated** in patients with narrow-angle glaucoma, shock. Use with **caution** if patient is receiving cimetidine, theophylline, or other anesthetic agents.
Minocycline (Minocin and others)	Tabs: 50, 100 mg Caps: 50, 100 mg Oral susp: 50 mg/5 ml (60 ml) Inj: 100 mg	*Children:* (8–12 yr) Initial: 4 mg/kg/dose × 1 PO/IV Maintenance: 4 mg/kg/24 hr ÷ Q12 hr **Max dose:** 200 mg/24 hr *Adolescents and adults:* Initial: 200 mg/dose × 1 PO/IV Maintenance: 200 mg/24 hr ÷ Q12 hr	Nausea, vomiting, allergy, photophobia, injury to developing teeth. High incidence of vestibular dysfunction. Hepatic metabolism and renal excretion. $T_{1/2}$ = 18 hr. **Do not take** with milk or dairy products.

Mithramycin (Mithracin, Plicamycin)	Inj: 2.5 mg	*Hypercalcemia with malignancies:* 25 µg/kg/dose in 1 L D₅W or NS over 4–8 hr IV QD × 1–4 days. Repeat at weekly intervals if necessary **or** maintain 1–3 doses weekly.	Bone marrow suppression, hemorrhagic diathesis with coagulopathy, cellulitis on extravasation, nausea, vomiting, electrolyte imbalances, hepatotoxicity, renal toxicity. **Contraindicated** in bleeding diathesis, bone marrow suppression.
Morphine sulfate (various brand names)	Oral Sol: 2, 4, 20 mg/ml (30, 120 ml) Tabs: 10, 15, 30 mg Controlled-release tabs: 15, 30, 60, 100 mg Inj: 1, 2, 4, 5, 8, 10, 15 mg/ml	*Analgesia/tetralogy (cyanotic) spells:* Neonates: 0.05–0.2 mg/kg/dose IM, slow IV, SC Q4 hr Child: 0.1–0.2 mg/kg/dose SC, IV, or IM Q2–4 hr PRN. **Max dose:** 15 mg/dose Adults: PO: 10–30 mg Q4 hr PRN IV: 2–15 mg/dose Q2–6 hr PRN *Continuous IV:* 0.025–2 mg/kg/hr; begin with lower dose and titrate to effect.	Dependence, CNS and respiratory depression, nausea, vomiting, constipation, hypotension, bradycardia, increased ICP, miosis, biliary or urinary tract spasm, allergy may occur. Naloxone may be used to reverse effects, especially respiratory depression. Neonates may require higher doses due to decreased amounts of active metabolites. Refer to Chapter 27 for equianalgesic dosing.

(Continued.)

Drug	How Supplied	Dose and Route	Remarks
Mupirocin (Bactroban)	Ointment: 2% (15 gm)	Apply to affected area TID for 3–5 days.	May cause minor local burning, itching, stinging, or pain.
Nafcillin (Unipen, Natcil, Nallpen, and others)	Tabs: 500 mg Caps: 250 mg Oral Sol: 250 mg/5 ml Inj: 0.5, 1.0, 1.5, 2.0, 4.0 gm Contains 2.9 mEq Na/gm	*Newborn IV or IM:* ≤2 kg: ≤7 days: 50 mg/kg/24 hr ÷ Q12 hr >7 days: 75 mg/kg/24 hr ÷ Q8 hr >2 kg: ≤7 days: 50 mg/kg/24 hr ÷ Q8 hr >7 days: 75 mg/kg/24 hr ÷ Q6 hr *Infants and children:* PO: 50–100 mg/kg/24 hr ÷ Q6 hr IM: 100–200 mg/kg/24 hr ÷ Q12 hr IV: 100–200 mg/kg/24 hr ÷ Q6 hr *Adults:* PO: 250–1000 mg Q4–6 hr IV or IM: 500–2000 mg Q4–6 hr **Max dose:** 12 gm/24 hr	Allergic cross-sensitivity with penicillin. Oral route not recommended due to poor absorption. High incidence of phlebitis with IV dosing.

Naloxone (Narcan)	Inj: 0.4, 1 mg/ml Neonatal inj: 0.02 mg/ml	*Children: <20 kg:* 0.01–0.1 mg/kg/dose IM/ IV/SC. Repeat as necessary Q3–5 min *≥20 kg:* or > 5 yrs. 2 mg/dose. Repeat as necessary Q3–5 min May give 10-fold higher dose if needed for diagnosis or therapy *Continuous infusion:* After titrating initial dose to effectiveness, add 75–100% of last effective dose to 1 hr of maintenance IV fluid to run over 1 hr. May wean in 50% increments over next 6–12 hr. (May need to wean over as long as 48 hr for methadone.) If symptoms recur, rebolus and go back to 100%.	Does not cause respiratory depression. Short duration of action may necessitate multiple doses. For very large ingestions 200 µg/kg doses have been necessary. Will produce narcotic withdrawal syndrome in patients with chronic dependence. Use with **caution** in patients with chronic cardiac disease. Abrupt reversal of narcotic depression may result in nausea, vomiting, diaphoresis, tachycardia, hypertension, and tremulousness.
Naproxen (Naprosyn, Anaprox)	Tabs: 250, 375, 500 mg Susp: 125 mg/5 ml Naproxen sodium (Anaprox) 275 mg = 250 mg base	(All doses based on naproxen base) *JRA* 10 mg/kg/24 hr ÷ Q12 hr PO	May cause GI bleeding, heartburn, headache, fatigue, drowsiness, vertigo, abdominal pain. Use with

(Continued.)

Drug	How Supplied	Dose and Route	Remarks
Naproxen *(continued.)*.	(Naprosyn)	*Rheumatoid arthritis, ankylosing spondylitis:* Adults: 250–500 mg BID. **Max dose:** 1500 mg/24 hr. *Dysmenorrhea:* 500 mg × 1, then 250 mg Q6–8 hr; **Max dose:** 1250 mg	**caution** in patients with GI disease, cardiac disease, renal or hepatic impairment. See Ibuprofen.
Neomycin sulfate (Mycifradin)	Tabs: 500 mg Sol: 125 mg/5 ml (contains parabens) Inj: 500 mg Topical: 3.5 mg/gm	*Prematures and newborns:* 50 mg/kg/24 hr ÷ Q6 hr PO *Infants and children:* 50–100 mg/kg/24 hr ÷ Q6 hr PO Adult: 50 mg/kg/24 hr ÷ Q6 hr PO *Hepatic encephalopathy:* Acute: 2.5–7.0 gm/m²/24 hr ÷ Q6 hr PO × 5–7 days. Chronic: 2.5 gm/m²/24 hr PO ÷ QID *Bowel prep:* Children: 90 mg/kg/24 hr PO Q4 hr × 3 days	Follow for renal or ototoxicity. **Contraindicated** in ulcerative bowel disease or intestinal obstruction. Parenteral use not recommended. Oral absorption is limited, but levels may accumulate. May cause itching, redness, edema, or failure to heal if applied topically.

		Adults: 1 gm Q1 hr × 4 doses, then 1 gm Q4 hr × 5 doses. (Many other regimens exist.)	
Neosporin (Polymyxin B sulfate-bacitracin zinc-neomycin sulfate)	Ointment: 3.5 mg neomycin, 400 U bacitracin, 5000 U polymyxin B/gm Cream: 3.5 mg neomycin, 10,000 U polymyxin B/gm	Apply to minor cuts and burns Q8 hr	Do not use for extended periods. May cause superinfection, delayed healing. See Neomycin.
Neostigmine (Prostigmin)	Tabs: 15 mg (bromide) Inj: 0.25, 0.5, 1 mg/ml (methylsulfate)	*Myasthenia gravis-Diagnosis:* Children: 0.04 mg/kg IM × 1 Adults: 0.022 mg/kg IM × 1 *Treatment:* Children: IM, IV, SC: 0.01–0.04 mg/kg/dose Q2–3 hr PRN PO: 2 mg/kg/24 hr ÷ Q3–4 hr Adults: IM, IV, SC: 0.5–2.5 mg/dose Q3–4 hr PRN PO: 15 mg/dose Q3–4 hr *Reversal of nondepolarizing neuromuscular blocking agents:*	Titrate for each patient, but avoid excessive cholinergic effects. **Caution** in asthmatics. **Contraindicated** in GI and urinary obstruction. May cause cholinergic crisis, bronchospasm, salivation, nausea, vomiting, diarrhea, miosis, diaphoresis, lacrimation, bradycardia, hypotension, fatigue, confusion, respiratory depression, seizures. **Antidote:** Atropine 0.01–0.04 mg/kg/dose.

(Continued.)

Drug	How Supplied	Dose and Route	Remarks
Neostigmine *(continued.)*.		Infants: 0.025–0.1 mg/kg/dose IV with atropine or glycopyrrolate Children: 0.025–0.08 mg/kg/dose IV with atropine or glycopyrrolate Adults: 0.5–2.0 mg/dose IV with atropine or glycopyrrolate **Max dose:** 2.5 mg/dose	
Nifedipine (Adalat, Procardia, Procardia XL, and others)	Caps: 10, 20 mg Sustained-release tabs: 30, 60, 90 mg	These doses have been used in *children:* Hypertension: 0.25–0.5 mg/kg/dose Q6–8 hr PRN PO or sublingual Hypertrophic cardiomyopathy: 0.5–0.9 mg/kg/24 hr ÷ Q6–8 hr PO *Adults:* Start with 10 mg/dose PO TID, then 10–30 mg TID-QID titrating to effect. **Max dose:** 180 mg/24 hr	May cause severe hypotension, peripheral edema, flushing, tachycardia, headaches, dizziness, nausea, palpitation, syncope. For sublingual administration, capsule must be punctured and liquid expressed into mouth (0.175 ml ~5 mg). Use with **caution** in patients with aortic stenosis, CHF.

Nitrofurantoin (Furadantin, Macrodantin, and others)	Tabs: 50, 100 mg Caps (Macrocrystal): 25, 50, 100 mg Susp: 25 mg/5 ml	*Children >1 mo:* 5–7 mg/kg/24 hr ÷ Q6 hr PO Prophylaxis: 1–2 mg/kg QHS PO **Max dose:** 400 mg/24 hr *Adults:* 50–100 mg/dose Q6 hr PO Prophylaxis: 50–100 mg/PO QHS	Large variety of hypersensitivity reactions. May cause nausea, vomiting, diarrhea, cholestatic jaundice, headache, polyneuropathy. **Contraindicated** in severe renal disease, G6PD deficiency, and in infants <1 mo of age. Dose may need reduction with prolonged use (>2 wk). Give with food or milk.
Nitroglycerin (Tridil, Nitro-Bid, Nitrostat, and others)	Injection: 0.5, 0.8, 5.0 mg/ml Sublingual tabs: 0.15, 0.3, 0.4, 0.6 mg.	*Children:* Begin with 0.25–0.5 μg/kg/min; titrate to effect. **Max dose:** 5 μg/kg/min *Adults:* 5 μg/kg/min IV, then increase by 5 μg/kg/min up to 20 μg/kg/min; titrate to effect. Sublingual: 0.2–0.6 mg Q5 min for **max** of 3 doses in 15 min To prepare infusion: See inside front cover	In small doses (1–2 μg/kg/min) acts mainly on systemic veins and decreases preload. At 3–5 μg/kg/min acts on systemic arterioles to decrease resistance. Must use polypropylene infusion sets to avoid plastic adsorbing drug. May cause headache, flushing, GI upset, blurred vision, methemoglobinemia. Use with **caution** in severe renal impairment, increased ICP, hepatic failure.

(Continued.)

Drug	How Supplied	Dose and Route	Remarks
Nitroprusside (Nipride and others)	Inj: 50 mg	Dilute with D₅W and protect from light Dose: 0.5–10 µg/kg/min Titrate to effect; usual dose is 3–4 µg/kg/min *Continuous infusion:* See inside front cover for details.	Must be monitored with arterial line. Produces profound hypotension, metabolic acidosis, and CNS symptoms when overdosed. Nitroprusside is nonenzymatically converted to cyanide, which is metabolized to thiocyanate. Monitor thiocyanate levels if used >48 hr. **Levels should be <12 mg/L.**
Norfloxacin (Noroxin, Chibroxin)	400 mg tabs Ophthalmic drops: 0.3 (5 ml)	Adults: 400 mg PO Q12 hr *N. gonorrheae:* 800 mg once, followed by doxycycline. Ophthalmic: 1–2 drops Q2 hr QID.	Not recommended for children; may cause arthropathy in immature animals. May increase serum theophylline levels. May prolong PTs for patients on warfarin. See Ciprofloxacin for common side effects and drug interactions.
Nystatin (Mycostatin, Nilstat, and others)	Tabs: 500,000 U Troches/pastilles: 200,000 U Susp: 100,000 U/ml (60,473 ml)	*Oral:* Pre-term infants: 0.5 ml (50,000 U) to each side of mouth QID	May produce diarrhea and GI side effects. Treat until 48–72 hr after resolution of symptoms. Drug is poorly absorbed through the GI tract.

	Topical (powder, ointment, cream): 100,000 U/gm (15, 30 gm) Vaginal tabs: 100,000 U	Term infants: 1 ml (100,000 U) to each side of mouth QID Children/adults: 4–6 ml (400,000–600,000 U); swish and swallow QID *Vaginal:* 1 tab QHS × 10 days. *Topical:* Apply BID-QID.	
Octreotide acetate (Sandostatin)	Inj: 0.05, 0.1, 0.5 mg/ml	*Antidiarrheal (GI tumor):* 1–10 μg/kg/24 hr SC ÷ QD–Q12 hr	Cholelithiasis, hyperglycemia, hypoglycemia, nausea, diarrhea, abdominal discomfort, headache, pain at injection site may occur. Cyclosporine levels may be reduced in patients receiving this drug.
Ondansetron (Zofran)	Inj: 2 mg/ml (20 ml)	*Children >3 yr-adults:* 0.15 mg/kg/dose IV × 3 doses (1st dose 30 min prior to emetogenic chemotherapy; subsequent doses at 4 and 8 hr after initial dose)	Bronchospasm, tachycardia, hypokalemia, seizures, headaches, lightheadedness, constipation or diarrhea, and transient increases in AST, ALT, and bilirubin may occur. Drug has been used successfully by the oral route of administration, using the IV dosage.

(Continued.)

Drug	How Supplied	Dose and Route	Remarks
Oxacillin (Bactocil, Prostaphlin)	Caps: 250, 500 mg Oral Sol: 250 mg/5 ml Inj: 0.25, 0.5, 1.0, 2.0, 4.0, 10.0 gm 1 gm of drug contains 2.8–3.1 mEq Na	*Children:* 50–100 mg/kg/24 hr ÷ Q6 hr PO *Adults:* 500–1000 mg/dose Q4–6 hr PO; for neonatal and IV dosing see Nafcillin	Same as Methicillin: allergy, diarrhea, nausea, vomiting, leukopenia, elevated AST.
Oxtriphylline (Choledyl)	Many preparations (64% theophylline) Tabs: 100, 200 mg Extended release tabs: 400, 600 mg Elixir: 100 mg/5 ml (20% alcohol) Syrup: 50 mg/5ml	*See doses under Theophylline and convert:* 16 mg theophylline = 25 mg oxtriphylline	Same as Theophylline, which see.
Oxybutynin chloride (Ditropan, Dridase)	Tabs: 5 mg Syrup: 5 mg/5 ml (473 ml)	*Child ≤5 yr:* 0.4–0.8 mg/kg/24 hr ÷ BID-QID PO *Child >5 yr:* 10–15 mg/24 hr ÷ BID-TID PO *Adult:* 10–20 mg/24 hr ÷ BID-QID PO	Atropine-like side effects. **Contraindicated** in glaucoma, GI obstruction, megacolon, myasthenia gravis, severe colitis, hypovolemia.
Oxycodone (Roxicodone)	Sol: 1 (8% alcohol) and 20 mg/ml Tabs: 5 mg	*Dose based upon oxycodone salt:* Children: 0.05–0.15 mg/kg/dose Q4–6 hr PRN up to 10 mg/dose Adults: 5 mg Q6 hr	Abuse potential, dizziness, constipation, urinary retention, and hypersensitivity may

Oxycodone and acetaminophen
(Tylox, Roxilox, Percocet)

Combination product with acetominophen:
Caps: acetominophen 500 mg/oxycodone HCl 5 mg
Sol: acetominophen 325 mg and oxyocodone HCl 5 mg/5 ml (0.4% alcohol)
Tabs: Acetominophen 325 mg and oxycodone HCl 5mg; acetominophen 500 mg and oxycodone HCl 5 mg

Oxycodone and aspirin
(Percodan, Percodan-Demi, Roxiprin, Codoxy)

Combination product with aspirin:
Tabs: aspirin 325 mg, oxycodone HCl 4.5 mg, and oxycodone tereph 0.38 mg; aspirin 325 mg, oxycodone HCl 2.25 mg and oxycodone tereph 0.19 mg

occur. Naloxone is the antidote. See Chapter 27 for equianalgesic conversion chart. **Contraindicated** in patients with severe respiratory depression.

(Continued.)

Drug	How Supplied	Dose and Route	Remarks
Pancreatic enzymes See Chapter 26 for description and contents of lipase, protease, and amylase	See Chapter 26	Initial doses: (actual requirements are patient-specific) *Powder:* <1 yr: 1/8 tsp (0.35 gm) with feedings *Enteric-coated microspheres and microtabs:* <1 yr: 2000 U lipase with meals or feedings 1–6 yr: 4000–8000 U lipase with meals and 4000 U with snacks 7–12 yr: 4000–12,000 U lipase with meals and snacks Adults: 4000–16,000 U lipase with meals and snacks	May cause occult GI bleeding, allergic reactions to porcine proteins, hyperuricemia, and hyperuricosuria with high doses. Dose should be titrated to eliminate diarrhea and to minimize steatorrhea. Do not chew microspheres or microtabs. Concurrent administration with H$_2$ antagonists may enhance enzyme efficacy.
Pancuronium bromide (Pavulon)	Injection: 1, 2 mg/ml (contains 1% benzyl alcohol)	*Neonate:* Initial: 0.02 mg/kg/dose IV. May repeat × 2 Q5–10 min PRN Maintenance: 0.03–0.09 mg/kg/dose IV Q1/2–Q4 hr PRN *>1 mo-adult:* Initial: 0.04–0.1 mg/kg/dose IV	Must be prepared to intubate within 2 min of induction. Drug effects accentuated by hypothermia, acidosis, neonatal age, decreased renal function, halothane, succinylcholine, hypokalemia, and aminoglycoside antibiotics. May cause

	Maintenance: 0.015–0.1 mg/kg/dose IV Q30–60 min *Defasciculating dose:* 0.005–0.01 mg/kg/dose IV. Individualize dosage according to patient's response	tachycardia, mild salivation, and rash. **Antidote:** neostigmine (with atropine or glycopyrrolate).
Paraldehyde (Paral)	Oral or rectal liquid: 1gm/ml (30 ml)	*Sedative:* 0.15 ml (150 mg)/kg/dose PO (diluted in milk or fruit juice) or PR (diluted with equal volume of cottonseed or olive oil) **Max dose:** 5 ml. *Anti-convulsant:* 0.3 ml (300 mg)/kg/dose in 1:1 dilution with cottonseed or olive oil Q2–4 hr PR. **Max dose:** 5 ml.	**Do not use** discolored or "vinegar scented" solutions. Avoid exposure to plastics, air, and light. **Contraindicated** in hepatic or pulmonary disease. Overdose may cause cardiorespiratory depression. Parenteral dosage form is no longer commercially available in the U.S. Less frequently used as an anti-convulsant.
Paregoric (camphorated opium tincture)	Camphorated tincture: 2 mg (morphine equivalent)/5 ml (some preparations contain up to 45% alcohol)	*Analgesia:* Children: 0.25–0.5 ml/kg/dose PO QD-QID Adults: 5–10 ml/dose PO QD-QID	Same side effects as morphine (constipation, lethargy, etc.). After symptoms are controlled for several days, dose for opiate withdrawal should be

(Continued.)

Drug	How Supplied	Dose and Route	Remarks
Paregoric *(continued.).*		*Neonatal opiate withdrawal:* Initial: 0.2–0.3 ml/dose Q3–4 hr Increment: 0.05 ml/dose until symptoms abate. Rare to exceed 0.7 ml/dose. **Max dose:** 1–2 ml/kg/24 hr. *Diarrhea:* 0.25–0.5 ml/kg/dose QD–QID	decreased gradually over a 2–4 wk period (e.g., by 10% Q2–3 days). **Note:** Deodorized opium tincture contains **10 mg morphine/ml** and is **25 times stronger** than the camphorated product.
Pemoline (Cylert)	Tabs: 18.75, 37.5, 75 mg Chewable tabs: 37.5 mg	*Children >6 yr:* Initial: 37.5 mg QAM PO Increment: 18.75 mg/24 hr at weekly intervals Maintenance: 0.5–3 mg/kg/24 hr (effective dose range: 56.25–75 mg/24 hr) **Max dose:** 112.5 mg/24 hr	May cause insomnia, anorexia, hypersensitivity, depression, abdominal pain, hepatotoxicity; drug dependence. Use with **caution** in renal disease. **Contraindicated** in hepatic insufficiency. Effect may not be seen until 3–4 wk of therapy. Long-term use associated with growth inhibition. **Not recommended for children <6 yr old.**

| **Penicillamine**
(Cuprimine, Depen) | Tabs: 250 mg
Caps: 125, 250 mg | *Lead chelation therapy:* See
Poisonings, Chapter 3
Wilson's disease:
Infants <6 mo: 250 mg/dose
QD PO
Children <12 yr: 250 mg/dose
BID-TID PO
Adults: 250 mg/dose QID PO
Max dose: 2 gm/24 hr
Arsenic poisoning: 100
mg/kg/24 hr PO ÷ Q6 hr × 5
days. **Max dose:** 1 gm/24 hr
Cystinuria:
Infants/young children: 30
mg/kg/24 hr ÷ Q6 hr PO
Older children/adults: 1–4
gm/24 hr ÷ Q6 hr PO
Primary biliary cirrhosis:
Initial: 250 mg/24 hr PO;
increase by 250 mg Q2 wk
to a total of 1gm/24 hr
(given as 250 mg QID) | Dose should be given 1 hr
before or 2 hr after meals.
Must be in lead-free
environment, as can increase
absorption of lead if present in
GI tract. Follow CBC, LFTs,
and urine. Can cause
cataracts, fever, rash, nausea,
vomiting, lupus-like syndrome,
leukopenia, leukocytosis,
eosinophilia,
thrombocytopenia. May
reduce serum digoxin levels.
Avoid concomitant
administration with iron,
antacids, and food. Patients
treated for Wilson's disease or
cystinuria should be treated
with pyridoxine 25 mg/24 hr.
Titrate urinary copper
excretion to >1 mg/24 hr for
patients with Wilson's
disease. |

(Continued.)

Drug	How Supplied	Dose and Route	Remarks
Penicillin G preparations- potassium and sodium	*Potassium:* Tabs: 250,000, 400,000, 500,000, 800,000 U Sol: 200,000, 400,000 U/5 ml (100,200 ml) Inj: 0.2, 0.5,1, 5, 10, 20 million U. *Sodium:* Inj: 5 million U 250 mg = 400,000 U.	*Newborn IV or IM:* *0–4 wk, <1200 gm:* 50,000–100,000 U/kg/24 hr ÷ Q12 hr *≤5 days:* <2 kg: 50,000–100,000 U/kg/24 hr ÷ Q12 hr >2 kg: 75,000–150,000 U/kg/24 hr ÷ Q8 hr *>7 days:* <2 kg: 75,000–225,000 U/kg/24 hr ÷ Q8 hr >2 kg: 100,000–200,000 U/kg/24 hr ÷ Q6 hr *Congenital syphilis:* <7 days: 100,000 U/kg/24 hr ÷ Q12 hr 7–28 days: 150,000 U/kg/24 hr ÷ Q8 hr >28 days: 200,000 U/kg/24 hr ÷ Q6 hr Treat for 10–14 days	Contains 1.7 mEq of K and 0.3 mEq Na per 1 million U of penicillin G K. 1 million U of penicillin G Na contains 2 mEq Na. Oral penicillin G should be taken 1–2 hr before or 2 hr after meals. Side effects: anaphylaxis, hemolytic anemia, interstitial nephritis, Herxheimer reaction. $T_{1/2}$ = 30 min; may be prolonged by concurrent use of probenecid. For meningitis, use higher daily dose at shorter dosing intervals. Adjust dose in renal impairment; see Chapter 28 for details.

	Children: IV or IM: 100,000–400,000 U/kg/24 hr ÷ Q4–6 hr **Max dose:** 24 million U/24 hr PO: 40,000–80,000 U/kg/24 hr ÷ Q6–8 hr or 25–50 mg/kg/24 hr ÷ Q6–8 hr Adults: IV or IM: 2–24 million U/24 hr ÷ Q4–6 hr PO: 200,000–800,000 U/dose ÷ Q6–8 hr **or** 125–500 mg/dose Q6–8 hr.	
Penicillin G preparations- benzathine (Permapen, Bicillin L-A)	Inj: 300,000, 600,000 U/ml (may contain parabens and povidone) *Syphilis, early acquired:* Infants and children: 50,000 U/kg × 1 IM. **Max dose:** 2.4 million U. Adults: 1.2 million U × 1 IM *Syphilis >1 yr:* Infants and children: 50,000 U/kg IM Q wk × 3 doses **Max dose:** 2.4 million U/dose	Same as for Penicillin G. Provides sustained levels for 2–4 wk. Do **not** administer IV.

(Continued.)

Drug	How Supplied	Dose and Route	Remarks
Penicillin G *(continued.)*		Adults: 2.4 million U IM Q wk × 3 doses *Group A streptococci:* Infants/children: 25,000 U/kg × 1 IM **Max dose: 1.2 million U/dose.** Adults: 1.2 million U × 1 IM *Rheumatic fever prophylaxis:* Infants/children: 25,000 U/kg IM Q3–4 wk. **Max dose:** 1.2 million U/dose Adults: 1.2 million U IM Q3–4 wk, or 600,000 U IM Q2 wk.	
Penicillin G preparations-procaine (Duracillin A.S., Wycillin, Cysticillin A.S., Pfizerpen-AS)	Inj: 300,000, 500,000, 600,000 U/ml (may contain parabens, phenol, povidone, and formaldehyde)	*Infants and children:* 25,000–50,000 U/kg/24 hr ÷ Q12–24 hr IM. **Max dose:** 4.8 million U/24 hr *Adults:* 0.6–4.8 million U/24 hr ÷ Q12–24 hr IM *Congenital syphilis:* 50,000 U/kg/24 hr ÷ Q12–24 hr × 10–14 days	Provides sustained levels for 2–4 days. May cause sterile abscess at injection site. Contains 120 mg procaine/300,000 U. This may cause allergic reactions, CNS stimulation, seizures. Use with **caution** in neonates. Do **not** administer IV. Larger dose volumes may be administered in 2 injection sites.

	Syphilis: >12 yr-adult: 600,000 U QD IM × 8–15 days *Gonorrhea (acute, uncomplicated):* Infants/children: Probenecid 25 mg/kg PO (**max dose:** 1 gm) 30 min prior to 100,000 U/kg procaine penicillin IM × 1 Adults: Probenecid 1 gm PO 30 min prior to 4.8 million U procaine penicillin IM × 1	This preparation provides early peak levels in addition to prolonged levels of penicillin in the blood.
Penicillin G preparations-penicillin G benzathine and penicillin G procaine (Bicillin C-R, Bicillin C-R 900/300)	Tubex: 300,000 U penicillin G Procaine + 300,000 U penicillin G benzathine/ml or 150,000 U penicillin G procaine + 150,000 or 450,000 U penicillin G benzathine/ml	*Acute streptococcal infections:* <14 kg: 600,000 U × 1 IM 14–27 kg: 900,000–1.2 million U × 1 IM >27 kg: 2.4 million U × 1 IM
Penicillin V potassium (Pen Vee K, V-Cillin K and others)	Tabs: 125 mg (200,000 U), 250 mg (400,000 U), 500 mg (800,000 U), Oral Sol: 125, 250 mg/5 ml (100, 200 ml)	Children: 25–50 mg/kg/24 hr ÷ Q6 hr PO **Max dose:** 3 gm/24 hr Adults: 250–500 mg/dose PO Q6 hr	GI absorption is better than penicillin G. **Note:** Must be taken 1 hr before or 2 hr after meals. Complete 10 day course for streptococcal pharyngitis to prevent rheumatic fever.

(Continued.)

Drug	How Supplied	Dose and Route	Remarks
Penicillin V Potassium *(continued.).*		*Secondary rheumatic fever/pneumococcal prophylaxis:* ≤5 yr: 125 mg PO BID >5 yr: 250 mg PO BID	
Pentamidine isethionate (Pentam 300, NebuPent)	Inj: 300 mg (Pentam 300) Inhalation: 300 mg (NebuPent)	*IM or IV:* *T. gambiense:* 4 mg/kg/24 hr QD × 10 days *P. carinii:* 4 mg/kg/24 hr QD × 12–14 days *L. donovani:* 2–4 mg/kg/24 hr QD × 15 days. Risks of therapy >14 days is not well defined; some recommend 10–21 days. *Pneumocystis prophylaxis:* *Inhalation:* >5 yr: 300 mg in 6 ml H_2O. Give via Respirgard II jet nebulizer Q mo. *IM/IV:* 4 mg/kg Q mo or Q2 wk	May cause hypoglycemia, transient hypotension, tachycardia, nausea, vomiting, mild hepatotoxicity, megaloblastic anemia, pancreatitis, granulocytopenia, hypocalcemia, and renal toxicity. Infuse IV over 1 hr to reduce risk of hypotension. **Sterile abscess** may occur at IM injection site.

Pentobarbital
(Nembutal, others)

Caps: 50, 100 mg
Elixir: 18.5 mg/5 ml
Suppository: 30, 60, 120, 200 mg
Inj: 50 mg/ml

Hypnotic:
PO, PR:
2 mo–1 yr: 30 mg QHS
1–4 yr: 30-60 mg QHS
5–12 yr: 60 mg QHS
12–14 yr: 60–120 mg QHS
or
≤4 yr: 3–6 mg/kg QHS
>4 yr: 1.5–3.0 mg/kg QHS
Adult: 100–200 mg QHS IM
Child: 2–6 mg/kg/dose. **Max dose:** 100 mg
Adult: 150–200 mg/dose

Sedative:
Child: 2–6 mg/kg/24 hr PO/PR/IM ÷ TID
IV: 1–3 mg/kg slowly until asleep
Max dose: 100 mg/24 hr.
Adult: 20–40 mg/dose PO/PR BID-QID

Barbiturate coma:
Initial: 10–15 mg/kg over 1–2 hr

No advantage over phenobarbital for control of seizures. Adjunct in treatment of ICP. May cause drug-related isoelectric EEG. Do not administer for >2 wk in treatment of insomnia.
Contraindicated in liver failure.
Onset of action: PO/PR: 15–60 min; IM: 10–15 min; IV: 1 min.
Administer IV at a rate of <50 mg/min.
Suppositories should not be divided.
Therapeutic serum levels:
Sedation: 1–5 mg/L;
Hypnosis: 5–15 mg/L;
Coma: 20–40 mg/L.

(Continued.)

Drug	How Supplied	Dose and Route	Remarks
Pentobarbital *(continued).*		Maintenance: Start at 1 mg/kg/hr; increase to 2–3 mg/kg/hr to maintain EEG burst suppression.	
Permethrin (Elimite, Nix)	Cream 5% (Elimite) Liquid cream rinse: 1% (Nix)	*Head lice:* >2 mo: saturate hair and scalp with medication after shampooing, rinsing, and towel-drying hair. Leave on 10 min, then rinse. May repeat in 7 days. *Scabies:* Apply cream head to toe and wash off with water after 8–14 hr.	Avoid contact with eyes during application. Shake well before using. May cause pruritus, hypersensitivity, burning, stinging, erythema, and rash.
Phenazopyridine (Pyridium)	Tabs: 100,200 mg	*Children 6–12 yr:* 12 mg/kg/24 hr ÷ TID until symptoms of lower urinary tract irritation are controlled *Adults:* 200 mg TID until symptoms are controlled	May cause GI problems, or renal insufficiency. May cause methemoglobinemia, hemolytic anemia. Colors urine orange; stains clothing. May also stain contact lenses. Give after meals.

| **Phenobarbital** (Luminal) | Tabs: 8, 15, 16, 30, 32, 60, 65, 100 mg
Caps: 16 mg
Elixir: 15, 20 mg/5 ml
Inj: 30, 60, 65, 130 mg/ml (some injectable products may contain benzyl alcohol and propylene glycol) | *Sedation:* Child: 6 mg/kg/24 hr PO ÷ TID
Adults: 30–120 mg/24 hr PO ÷ BID-TID
Pre-op sedation:
PO/IM/IV: 1–3 mg/kg × 1, 1.0–1.5 hr prior to procedure.
Status epilepticus:.
Loading dose (IV):
  Neonate: 15–20 mg/kg in single or divided dose.
  Infants/children/adults:
  15–18 mg/kg in single or divided dose. May give additional 5 mg/kg Q15–30 min up to a maximum of 30 mg/kg.
Maintenance dose (PO/IV):
  Neonate: 3–4 mg/kg/24 hr ÷ QD-BID; increase to 5 mg/kg/24 hr if needed.
  Infants: 5–6 mg/kg/24 hr ÷ QD-BID
  1–5 yr: 6–8 mg/kg/24 hr ÷ QD-BID | IV administration may cause respiratory arrest or hypotension. **Contraindicated** in hepatic or renal disease and porphyria. $T_{1/2}$ approximately 96 hr in children. Therefore, shorter-acting barbiturates are preferred for sedation. Paradoxical reaction in children (not dose-related) may cause hyperactivity, irritability, insomnia.
Therapeutic levels: 15–40 mg/L. Induces liver enzymes, thus decreases blood levels of many drugs (e.g., anticonvulsants). **IV push not to exceed 1 mg/kg/min.** |

(Continued.)

Drug	How Supplied	Dose and Route	Remarks
Phenobarbital (*continued.*).		6–12 yr: 4–6 mg/kg/24 hr ÷ QD-BID >12 yr: 1–3 mg/kg/24 hr ÷ QD-BID **Max dose:** 1–2 gm. *Hyperbilirubinemia:* <12 yr: 3–8 mg/kg/24 hr PO ÷ BID-TID. Doses up to 12 mg/kg/24 hr have been used.	
Phenylephrine HCl (Neo-Synephrine and others)	Nasal drops: 0.125, 0.16, 0.2, 0.25% (15, 30 ml) Nasal spray: 0.25, 0.5, 1% (15, 30 ml) Nasal gel: 0.5% Ophthalmic Sol: 0.12% (15 ml), 2.5% (15 ml), 10% (5 ml) Inj: 10 mg/ml (1%)	*Hypotension:* Children: IM/SC: 0.1 mg/kg/dose Q1–2 hr PRN IV; **max dose: 5 mg** IV bolus: 5–20 μg/kg/dose Q10–15 min PRN IV drip: 0.1–0.5 μg/kg/min; titrate to effect Adults: IM or SC: 2–5 mg/dose Q1–2 hr PRN; **max dose: 5 mg** IV bolus: 0.1–0.5 mg/dose Q10–15 min PRN IV drip: 1–4 μg/kg/min; titrate to effect	Use **cautiously** in presence of hypertension, arrhythmias, hyperthyroidism, hyperglycemia. May cause tremor, insomnia, palpitations. Metabolized by MAO. **Contraindicated** in pheochromocytoma and severe hypertension. Nasal decongestants may cause rebound congestion with excessive use (>3 days). Injectable product may contain sulfites. **Note:** Phenylephrine is found in a

To prepare infusion: See inside front cover.

Paroxysmal supraventricular tachycardia (give IV push over 20–30 sec):

Children: 5–10 μg/kg/dose

Adults: 0.25–0.5 mg/dose; may double and repeat dose Q5 min until desired systolic BP is reached

Nasal decongestant (give up to 3 days):

<6 yr: 2–3 drops of 0.125% Sol Q4 hr PRN

6–12 yr: 2–3 drops or 1–2 sprays of 0.25% Sol Q4 hr PRN

>12 yr-adult: 2–3 drops or 1–2 sprays of 0.25 or 0.5% Sol Q4 hr PRN

Pupillary dilation: 2.5% Sol; 1 drop in each eye 15 min before exam

variety of combination cough and cold products, such as Comhist and Naldecon.

(Continued.)

Drug	How Supplied	Dose and Route	Remarks
Phenytoin (Dilantin)	Chewable tabs: 50 mg (Infatab) Prompt caps: 30, 100 mg Extended-release caps: 30, 100 mg Susp: 30, 125 mg/5 ml (240 ml)	*Status epilepticus:* See Chapter 2. Loading dose: 15–20 mg/kg IV **Max dose:** 1000 mg/24 hr *Maintenance for seizure disorders:* Neonates: start 5 mg/kg/24 hr PO/IV ÷ Q12 hr; usual range 5–8 mg/kg/24 hr PO/IV ÷ Q8–12 hr. Infants/children: start 5 mg/kg/24 hr ÷ QD-Q12 hr PO/IV; usual range: 6 mo–3 yr: 8–10 mg/kg/24 hr 4–6 yr: 7.5–9 mg/kg/24 hr 7–9 yr: 7–8 mg/kg/24 hr 10–16 yr: 6–7 mg/kg/24 hr. Doses are divided Q8–12 hr **Note:** Prompt caps should not be used for QD dosing (use extended-release caps).	**Contraindicated in patients with heart block or sinus bradycardia.** Avoid IM administration. Oral absorption reduced in neonates. $T_{1/2}$ is variable (7–42 hr) and dose-dependent. Useful in ventricular tachycardia and digitalis-induced arrhythmias (esp. PAT with block). Not FDA approved for ventricular arrhythmias. Side effects: gingival hyperplasia, hirsutism, dermatitis, blood dyscrasia, ataxia, SLE-like and Stevens-Johnson syndromes, lymphadenopathy, liver damage, and nystagmus. For seizure disorders, **therapeutic levels: 10–20 mg/L (free and bound phenytoin) OR 1–2 mg/L (free only). IV push not to exceed 0.5 mg/kg/min.** Drug is highly protein-bound; free

	Adults: 300–400 mg/24 hr ÷ QD-Q12 hr IV/PO *Anti-arrhythmic* *Load (all ages):* 1.25 mg/kg IV Q5 min up to a total of 15 mg/kg *Maintenance:* Children: IV/PO: 5–10 mg/kg/24 hr ÷ Q12 hr Adults: 250 mg PO QID × 1 day, then 250 mg PO Q12 hr × 2 days, then 300–400 mg/24 hr ÷ QD–Q6 hr.	fraction of drug will be increased in patients with hypoalbuminemia. PO: measure level just before dose. Many drug interactions: levels may be increased by cimetidine, chloramphenicol, INH, sulfonamides, trimethoprim, etc. Levels may be decreased by some anti-neoplastic agents and theophylline. Phenytoin induces hepatic microsomal enzymes leading to decreased effectiveness of oral contraceptives, quinidine, etc.
Phosphorus Supplements: sodium phosphate (NeutraPhos); potassium phosphate (NeutraPhos-K); Na + K phosphate	Oral dosage forms (to be reconstituted in 75 ml H$_2$0 per capsule/packet.) *Na phosphate (NeutraPhos):* Caps, powder: 7 mEq Na, 7 mEq K, 250 mg (8 mM) P *K phosphate (NeutraPhos-K):* Caps, powder: 14.25 mEq K, 250 mg (8 mM) P	*Acute hypophosphatemia:* 5–10 mg/kg/dose IV over 6 hr *Maintenance (may divide doses):* Children: IV: 15–45 mg/kg/24 hr PO: 30–90 mg/kg/24 hr Adults: IV: 1.5–2 gm/24 hr	May cause tetany, hyperphosphatemia, hyperkalemia, hypocalcemia. IV administration may cause hypotension, renal failure, or myocardial infarction. PO dosing may cause nausea, vomiting, abdominal pain, or diarrhea. Use with **caution** in

(Continued.)

Drug	How Supplied	Dose and Route	Remarks
	Na + K phosphate: Tabs: 250 mg (8 mM) P, 13 mEq Na, 1.1 mEq K *Euro-KP neutral tabs:* 10.9 mEq Na, 1.27 mEq K 250 (8 mM) P. Inj (Na): 94 mg (3 mM) P + 4 mEq Na/ml (K): 94 mg (3 mM) P + 4.4 mEq K/ml	PO: 3–4.5 gm/24 hr **Max IV infusion rate:** 0.2 mM/kg/hr of phosphate. When potassium salt is used, rate will be limited by maximum potassium infusion rate	patients with renal impairment.
Physostigmine salicylate (Antilirium)	Inj: 1 mg/ml	For antihistamine overdose or anticholinergic poisoning, see Chapter 3.	**Physostigmine antidote:** Atropine always should be available.
Pilocarpine HCl (Akarpine, Isopto Carpine, Piligan, and others)	Ophthalmic Sol: 0.25, 0.5, 1, 2, 3, 4, 5, 6, 8, 10%	*For elevated intraocular pressure:* 1–2 drops in each eye 4–6 ×/24 hr; adjust concentration and frequency as needed.	May cause stinging, burning, lacrimation, headache, retinal detachment. Use with **caution** in patients with corneal abrasion.
Piperacillin (Pipracil)	Inj: 2, 3, 40 gm	*Neonates:* 200 mg/kg/24 hr IV ÷ Q12 hr *Children >12 yr:* cystic fibrosis: 300–600 mg/kg/24 hr ÷ Q4–6 hr IV or deep IM	Similar to penicillin. Piperacillin has been used in children <12 yr at dosages of 75–300 mg/kg/24 hr, although currently it is not approved by the FDA for this age group. Contains 1.85 mEq Na/gm.

Others: 200–300 mg/kg/24 hr ÷
Q4–6 hr IV or deep IM
Max dose: 24 gm/24 hr
Adults: 3–4 gm/dose IV Q4–6
hr **or** 2–3 gm/dose IM
Q6–12 hr. **Max dose:** 24
gm/24 hr.

Piperazine (Antepar, Bryrel)	Tabs: 250, 500 mg Syrup: 500 mg/5 ml	*Enterobius vermicularis* (pinworm): Adults and children: 65 mg/kg/24 hr PO QD × 7 days. **Max dose:** 2.5 gm/24 hr. May repeat in 1 wk if necessary. *Ascaris lumbricoides* (roundworm): Children: 75 mg/kg/24 hr PO QD × 2 days. Adult: 3.5 gm PO QD × 2 days **Max dose:** 3.5 gm/24 hr	**Contraindicated** in epilepsy. Large doses may cause vomiting, urticaria, muscle weakness, blurred vision, and GI irritation. Pyrantel pamoate and piperazine have antagonistic modes of action and should not be administered concomitantly. Use **caution** when administering with chlorpromazine.

(Continued.)

Drug	How Supplied	Dose and Route	Remarks
Polyethylene glycol-electrolyte solution (GoLYTELY, CoLyte)	Powder for oral solution: (GoLYTELY): polyethylene glycol 3350 236 gm, Na sulfate 22.74 gm, Na bicarbonate 6.74 gm, NaCl 5.86 gm, KCl 2.97 gm	Children: Oral: 25–40 ml/kg/hr until rectal effluent is clear Nasogastric: 20–30 ml/min up to 4 L	Effect should occur within 1–2 hr. Solution generally more palatable if chilled. Monitor electrolytes, BUN, serum glucose, and urine osmolality with prolonged administration. **Contraindicated** in toxic megacolon, gastric retention, colitis, bowel perforation.
Polymyxin B sulfate and bacitracin (Ak-poly-BAC, Ocumycin, Polysporin)	Ophthalmic ointment: Bacitracin 500 U and polymyxin B 10,000 U/gm (3.5, 3.75 gm) Topical ointment: Bacitracin 500 U and polymyxin B 10,000 U/gm (15, 30 gm) Topical powder (10 gm) Topical spray (90 gm)	Ophthalmic: Apply to affected eye 4–6 × /24 hr Topical: Apply ointment or powder to affected area QD-TID	Do not use ophthalmic ointment for longer than 1 wk. Do not use topical ointment in the eyes. Side effects: rash, itching, burning, conjunctival erythema, anaphylactoid reaction, swelling.
Polymyxin, neosporin, hydrocortisone (Cortisporin, Oticort, and others)	Otic Sol, susp: Neomycin sulfate 5 mg, bacitracin 400 U, polymyxin B sulfate 10,000 U, and hydrocortisone 10 mg/ml (10 ml)	*Otitis externa:* 3–4 drops 3–4 × /day × 7–10 days	**Contraindicated** in patients with perforated tympanic membranes. Not to be used in patients with active herpes simplex, vaccinia, or varicella. May cause cutaneous sensitization.

| Potassium iodide
(Iosat, Pima, Potassium Iodide Enseals, Thyro-Block) | Tabs: 130, 300 mg
Syrup: 325 mg/5 ml (500 ml)
Sol: 500 mg/15 ml (500 ml)
Saturated Sol (SSKI): 1000 mg/ml (30, 240 ml) | *Thyrotoxicosis:*
Children: 200–300 mg/24 hr
  PO ÷ BID-TID
Adults: 300–900 mg/24 hr PO
  ÷ TID
Sporotrichosis:
Initial:
  Preschool: 50 mg/dose PO
    TID
  Children: 250 mg/dose PO
    TID
  Adults: 500 mg/dose PO
    TID
  Increment: Increase 50
    mg/dose daily
  Max dose:
  Preschool: 500 mg/dose
    TID
  Child/adult: 1–2 gm/dose
    TID | **Contraindicated** in pregnancy. GI disturbance, metallic taste, rash, salivary gland inflammation, headache, lacrimation, and rhinitis are symptoms of iodism. Give with milk or water after meals. Continue sporotrichosis treatment for 4–6 wk after lesions have completely healed. Increase dose until either maximum dose is achieved or signs of iodism appear. |
| Potassium supplements
(Many brand names) | *Potassium chloride:*
40 mEq K = 3 gm KCl
Sustained-release caps: 8, 10
  mEq
Tabs: 2.5, 4, 13.4 mEq | Starting dose should be determined by considering maintenance, losses, and desired replacement. See Chapter 10. | PO administration may cause GI disturbance and ulceration. IV administration may cause irritation, pain, or phlebitis at the infusion site. Rapid or |

(Continued.)

Drug	How Supplied	Dose and Route	Remarks
Potassium supplements *(continued.)*.	Sustained-release tabs: 6.7, 8, 10, 20 mEq Powder: 15, 20, 25 mEq/packet Sol: 10% (6.7 mEq/5 ml) 15% (10 mEq/5 ml), 20% (13.3 mEq/5 ml) Conc. inj: 2 mEq/ml *Potassium gluconate:* 40mEq K = 9.4 gm K gluconate Tabs: 2, 5 mEq Elixir: 20 mEq/15 ml *Potassium acetate* 40 mEq K = 3.9 gm K acetate Inj: 4mEq/ml	*Children:* 1–4 mEq/kg/24 hr PO ÷ BID-QID as required to maintain normal serum potassium. *Adults:* 10–15 mEq/dose PO TID-QID **Max infusion rate:** 0.5–1 mEq/kg/hr. **Max peripheral IV Sol concentration:** 40 mEq/L. *Normal daily requirements* Newborn: 2–6 mEq/kg/24 hr Children: 2–3 mEq/kg/24 hr Adult: 40–80 mEq/24 hr	central IV infusion may cause cardiac arrhythmias. Patients receiving infusion >0.5 mEq/kg/hr should be placed on an ECG monitor. Oral liquid supplements should be diluted in water or fruit juice prior to administration. Sustained-release tablets must be swallowed and not dissolved in the mouth.
Praziquantel (Biltricide, Droncit)	Tab: 600 mg	Children and adults: *Schistosomiasis:* 20 mg/kg/dose Q4–6 hr × 1 day *Flukes:* 25 mg/kg/dose Q8 hr × 1–2 days	Take with food. Do not chew tablets owing to bitter taste. May cause dizziness, drowsiness. **Contraindicated** in ocular cysticercosis.

	Cysticercosis: 50 mg/kg/24 hr ÷ Q8 hr × 14 days *Tapeworms:* 10–20 mg/kg/dose × 1 dose	Use with **caution** in patients with severe hepatic disease.
Prazosin HCl (Minipress)	Caps: 1, 2, 5 mg	
	Children: Initial: 5 µg/kg PO test dose Maintenance: 25–150 µg/kg/24 hr ÷ Q6 hr *Adults:* 1 mg PO BID-TID initially. Increase slowly to **max dose** of 20 mg/24 hr PO ÷ BID-TID	Not FDA approved for children. May cause syncope, tachycardia, hypotension, dizziness, nausea, headache, drowsiness, fatigue, anticholinergic effects. Marked orthostatic hypotension, syncope, and loss of consciousness may occur with 1st dose.
Prednisolone (Delta-Cortef, Prelone, Pediapred, and others)	Tabs: 5 mg Syrup: 5 mg/5ml (Pediapred), 15 mg/5ml (Prelone) (both contain some alcohol) Opthalmic susp: 0.125% (5,10 ml), 1% (5,10 ml) Inj: Acetate (25, 50 mg/ml), phosphate (20 mg/ml)	See Prednisone See Chapter 26. Equivalent glucocorticoid and mineralocorticoid potencies as prednisone.

(Continued.)

Drug	How Supplied	Dose and Route	Remarks
Prednisone (many brand names)	Tabs: 1, 2.5, 5, 10, 20, 50 mg Solution: 5 mg/5 ml Conc Sol: 5 mg/ml Syrup: 5 mg/ml	*Anti-inflammatory or immunosuppresive:* 0.5–2 mg/kg/24 hr **or** 25–60 mg/m² /24 hr ÷ Q6–12 hr PO *Asthma:* Acute exacerbation: 0.5–2.0 mg/kg/24 hr up to 20–40 mg/24 hr PO × 3–5 days. *Chronic refractory* asthma: 5–10 mg/dose QD or 10–30 mg QOD PO. Attempt to taper/wean to aerosol corticosteroid. *Nephrotic syndrome:* Initial: 2 mg/kg/24 hr ÷ TID-QID PO (**max dose:** 80 mg/24 hr) until urine is protein-free × 5 days or for **max** of 28 days. If proteinura persists, dose may be changed to 4 mg/kg/dose (**max dose:** 120 mg/24 hr) QOD for an additional 28 days.	See Chapter 26. Methylprednisolone preferable in hepatic disease, since prednisone must be converted to methylprednisolone in the liver. Long-term low maintenance doses may be beneficial in relapsing nephrotic syndrome.

	Maintenance: 2 mg/kg/dose QOD × 28 days. Then taper over 4–6 wk. *Physiologic replacement:* 4–5 mg/m²/24 hr ÷ BID PO	
Primaquine phosphate	Tab: 26.3 mg (15 mg base)	Contraindicated in granulocytopenic patients and patients receiving quinacrine. Use with **caution** in G6PD deficiency. May cause hemolytic anemia, leukopenia, leukocytosis, methemoglobinemia.
	Children: 0.3 mg base/kg/dose × 14 days. **Max dose:** 15 mg/day **or** 0.9 mg base/kg/dose Q wk × 8 wk *Adults:* 15 mg base/dose QD × 14 days **or** 45 mg base/dose Q wk × 8 wk	
Primidone (Mysoline, Neurosyn)	Tabs: 50, 250 mg Susp: 250 mg/5 ml	Primidone is metabolized to phenobarbital and has the same toxicities: sedation, nausea, rash, leukopenia, lupus-like syndrome. Follow both primidone and phenobarbital levels. **Therapeutic level: 8–12 mg/L** of primidone or **15–40 mg/L** of phenobarbital. Use with **caution** in renal or hepatic disease and pulmonary insufficiency.
	<8 yr: Initial: 125 mg/24 hr QD PO Weekly increment: 125 mg Maintenance: 10–25 mg/kg/24 hr ÷ TID-QID PO *≥8 yr–adults:* Initial: 250 mg/24 hr QD PO Weekly increment: 250 mg Maintenance: 0.75–1.5 gm/24 hr ÷ TID-QID PO **max dose: 2 gm/24 hr**	

(Continued.)

Drug	How Supplied	Dose and Route	Remarks
Probenecid (Benemid)	Tabs: 500 mg	Use with penicillin: *Children (2–14 yr):* 25 mg/kg PO X 1, then 40 mg/kg/24 hr ÷ QID *Adult dose (>50kg):* 500 mg PO QID: for gonorrhea give 1 gm probenecid PO 30 min before penicillin or ampicillin. *Hyperuricemia:* 250 mg PO BID × 1 wk, then 500 mg twice weekly, up to 2–3 gm/24 hr	Inhibits renal tubular transport of organic acids, penicillin, cephalosporins. Increases uric acid excretion. Alkalinize urine in patients with gout. Use with **caution** in peptic ulcer. May cause headache, rash, GI symptoms, hypersensitivity, anemia. **Contraindicated** in infants <2 yr and patients with renal insufficiency.
Procainamide (Pronestyl, Procan SR)	Tabs: 250, 375, 500 mg Slow-release tabs: 250, 500, 750, 1000 mg Caps: 250, 375, 500 mg Inj: 100, 500 mg/ml	*Children:* IM: 20–30 mg/kg/24 hr ÷ Q4–6 hr. **Max dose:** 4 gm/24 hr (peak effect in 1 hr) IV: Load: 2–6 mg/kg/dose over 5 min. Maintenance: 20–80 μg/kg/min by continuous infusion; **Max dose:** 100 mg/dose or 2 gm/24 hr PO: 15–50 mg/kg/24 hr ÷ Q3–6 hr; **Max dose:** 4 gm/24 hr	**Contraindicated** in myasthenia gravis, complete heart block. May cause lupus-like syndrome, positive Coombs', thrombocytopenia, arrhythmias, GI complaints, confusion. Monitor BPs, ECG when using IV. QRS widening >0.02 sec suggests toxicity. **Therapeutic levels: 4–10 mg/L of procainamide or 10–30 mg/L of procainamide and NAPA levels combined.**

Adults: IM: loading: 1 gm/dose × 1

Maintenance: 250 mg/dose Q3 hr

IV: loading: 100–200 mg/dose; repeat Q5 min PRN to **max dose** of 1000 mg.

Maintenance: 1–6 mg/min by continuous infusion. PO: 250–500 mg/dose Q3–6 hr. Usual dose 50 mg/kg/24 hr or 2–4 gm/24 hr.

| **Prochlorperazine** (Compazine) | Tabs: 5, 10, 25 mg
Slow-release caps: 10, 15, 30 mg
Syrup: 5 mg/5 ml (120 ml)
Suppository: 2.5, 5, 25 mg
Inj: 5 mg/ml | *Children (>10 kg or >2 yr):* PO or PR: 0.4 mg/kg/24 hr ÷ TID-QID
IM: 0.1–0.15 mg/kg/dose TID-QID
Adults: PO: 5–10 mg/dose TID-QID
PR: 25 mg/dose BID
IM: 5–10 mg/dose Q4–6 hr | Toxicity as for other phenothiazines (see chlorpromazine).
Extrapyramidal reactions or orthostatic hypotension may occur. **Do not use** IV route in children <10 kg or <2 yr. Use only in management of **known** prolonged vomiting of **known** |

(Continued.)

Drug	How Supplied	Dose and Route	Remarks
		Max IV/IM dose: 40 mg/24 hr IV: 5–10 mg/dose (**Max dose:** 10 mg/dose) may repeat × 1	etiology.
Promethazine (Phenergan, Provigan)	Tabs: 12.5, 25, 50 mg Syrup: 6.25 mg/5 ml, 25 mg/5 ml Suppository: 12.5, 25, 50 mg Inj: 25, 50 mg/ml	*Antihistaminic:* Children: 0.1 mg/kg/dose Q6 hr and 0.5 mg/kg/dose QHS PO PRN Adults: 12.5 mg PO TID and 25 mg QHS *Nausea and vomiting:* Children: 0.25–0.5 mg/kg/dose PO, IV, IM or PR Q4–6 hr PRN Adults: 12.5–25 mg Q4–6 hr PRN *Motion sickness:* (1st dose 0.5–1. hr before departure): Children: 0.5 mg/kg/dose Q12 hr PO PRN Adults: 25 mg PO BID	Toxicity similar to other phenothiazines (see Chlorpromazine). Use only in management of prolonged vomiting of **known** etiology.
Propranolol (Inderal)	Tabs: 10, 20, 40, 60, 80, 90 mg Extended-release caps: 60, 80, 120,160 mg Sol: 20, 40 mg/5 ml Conc. Sol: 80 mg/ml Susp*: 1 mg/ml Inj: 1 mg/ml	*Arrhythmias:* Children IV: 0.01–0.1 mg/kg/dose slow IV push; repeat Q6–8 hr PRN; **Max dose:** 1 mg/dose. PO: 0.5–4 mg/kg/24 hr ÷ Q6–8 hr PO; **Max dose:** 60 mg/24 hr.	**Contraindicated** in asthma and heart block. Use with caution in presence of obstructive lung disease, heart failure, renal or hepatic disease. May cause hypoglycemia, hypotension, nausea,

Adults IV: 1 mg/dose Q5 min up to **total** 5 mg; PO 40–320 mg/24 hr ÷ BID-TID

Hypertension: Children: Initial: 0.5–1.0 mg/kg/24 hr PO ÷ Q6–12 hr **max dose:** 2 mg/kg/24 hr.

Adults: Initial: 40 mg/dose PO BID Increment: 10–20 mg/dose at 3–7 day intervals. **Max dose:** 320–480 mg/24 hr PO ÷ BID-TID

Migraine prophylaxis: Children: ≤35 kg: 10–20 mg PO TID >35 kg: 20–40 mg PO TID Adults: Initial: 80 mg/24 hr ÷ Q6–8 hr PO. Usual effective dose range: 160–240 mg/24 hr. **Max dose:** 320 mg/24 hr

vomiting, depression, weakness, impotence, bronchospasm, heart block. **Therapeutic levels: 30–100 ng/ml.** Concurrent administration with barbiturates, indomethacin, or rifampin may cause decreased activity of propranolol. Concurrent administration with cimetidine, hydralazine, chlorpromazine, or verapamil may lead to increased activity of propranolol. **Note:** Bioavailability is 30–60% of dose.

---

*Indicates suspensions not commercially available; need to be extemporaneously compounded by a pharmacist. See references 6 and 7 for specific formulations.
(Continued.)

Drug	How Supplied	Dose and Route	Remarks
Propranolol *(continued.).*		*Tetralogy spells:* 0.15–0.25 mg/kg/dose IV slowly. May repeat in 15 min × 1 (**max single dose:** 10 mg), then 1–2 mg/kg/dose Q6 hr PO PRN. *Thyrotoxicosis:* Neonate: 2 mg/kg/24 hr PO ÷ Q6 hr Adolescents/adults: IV: 1–3 mg/dose × 1 over 10 min PO: 10–40 mg Q6 hr	
Propylthiouracil (PTU)	Tabs: 50 mg	*Children:* Initial: 5–7 mg/kg/24 hr ÷ Q8 hr PO **or** 6–10 yr: 50–150 mg/24 hr ÷ Q8 hr PO >10 yr: 150–300 mg/24 hr ÷ Q8 hr PO Maintenance: Adjust to patient response. Usually 1/3–2/3 the initial dose beginning when the patient is euthyroid. *Adults:* Initial: 300–450 mg/24 hr ÷ Q8 hr PO Maintenance: 100–150 mg/24 hr ÷ Q8 hr	May cause blood dyscrasias, fever, liver disease, dermatitis, urticaria, malaise, CNS stimulation or depression, arthralgias. Monitor thyroid function. Dosages should be adjusted as required to achieve and maintain T_3, T_4, TSH levels in normal ranges. 100 mg PTU = 10 mg methimazole.

Prostaglandin E₁ (PGE₁, Alprostadil, Prostin VR)	Inj: 500 μg/ml	*Neonates:* Initial: 0.05 – 0.1 μg/kg/min. Advance to 0.2 μg/kg/min if necessary. Maintenance: When increase in PaO₂ is noted, decrease immediately to lowest effective dose.	For palliation only. Continuous vital sign monitoring essential. May cause apnea, fever, seizures, flushing, bradycardia, hypotension, and diarrhea. Decreases platelet aggregation.
Protamine sulfate	Inj: 10 mg/ml Inj: 50 mg/vial	*Heparin antidote:* 1 mg will neutralize approximately 90 U (bovine source) or 100 U (porcine source) of heparin. For IV heparin, base dose on amount received in previous 2 hr. **Max dose:** 50 mg IV; rate not to exceed 5 mg/min.	Actual dosage depends on route of administration and time elapsed since heparin dose. Can cause hypotension, bradycardia, dyspnea, and anaphylaxis. Rarely, heparin rebound has occurred.
Pseudoephedrine (Sudafed, Novafed, and others)	Tabs: 30, 60 mg Sustained-release caps: 120 mg Syrup: 15, 30 mg/5 ml (120 ml) Drops: 7.5 mg/0.8 ml	*Children ≤12 yr:* 4 mg/kg/24 hr ÷ Q6 hr PO *Children >12 yr and adults:* 30–60 mg/dose Q6–8 hr PO **Max dose:** 240 mg/24 hr *Sustained release:* >12 yr–adults: 120 mg PO Q12 hr	Use with **caution** in hypertension, hyperglycemia, cardiac disease. May cause nervousness, restlessness, insomnia, arrhythmias.

(Continued.)

Drug	How Supplied	Dose and Route	Remarks
Psyllium (Metamucil, Fiberall, Seraton and many others)	Granules: 2.5, 4.0 gm/tsp Effervescent powder: 3.4 gm/heaping tsp Powder: psyllium 50%, dextrose 50% Chewable squares: 3.4 gm Wafer: 1.7, 3.4 gm	*Children (6–11 yr):* 0.5–1.0 rounded tsp/dose QD-TID. **Max dose:** 15 gm/24 hr ≥*12 yr:* 1–2 rounded tsp/dose QD-QID. **Max dose:** 30 gm/24 hr	**Contraindicated** in cases of fecal impaction or GI obstruction. Should be taken with a full glass of liquid. **Onset** of action 12–72 hr.
Pyrantel pamoate (Antiminth)	Susp: 250 mg/5 ml (60 ml)	*Ascariasis (roundworm), hookworm:* In children and adults: 11 mg/kg PO as single dose. **Max dose:** 1 gm. *Enterobius (pinworm):* 11 mg/kg/dose PO. **Max dose:** 1 gm. Repeat after 2 wk.	Nausea, vomiting, anorexia, transient AST elevations, headaches, rash. Use with **caution** with liver dysfunction.
Pyrazinamide (pyrazinoic acid amide)	Tab: 500 mg	*Tuberculosis:* Children: 15–30 mg/kg/24 hr ÷ QD-BID **Max dose:** 2 gm/24 hr Adults: 15–30 mg/kg/24 hr ÷ TID-QID **Max dose:** 2 gm/24 hr	**Contraindicated** in severe hepatic damage. Hepatotoxicity is most common side effect. Hyperuricemia, maculopapular rash, arthralgia, fever, acne, porphyria, dysuria, photosensitivity may occur. Use with **caution** in patients with renal failure, gout, or diabetes mellitus.

Pyrethrins (A-200 Pyrinate, Pyrinal, Pronto, RID)	Available as gel, shampoo, and liquid, all in combination with piperonyl butoxide	*Pediculosis* Apply to hair or affected body area for 10 min, then wash thoroughly; may repeat in 7–10 days.	For topical use only. Avoid eye or facial contact and PO intake. Avoid repeat applications in <24 hr.
Pyridostigmine bromide (Mestinon, Regonol)	Syrup: 60 mg/5ml (480 ml) Tab: 60 mg Slow-release tab: 180 mg Inj: 5 mg/ml	*Myasthenia gravis:* Children: 7 mg/kg/24 hr in 5–6 divided doses PO. IV/IM 0.05–0.15 mg/kg/dose Max single dose 10 mg. Adult: PO: immediate release. IV/IM 2–5 mg/dose Q2–3hr 60 mg TID. **Max dose:** 1.5 gm/24 hr. PO sustained release: 180–540 mg QD-BID	Changes in oral dosages may take several days to show results. Use with **caution** in patients with epilepsy, asthma, bradycardia, hyperthyroidism, arrhythmias, or peptic ulcer. May cause nausea, vomiting, diarrhea, rash, headache, and muscle cramps. Atropine is the antagonist.
Pyridoxine (vitamin B₆)	Tabs: 10, 25, 50, 100, 200, 250, 500 mg Slow-release tabs: 500 mg Caps: 500 mg Slow-release caps: 100, 500 mg Inj: 100 mg/ml	*Deficiency:* 5–10 mg/24 hr × several wk *Drug-induced neuritis:* 1–2 mg/kg/24 hr for prophylaxis or 10–50 mg/24 hr as treatment. *Sideroblastic anemia:* 200–600 mg/24 hr × 1–2 mo *Pyridoxine-dependent seizures:* 10–100 mg/dose, rapid IV or IM	May be given IV, IM, or SC when oral administration is not feasible. Chronic administration has been associated with adverse neurologic effects. Nausea, headache, increased AST, decreased serum folic acid level, and allergic reaction may occur.

(Continued.)

Drug	How Supplied	Dose and Route	Remarks
Pyrimethamine (Daraprim)	Tabs: 25 mg Susp*: 2 mg/ml	*Toxoplasmosis* (administer with sulfadiazine or trisulfapyrimidines): Children: Loading: 2 mg/kg/24 hr PO ÷ QD-BID × 3 days. **Max dose:** 100 mg/24 hr Maintenance: 1 mg/kg/24 hr PO ÷ QD-BID × 4 wk. **Max dose:** 25 mg/24 hr Adults: 25 mg/24 hr PO for 3–4 wk	Blood dyscrasias, glossitis, leukopenia, folic acid deficiency, rash, seizures. After 3–4 days of continuous therapy, it is advisable to give leucovorin (2–15 mg/24 hr QD) to prevent hematologic complications.
Pyrimethamine with sulfadoxine (Fansidar)	Tabs: 25 mg pyrimethamine and 500 mg sulfadoxine	*Malaria suppression/ prophylaxis:* Pyrimethamine 0.5 mg/kg/dose and sulfadoxine 10 mg/kg/dose PO (**max dose:** 1 tab) Q wk from 1–2 wk before until 6 wk after exposure	Complications include those of pyrimethamine, as well as crystalluria, hypersensitivity, fever, rash, hepatitis, vasculitis, anemia, thrombocytopenia, and Stevens-Johnson syndrome.
Quinacrine HCl (Atabrine, Mepacrine HCl)	Tabs: 100 mg	*Giardiasis:* 6 mg/kg/24 hr ÷ Q8 hr PO × 5–7 days. **Max dose:** 300 mg/24 hr.	May cause GI symptoms, dermatosis, myelosuppression, psychosis, retinal depigmentation,

seizures, and headache. May
cause temporary yellow skin
color (not jaundice). Use with
caution in patients with G6PD
deficiency, renal cardiac or
hepatic disease. **Do not use**
concurrently with primaquine.

Tapeworm:
5–10 yr: 100 mg Q10 min PO
× 4 doses
11–14 yr: 200 mg Q10 min
PO × 3 doses

Malaria, acute attacks:
1–4 yr: 100 mg TID × 1 day
followed by 100 mg QD × 6
days.
4–8 yr: 200 mg TID × 1 day
followed by 100 mg BID ×
6 days.
>8 yr: 200 mg with 1 gm of
NaHCO₃ Q6 hr × 5 doses
followed by 100 mg TID ×
6 days. **Max dose:** 2.8
gm/wk.

Suppression:
<8 yr: 50 mg QD for 1–3 mo.
≥8 yr: 100 mg QD for 1–3
mo.

Quinidine	*Gluconate:* (62% quinidine)	Test dose: 2 mg/kg PO. **Max**	Toxicity indicated by increase of
(many brand names)	Tabs: 330 mg	**dose:** 200 mg	QRS interval by ≥0.02 sec
	Slow-release tabs: 324 mg	*Therapeutic dose:*	(skip dose or stop drug). May
	Inj: 80 mg/ml	Children: IV **(not**	cause GI symptoms,
	Sulfate: (83% quinidine)	**recommended):** 2–10	hypotension, tinnitus, TTP,

*Indicates suspensions not commercially available; need to be extemporaneously compounded by a pharmacist. See references 6 and
7 for specific formulations.

(Continued.)

Drug	How Supplied	Dose and Route	Remarks
Quinidine *(continued.)*.	Tabs: 100, 200, 300 mg Slow-release tabs: 300 mg Caps: 300 mg Inj: 200 mg/mg Susp*:10 mg/ml	mg/kg/dose Q3–6 hr PRN (gluconate) PO: 15–60 mg/kg/24 hr ÷ Q6 hr (sulfate) Adults: IM: 400 mg/dose Q4–6 hr IV: 200–400 mg/dose PO: 100–600 mg/dose Q4–6 hr; begin at 200 mg/dose and titrate to desired effect (gluconate or sulfate) *Malaria:* Adult: Load 10 mg base/kg IV over 1 hr, then 0.02 mg/kg/min continuous infusion until oral dose can be started Children: 10 mg base/kg, then 5 mg/kg 6 hr later, then 5 mg/kg/24 hr at 24 and 48 hr. **Max dose:** 600 mg base.	rash, heart block, blood dyscrasias. Can cause increase in digoxin levels if these drugs are used concomitantly. Amiodarone or cimetidine may enhance the drug's effect. Barbituates, phenytoin, or rifampin may reduce the drug's effect. When used alone, may cause 1:1 conduction in atrial flutter leading to ventricular fibrillation. May get idiosyncratic ventricular tachycardia with low levels, especially when initiating therapy. **Therapeutic levels: 3–7 mg/L.** Sustained release tabs may be given Q8–12hr.

Quinine sulfate	Tabs: 162.5, 260 mg Caps: 130, 200, 300, 325 mg	*Malaria:* 25 mg/kg/24 hr ÷ Q8 hr PO × 3 days. **Max dose:** 650 mg/dose *Babesia:* 25 mg/kg/24 hr ÷ Q8 hr PO × 7 days. **Max dose:** 650 mg/dose.	May cause cinchonism (tinnitus, headache, nausea, abdominal pain, visual disturbance), blood dyscrasias, arrhythmias, hypotension, hemolysis. **Contraindicated** in pregnancy, G6PD deficiency, hypersensitivity. Use with **caution** in patients with myasthenia gravis.
Ranitidine HCl (Zantac)	Tabs: 150, 300 mg Syrup: 15 mg/ml (7.5% alcohol) Inj: 25 mg/ml	*Children:* PO: 2–4 mg/kg/24 hr ÷ Q12 hr IV: 1–2 mg/kg/24 hr ÷ Q6–8 hr *Adults:* PO: 150 mg BID or 300 mg QHS IV: 50 mg Q6–8 hr	Usual adverse reactions include headache and GI disturbance, malaise, insomnia, sedation, arthralgia, hepatotoxicity. May increase levels of theophylline, warfarin.
Ribavirin (Virazole)	Aerosol: 6 gm/100 ml	Administer by aerosol 12–18 hr daily for 3–7 days. The 6 gm ribavirin vial is diluted in 300 ml preservative-free sterile water to a final concentration of 20 mg/ml. Must be administered with Viratek Small Particle Aerosol Generator (SPAG-2).	Most effective if begun early in course of illness—generally in the first 3 days. Worsening respiratory distress, rash, conjunctivitis, mild bronchospasm, hypotension, anemia, and cardiac arrest have been described. See references 6 and 7 for specific formulations. *(Continued.)*

*Indicates suspensions not commercially available; need to be extemporaneously compounded by a pharmacist. See references 6 and 7 for specific formulations.

Drug	How Supplied	Dose and Route	Remarks
Rifampin (Rimactane, Rifadin)	Caps: 150, 300 mg liquid: 10 mg/ml (1%). Can be made according to directions found in package insert. Susp*: 15 mg/ml Inj: 600 mg.	*Children:* 10–20 mg/kg/24 hr IV/PO ÷ Q12–24 hr *Tuberculosis:* (see Chapter 17.) 10–20 mg/kg/dose up to **max dose** of 600 mg/dose PO QD or twice weekly. *Meningitis prophylaxis, N. meningitidis:* 0–1 mo: 10 mg/kg/24 hr ÷ Q12 hr × 2 days. >1 mo: 20 mg/kg/24 hr to **max dose** of 600 mg/dose ÷ Q12 hr PO × 2 days *H. influenzae:* 0–1 mo: 10 mg/kg/24 hr PO QD × 4 days >1 mo: 20 mg/kg/24 hr PO up to **max dose** of 600 mg/24 hr QD × 4 days	Causes red discoloration of body secretions (e.g., urine, saliva, and tears, which can permanently stain contact lenses). Induces hepatic microsomal enzymes; may need increased doses of digoxin, phenytoin, theophylline, etc. Reduces effectiveness of oral contraceptives; recommend other methods of birth control. Give 1 hr before or 2 hr after meals. Use with **caution** in liver disease. May cause gastrointestinal irritation, allergy, headache, fatigue, ataxia, confusion, fever, hepatitis, blood dyscrasias, and elevated BUN and uric acid. IV dose is similar to PO dose.

Scopolamine hydrobromide (Hyoscine, Transderm Scop, Isopto)	Inj: 0.3, 0.4, 0.86, 1 mg/ml Transdermal: 0.5 mg Opthalmic Sol: 0.25% (5 ml)	*Antiemesis:* Children: 6 µg/kg/dose SC, IM, or IV Adults: 0.2–1 mg/dose SC, IM, or IV *Transdermal:* Apply patch behind the ear at least 4 hr prior to exposure to motion; use for 72 hr *Ophthalmic:* Children refraction: 1 drop BID for 2 days before procedure. Children iridocyclitis: 1 drop up to TID.	Toxicities similar to atropine. May cause dry mouth, drowsiness, blurred vision. **Contraindicated** in urinary or GI obstruction and glaucoma. Transdermal route should **not** be used in children <12 yr. Systemic effects have been reported with both topical and ophthalmic preparations. Compress lacrimal ducts to minimize systemic effects.
Secobarbital (Seconal)	Caps: 50, 100 mg Inj: 50 mg/ml	*Sedation:* Children: 4–6 mg/kg/24 hr ÷ Q8 hr PO, IM, PR Adults: 20–40 mg/dose PO BID-TID **or** 200–300 mg/dose PO 2–3 hr preoperatively	See amobarbital. T$_{1/2}$=20–28 hr. The injectable preparation of secobarbital may be given rectally; (dilute to conc. of 10–15 mg/ml with warm tap water). Secobarbital suppositories are

*Indicates suspensions not commercially available; need to be extemporaneously compounded by a pharmacist. See references 6 and 7 for specific formulations.

(Continued.)

Drug	How Supplied	Dose and Route	Remarks
Secobarbitol *(continued.)*.		*Hypnosis:* Children: 3–5 mg/kg/dose IM Adults: IM or PO: 100–200 mg/dose IV: 50–250 mg/dose	no longer commercially available in the United States. **Max IV infusion rate** ≤50 mg/15 sec. Patient should be observed closely for 20–30 min after IM administration of large hypnotic doses.
Selenium sulfide (Selsun)	Lotion: 1% shampoo (120, 210, 300 ml). 2.5% (120 ml)	*Tinea versicolor:* Apply weekly × 4 wk to affected areas. *Tinea capitis:* Apply twice weekly for 2–4 wk.	May cause local irritation, rare discoloration of hair, hair loss. Lather and rinse from body areas after 5 min or from face after 10 min. Avoid eyes and genital area.
Senna (Senokot, Senna-Gen, and others)	Granules: 326 mg/tsp Liquid: 7%, 6.5% Rectal suppository: 652 mg Syrup: 218 mg/5 ml (60 ml, 240 ml) Tab: 187 mg, 217 mg, 600 mg	Children: 10–20 mg/kg/dose at bedtime; **Max dose:** 872 mg. Adults: Granules: 1 tsp at bedtime; **max dose:** 2 tsp BID. Syrup: 2–3 tsp at bedtime; **max dose:** 3 tsp BID. Tablet: 2 tabs (187 mg × 2) at bedtime; **max dose:** 4 tabs BID (187 mg × 4).	Effects occur within 6–24 hr after oral administration. May cause nausea, vomiting, diarrhea, abdominal cramps. May induce peristalsis by stimulating Auerbach's plexus (active metabolite).

Sodium polystyrene sulfonate (Kayexalate, SPS)	Powder: 454 gm (1 tsp = 3.5 gm) Susp: 15 gm/60 ml (contains 21.5 ml sorbitol/60 ml and 4.1mEq Na⁺ per gram)	*Children:* Practical exchange ratio is 1 mEqK per 1 gm resin. Calculate dose according to desired exchange. Usual dose: 1 gm/kg/dose Q6 hr PO or Q2–6 hr rectally *Adults:* 15–60 gm PO or 30–60 gm rectally Q6 hr **Note:** Suspension may be given PO or PR	1 mEq Na delivered for each mEq K removed. Use **cautiously** in presence of renal failure. May cause hypokalemia, hypomagnesemia, and hypocalcemia. **Do not** administer with antacids or laxatives containing Mg or Al. Systemic alkalosis may result.
Spectinomycin (Trobicin)	Inj: 2, 4 gm	*Children:* 40 mg/kg × 1 up to **max dose** of 2 gm/dose IM *Adults:* 2–4 gm IM as a single dose *Gonorrhea:* 40 mg/kg IM × 1	Not effective for syphilis. Used almost exclusively for *N. gonorrheae* infection. Vertigo, nausea, anorexia, malaise, chills, fever, urticaria may occur.
Spironolactone (Aldactone)	Tabs: 25, 50, 100 mg Susp*: 2 mg/ml	*Children:* 1–3.3 mg/kg/24 hr ÷ BID-QID PO *Adults:* 25–100 mg/24 hr ÷ BID-QID PO. **Max dose:** 200 mg/24 hr	**Contraindicated** in acute renal failure. May potentiate ganglionic blocking agents and other antihypertensives. May cause hyperkalemia, GI distress, rash, gynecomastia. See references 6 and 7 for specific formulations. *(Continued.)*

*Indicates suspensions not commercially available; need to be extemporaneously compounded by a pharmacist. See references 6 and 7 for specific formulations.

Drug	How Supplied	Dose and Route	Remarks
Spironolactone *(continued.)*.		*Primary hypoaldosteronism:* Child: 125–375 mg/m²/24 hr in divided doses. Adult: 100–400 mg/24 hr ÷ QD-BID	
Streptokinase (Kabikinase, Streptase)	Inj: 250,000, 750,000, 1,500,000 IU	DVT: Children: 3500–4000 U/kg over 30 min, followed by 1000–1500 U/kg/hr.	**Safety and efficacy have not been established in children. Contraindicated** with intracranial or intraspinal surgery, hx of internal bleeding. May cause hemorrhage, urticaria, itching, flushing, musculoskeletal pain.
Streptomycin sulfate	Inj: 0.5, 1, 5 gm	*Infants and children* (tuberculosis): 20–30 mg/kg/24 hr ÷ Q12 hr IM for 7–10 days **Max dose:** 2 gm/24 hr *Adults* (tuberculosis): 15 mg/kg/24 hr ÷ Q12 hr IM × 7–10 days. **Max dose:** 2 gm/24 hr	Reduce dose in presence of renal insufficiency. Drug is administered via deep IM injection only. IV administration not recommended due to increased risk of toxicity. Follow auditory status. May cause CNS depression or

	Enterococcal endocarditis: 1 gm Q12 hr × 2 wk followed by 500 mg Q12 hr × 4 wk *Streptococcal endocarditis:* 1 gm Q12 hr × 1 wk followed by 500 mg Q12 hr × 1 wk	other neurologic problems, myocarditis, serum sickness. **Therapeutic levels: peak 20–30 mg/L, trough: <5 mg/L.** Therapeutic levels are not achieved in CSF. For TB: use in conjunction with other anti-TB drugs. See Infectious Diseases, Chapter 17.
Succimer (Chemet, DMSA [dimercaptosuccinic acid])	Cap: 100 mg *Lead Chelation:* | Wt (kg)	Initial (mg/dose Q8 hr)
---	---
8–15	100
16–23	200
24–34	300
35–44	400
≥45	500 | Give initial dose for 5 days, followed by same dose Q12 hr for 14 days	Repeated courses may be necessary. Follow serum lead levels (see Chapters 3,14.) Min: 2 wk between courses, unless blood levels indicate more aggressive management. Side effects: GI symptoms, increased LFTs (10%), rash.
Succinylcholine (Anectine, Quelicin)	Inj: 20 mg/ml (10 ml), 50 mg/ml (10 ml), 100 mg/ml (5, 10 ml), 500, 1000 mg **Note:** Some preparations contain benzyl alcohol.	*Infants and children* Initial: 1–2 mg/kg/dose IV × 1 Maintenance: 0.3–0.6 mg/kg/dose IV at intervals of 5–10 min PRN
		Premedicate patient with atropine prior to administration. Duration of action: 10 min. Must be able to intubate patient within 1

(Continued.)

Drug	How Supplied	Dose and Route	Remarks
Succinylcholine (*continued*.).		Continuous infusion: **not** recommended. *Adults*: Initial: 0.3–1.1 mg/kg/dose IV × 1 Maintenance: 0.04–0.07 mg/kgIV at intervals of 5–10 min PRN; Continuous infusion: 0.5–10 mg/min (average dose 2.5 mg/min). Titrate dose to desired effect.	min. Side effects: bradycardia, hypotension, arrhythmia. **Beware** of prolonged depression in patients with liver disease, malnutrition, aminoglycoside therapy, hypothermia, pseudocholinesterase deficiency. May cause malignant hyperthermia.
Sucralfate (Carafate)	Tabs: 1 gm Susp*: 67, 200 mg/ml	*Children*: 40–80 mg/kg/24 hr ÷ Q6 hr *Adults*: 1 gm PO QID 1 hr AC and QHS	Safety and efficacy in children have **not** been established. May cause vertigo, constipation, dry mouth. Aluminum may accumulate in patients with renal failure.
Sulfacetamide sodium (Sulamyd and others)	Ophth Sol: 10%, 15%, 30% (5, 15 ml) Ophthalmic ointment: 10% (3.5 gm)	Ophthalmic ointment: Apply ribbon QID and QHS Drops: 1–2 drops Q2–3 hr to affected eye.	See sulfisoxazole. May cause local irritation, stinging, burning, toxic epidermal necrolysis (rarely).

Sulfadiazine (Microsulfon, and others)	Tabs: 500 mg Susp*: 100 mg/mL	*Children >2 mo:* Loading: 75 mg/kg/dose PO × 1 Maintenance: 150 mg/kg/24 hr ÷ Q6 hr PO. **Max dose:** 6 gm/24 hr *Adults:* Loading: 2–4 gm PO × 1 Maintenance: 1 gm Q4–6 hr PO *Congenital toxoplasmosis:* 85 mg/kg/24 hr PO ÷ Q6 hr with pyrimethamine 1 mg/kg PO QD × 6 mos. Supplement with folic acid 5 mg Q 3 days × 6 mos. *Malaria* (with quinine and pyrimethamine): Children: 100–200 mg/kg/24 hr ÷ QID PO × 5 days. **Max dose:** 2 gm/24 hr. Adults: 500 mg/dose QID PO × 5 days	May cause crystalluria (keep urine output high and alkaline), fever, rash, hepatitis, SLE-like syndrome, vasculitis, bone marrow depression, hemolysis in patients with G6PD deficiency, Stevens-Johnson syndrome. Use with **caution** in premature infants and newborns <2 mo because of risk of hyperbilirubinemia and ultimately kernicterus.

*Indicates suspensions not commercially available; need to be extemporaneously compounded by a pharmacist. See references 6 and 7 for specific formulations.

(Continued.)

Drug	How Supplied	Dose and Route	Remarks
Sulfadiazine *(continued)*.		*Toxoplasmosis:* with pyrimethamine Infants: 25 mg/kg/dose QID PO Children: 25–50 mg/kg/dose QID PO Adults: 2–8 gm/24 hr ÷ QID × 3–4 wk PO	
Sulfasalazine (Salicylazo-sulfapyridine, S.A.S., Azulfidine)	Tabs: 500 mg Enteric-coated Tabs:500 mg Oral Susp: 250 mg/5 ml	*Children >2 yr:* Initial: 40–60 mg/kg/24 hr ÷ Q4–6 hr PO Maintenance: 30 mg/kg/24 hr ÷ QID PO **Max dose:** 2 gm/24 hr *Adults* **(max dose:** 4 gm/24 hr): Initial: 3–4 gm/24 hr ÷ Q4–6 hr PO Maintenance: 2 gm/24 hr ÷ Q6 hr PO	Turns alkaline urine an orange-yellow color. May cause severe hypersensitivity reactions, blood dyscrasias, CNS changes, nausea, vomiting, anorexia, diarrhea, renal damage. Use with **caution** in G6PD deficiency.
Sulfisoxazole (Gantrisin)	Tabs: 500 mg Susp: 500 mg/5 ml (120 ml) Syrup: 500 mg/5 ml (472 ml) Ophthalmic Sol: 4% (15 ml)	*Children >2 mo:* Initial: 75 mg/kg/dose PO × 1 Maintenance: 150 mg/kg/24 hr ÷ Q4–6 hr PO **Max dose:** 6	**Contraindicated** in infants <2 mo, urinary obstruction, near-term pregnant or nursing mothers. Use with **caution** in

Ophthalmic ointment: 4% (3.5 gm)

presence of renal or liver disease, or G6PD deficiency. Maintain adequate fluid intake. See Sulfadiazine for toxicities.

gm/24 hr
Adults: Loading: 2–4 gm × 1 PO
Maintenance: 4–8 gm/24 hr ÷ Q4–6 hr PO **Max dose:** 8 gm/24 hr
Otitis media prophylaxis: 50–75 mg/kg/24 hr ÷ BID PO
Rheumatic fever prophylaxis:
≤30 kg: 500 mg/24 hr PO single dose
>30 kg: 1 gm/24 hr PO single dose
Ophthalmic Sol: 2–3 drops Q4–8 hr
Ophthalmic ointment: 1–3 × daily and at bedtime.

Surfactant, pulmonary
(Beractant, bovine lung surfactant, natural living surfactant) (Survanta)

Susp: 200 mg (8 ml)

Prophylatic therapy: 4 ml/kg/dose intratracheally as soon as possible; up to 4 doses may be given at intervals no shorter than Q6 hr during the first 48 hr of life.

All doses are administered intratracheally. If the suspension settles during storage, gently squirt the contents—**do not shake.** Each dose is divided into four

(Continued.)

Drug	How Supplied	Dose and Route	Remarks
Surfactant, pulmonary *(continued.)*.		*Rescue therapy:* 4 ml/kg/dose intratracheally, immediately following the diagnosis of respiratory distress syndrome (RDS).	1 ml/kg aliquots; administer 1 mg/kg in each of 4 different positions (slight downward inclination with head turned to the right, head turned to the left; slightly upward inclination with head turned to the right, head turned to the left). Transient bradycardia, O$_2$ desaturation, pallor, vasoconstriction, hypotension, endotracheal tube blockage, hypercarbia, hypercapnea, apnea, and hypertension may occur during the administration process. Other side effects may include pulmonary interstitial emphysema, pulmonary air leak, and post-treatment nosocomial sepsis.

Surfactant, pulmonary (colfosceril palmitate) (Dipalmitoylphosphatidylcholine, DPPC; synthetic lung surfactant) (Exosurf)	Intratracheal susp: 108 mg (10 ml)	*Prophylaxis therapy*: 5 ml/kg intratracheally as soon as possible; 2 additional doses (12 and 24 hr) following the initial dose are given to infants remaining on ventilators *Rescue therapy*: 5 ml/kg intratracheally as soon as the diagnosis of RDS is made. A second 5 ml/kg dose should be administered 12 hr later.	For intratracheal use only. Pulmonary hemorrhage, apnea, mucous plugging, and decrease in transcutaneous O_2 of >20% may occur. Drug needs to be reconstituted with preservative-free sterile water for injection. Suction infant prior to administration.
Terbutaline (Brethine, Bricanyl)	Tabs: 2.5, 5 mg Inj: 1 mg/ml inhaler: 200 μg/metered spray (300 doses per inhaler)	*PO*: ≤12 yr: Initial: 0.05 mg/kg/dose TID, increase as required. **Max dose**: 0.15 mg/kg/dose TID **or** total of 5 mg/24 hr >12 yr–adults: Initial: 2.5 mg/dose TID Maintenance: Usually 5 mg TID or 0.075 mg/kg/dose TID-QID	Nervousness, tremor, headache, nausea, tachycardia, arrhythmias, palpitations. Injectable product may be used for nebulization.

(Continued.)

Drug	How Supplied	Dose and Route	Remarks
Terbutaline *(continued.).*		*Nebulization:* <2 yr: 0.5 mg in 2.5 ml NS 2–9 yr: 1 mg in 2.5 ml NS >9 yr: 1.5 mg in 2.5 ml NS *SC:* ≤12 yr: 0.005–0.01 mg/kg/dose Q15–20 min × 3; **max dose:** 0.4 mg/dose. >12 yr–adults: 0.25 mg/dose Q15–30 min PRN × 1; **max dose:** 0.5 mg/4 hr period *Inhalation:* 2 inhalations Q4–6 hr	
Terfenadine (Seldane)	Tabs: 60 mg 60 mg terfenadine and 120 mg pseudoephedrine (SeldaneD)	*3–6 yr:* 15 mg BID PO *7–12 yr:* 30 mg BID PO *> 12 yr:* 60 mg BID PO	Significantly less sedative effect than other antihistamines. Ketoconazole and troleandomycin may result in prolonged QT wave/ventricular tachycardia
Tetracycline HCL (many brand names: Achromycin, Terramycin, Sumycin, Panmycin)	Tabs: 250, 500 mg Caps: 100, 250, 500 mg Suspension: 125 mg/5 ml (473 ml)	**Do not use in children <8 yr.** *Older children:* (**Max dose:** 2 gm/24 hr) PO: 25–50 mg/kg/24 hr ÷ Q6 hr	**Not recommended** in patients <8 yr due to tooth staining and decreased bone growth.

Ophthalmic ointment: 0.5%, 1% (3.5 gm)

Ophthalmic susp: 1% (4 ml)

Cream: 1%

Ointment: 3% (15, 30 gm)

Adults (**max dose:** 2 gm/24 hr)

PO: 1–2 gm/24 hr ÷ Q6 hr

Chlamydia genital infections:

500 mg Q6 hr PO (see Chapter 17.)

Ophthalmic: 2 drops into affected eye BID–QID

Also **not** recommended for use in pregnancy because these side effects may occur in the fetus. May cause nausea, GI upset, hepatotoxicity, stomatitis, rash, photosensitivity, fever and superinfection. **Do not give** with dairy products or with any divalent cations (i.e., Fe^{++}, Ca^{++}, Mg^{++}). Give 1 hr before or 2 hr after meals.

Theophylline (many brands)

Immediate release: theophylline

Sustained release: theophylline-SR

Many dosage forms exist; fill in space below as applicable to your practice:

Immediate release:

Tabs: 100, 200, 300 mg

Elixir: 80 mg/5 ml

Sol: 80 mg/15 ml

Sustained release:

Tabs: 100, 200, 300 mg

Immediate release:

Neonatal apnea:

Loading dose: 5 mg/kg/dose PO; then

Pre-term: (<36 wk) 1–2 mg/kg/24 hr PO ÷ Q8–12 hr

Term: 1 mo: 2–4 mg/kg/24 hr PO ÷ Q8–12 hr

Bronchospasm:

Loading dose (PO): 0.8 mg/kg/dose for each 2 mg/L desired increase in serum theophylline level

Drug metabolism varies widely with age, drug formulation, and route of administration. Most common side effects and toxicities are nausea, vomiting, anorexia, gastroesophageal reflux, nervousness, tachycardia, seizures, and arrhythmias. Serum levels should be monitored. **Therapeutic levels: bronchospasm: 10–20 mg/L; apnea: 7–13 mg/L. Note:** An alternative

(Continued.)

Drug	How Supplied	Dose and Route	Remarks
Theophylline *(continued.)*.		Maintenance (PO): 0–2 mo: 3–6 mg/kg/24 hr ÷ Q8 hr 2–6 mo: 6–15 mg/kg/24 hr ÷ Q6 hr 6–12 mo: 15–22 mg/kg/24 hr ÷ Q4–6 hr 1–9 yr: 22 mg/kg/24 hr ÷ Q4–6 hr 12–16 yr: 18 mg/kg/24 hr ÷ Q6 hr Adults: 13 mg/kg/24 hr ÷ Q6 hr **Max dose: 900 mg/24 hr** **Divide dosage BID or TID for sustained-release preparations.**	dosing regimen for infants 6 wk–1 yr: Dose (mg/kg/24 hr) = 0.2 × (age [wk]) + 5. Half-life is age-dependent: 30 hr (newborns); 6.9 hr (infants); 3.4 hr (children); 8.1 hr (adults). *Levels increased with:* allopurinol, cimetidine, erythromycin, propranolol, thiabendazole. *Levels decreased with:* isoproterenol, phenobarbital, phenytoin. Some elixir preparations may contain alcohol.
Thiamine (Aneurine HCl, thiaminium chloride HCl, vitamin B₁) (Betalin S, Biamine)	Tabs: 5, 10, 25, 50, 100, 250, 500 mg Inj: 100 mg/ml 200 mg/ml	*Dietary supplement:* Infants: 0.3–0.5 mg/24 hr Children: 0.5–1 mg/24 hr Adults: 1–2 mg/24 hr *Beriberi* (thiamine deficiency): Children: 10–25 mg/dose IM/IV QD (if critically ill) **or**	Multivitamin preparations contain amounts meeting RDA requirements. Allergic reactions and anaphylaxis may occur, especially with IV administration. **Therapeutic range: 1.6–4.0 mg/dL.** High

	10–50 mg/dose PO QD × 2 wk, followed by 5–10 mg/dose QD for 1 mo Adults: 5–30 mg/dose IM/IV TID for 2 wk, followed by 5–30 mg/24 hr ÷ QD or TID for 1 mo *Wernicke's encephalopathy syndrome:* 50 mg IV **and** 50 mg IM × 1, then 50 mg IM QD until patient resumes a normal diet. (Administer thiamine before starting glucose infusion.)	carbohydrate diets or IV dextrose diets may increase thiamine requirements. May cause false positive for uric acid and may also interfere with serum theophylline assay with large doses.
Thiopental sodium (Pentothal)	Inj: 250, 400, 500 mg; Vials: 0.5, 1.0 gm; Kits: 1, 2.5, 5.0 gm	*Cerebral edema:* 1.5–5.0 mg/kg/dose IV. Repeat PRN for increased ICP. *General anesthesia:* Induction: Children: 2 mg/kg × 1 IV Adults: 3–5 mg/kg × 1 IV Maintenance: Children: 1 mg/kg IV PRN Adults: 50–100 mg IV PRN	May cause respiratory depression, hypotension, anaphylaxis, decreased cardiac output. **Contraindicated** in acute intermittent porphyria. $T_{1/2}$: 3–8 hr in blood but effects on brain are very short-lived.

(Continued.)

Drug	How Supplied	Dose and Route	Remarks
Thioridazine (Mellaril)	Tabs: 10, 15, 25, 50, 100, 150, 200 mg Conc.: 30, 100 mg/ml (120 ml) Susp: 25, 100 mg/5 ml (120 ml)	*Children 2–12 yr:* 1– 2.5 mg/kg/24 hr ÷ Q6–12 hr, increase gradually *Adults:* Initially, 150– 300 mg/24 hr ÷ Q6–12 hr; increase gradually. **Max dose:** 800 mg/24 hr	Drowsiness, extrapyramidal reactions, autonomic symptoms, ECG changes, arrhythmias, paradoxical reactions, endocrine disturbances. Pigmentary retinopathy may be seen. More autonomic symptoms and less extrapyramidal effects than chlorpromazine.
Ticarcillin (Ticar)	Inj.: 1, 3, 6, 20, 30 gm	*Neonates (<1.2 kg):* 0–4 wk: 150 mg/kg/24 hr ÷ Q12 hr IV *1.2–2.0 kg:* 0–7 days: 150 mg/kg/24 hr ÷ Q12 hr IV >7 days: 225 mg/kg/24 hr ÷ Q8 hr IV *>2 kg:* 0–7 days: 225 mg/kg/24 hr ÷ Q8 hr IV >7 days: 300 mg/kg/24 hr ÷ Q8 hr IV	Each gram contains 5.2–6.5 mEq Na⁺. May cause decreased platelet aggregation, bleeding diathesis, hypernatremia, hypocalcemia, allergy, rash, increased AST. **Do not mix** with aminoglycoside in same solution.

	Children and adults: 200–300 mg/kg/24 hr ÷ Q4–6 hr IV or IM **Max dose:** 24–30 gm/24 hr *Uncomplicated UTI:* Child: 50–100 mg/kg/24 hr ÷ Q6–8 hr IM/IV Adult: 1 gm Q6 hr IM/IV **Max IM dose:** 2 gm/inj *Cystic fibrosis:* 300–600 mg/kg/24 hr ÷ Q4–6 hr IM/IV	Activity similar to ticarcillin except that beta-lactamase inhibitor broadens spectrum to include *S. aureus* and *H. influenzae.* May interfere with urine protein measurement.
Ticarcillin/clavulanate (Timentin)	Inj: 3.1 gm (3.0 gm ticarcillin and 0.1 gm clavulanate); contains 4.75 mEq Na⁺ and 00.15 mEq K⁺ per 1 gm drug	Dosing as with ticarcillin **Max dose:** 18–24 gm/24 hr

| **Tobramycin**
(Nebcin, Tobrex and others) | Inj: 10, 40 mg/ml
Ophthalmic ointment: 0.3% (3.5 gm)
Ophthalmic Sol: 0.3% (5 ml) | *Neonates:* 2.5 mg/kg/dose IV/IM | **Therapeutic levels: peak: 6–10 mg/L; trough:** <**2 mg/L.** Ototoxicity, nephrotoxicity, myelotoxicity, allergy. Ototoxic effects synergistic with furosemide. Higher doses are recommended in patients with cystic fibrosis, multiple sclerosis, or neutropenia. |

Dosing Interval

Gestational Age	Postnatal Age	
	<7 days	≥7 days
<28 wk	Q24 hr	Q18 hr
28–34 wk	Q18 hr	Q12 hr
>34 wk	Q12 hr	Q8 hr

(Continued.)

Drug	How Supplied	Dose and Route	Remarks
Tobramycin (continued).		*Child:* 6–7.5 mg/kg/24 hr ÷ Q8 hr IV/IM *Adults:* 3–5 mg/kg/24 hr ÷ Q8 hr IV/IM *Ophthalmic:* Apply thin ribbon of ointment to affected eye BID–TID; or 1–2 drops of solution to affected eye Q4 hr	
Tolazoline (Priscoline)	Inj: 25 mg/ml	*Test dose:* 1–2 mg/kg IV over 10 minutes, then *Constant infusion:* 1–2 mg/kg/hr IV. Dissolve 50 mg/kg × wt (kg) in 50 ml D_5W (ml/hr = mg/kg/hr)	Monitor BP, renal status, and bone marrow status. GI and pulmonary hemorrhage have been observed. For severe hypotension caused by this drug, use ephedrine or dopamine, **not** epinephrine or norepinephrine. For pulmonary hypertension, administer via upper extremity or scalp vein.
Tolmetin sodium (Tolectin)	Tabs: 200, 600 mg Caps: 400 mg	*Children:* Initial: 15 mg/kg/24 hr ÷ TID PO Increment: 5 mg/kg/24 hr PO at 1 wk intervals until therapeutic or adverse effects are observed	**Not** recommended for children <2 yr. May cause GI irritation or bleeding. CNS symptoms, false positive proteinuria. Take with food or milk. Each 200 mg contains 0.8 mEq Na.

Maintenance: 20–30
mg/kg/24 hr ÷ TID-QID PO
Max dose: 30 mg/kg/24 hr
Adults:
Initial: 400 mg TID PO
Maintenance: Titrate to
desired effect. Usually,
600–1800 mg/24 hr ÷ TID
PO

Tolnaftate (Tinactin, Aftate, and others)	Topical aerosol liquid: 1% (113 gm) Aerosol powder: 1% (100, 150 gm) Cream: 1% (15, 30, 45 gm) Gel: 1% (15 gm) Powder: 1% (45, 67.5, 70.9, 90 gm) Sol: 1% (10, 60 ml)	Apply 1–2 drops of solution or small amount of gel, liquid, cream or powder to affected areas BID for 2–6 wk.	May cause mild irritation and sensitivity. Avoid eye contact. Not for use with nail or scalp infections.
Triamcinolone (Aristocort, Kenacort, Kenalog, Azmacort)	Tabs: 1, 2, 4, 8, 16 mg Syrup: 2, 4 mg/5 ml (120 ml) Inj (repository): 40 mg/ml Inj (intralesional): 5, 25, 40 mg/ml Cream: 0.025% (15, 60 gm); 0.1% (15, 60, 240 gm; 5 lb); 0.5% (15, 240 gm)	*Intralesional inj:* 1 mg/site at intervals of 1 wk or more. May give separate doses in sites >1 cm apart. *Systemic use:* Use 1/6 of cortisone dose. *Topical:* Apply to affected areas BID–QID.	May cause dermal atrophy, telangiectasia, or hypopigmentation. **Do not use** topical preparations on face or genitalia. See Chapter 26. Rinse mouth thoroughly with water after each use of the oral inhalation dosage form.

(Continued.)

Drug	How Supplied	Dose and Route	Remarks
Triamcinolone *(continued.)*.	Ointment: 0.1% (15, 60, 240 gm; 5 lb); 0.5% (15, 240 gm); 0.1% (15, 60 ml) Lotion: 0.025% (60 ml); 0.1% (15, 60 ml) Inhaler: 100 μg/dose (20 gm)	*Oral inhalation:* 6–12 yr : 1–2 puffs TID-QID; **max dose: 12 puffs/24 hr** Adult: 2 puffs TID-QID; **Max dose: 16 puffs/24 hr**	
Trimethobenzamide HCL (Tigan)	Caps: 100, 250 mg Suppository: 100, 200 mg Inj: 100 mg/ml	*Children:* 15–40 kg: Oral: 100–200 mg/dose TID-QID Rectal (not for use in neonates): <15 kg: 100 mg TID-QID ≥15 kg: 100–200 mg TID-QID Inj: **Not** recommended for children. *Adults:* Oral: 250 mg/dose TID-QID Rectal: 200 mg TID-QID Inj: 200 mg IM TID-QID	CNS disturbances are common in children (extrapyramidal symptoms, drowsiness, confusion, dizziness, blood dyscrasias). **Avoid** use in patients with hepatotoxicity, acute vomiting, or allergic reaction. Suppository contains 2% benzocaine.
Trimethoprim-sulfamethoxazole	See Co-Trimoxazole		
Urokinase (Abbokinase, . Abbokinase Open Cath, Breokinase)	Inj: 5,000, 9,000, 250,000 U	*Deep vein thrombosis and pulmonary emboli:* 4400 U/kg over 10 min, followed by 4400 U/kg/hr for 12 hr.	Discontinue administration if signs of bleeding occur. Side effects include allergic reactions, fever, rash, and

bronchospasm.
Contraindicated for patients with active internal bleeding, intracranial neoplasm, arteriovenous malformation, or aneurysm, history of cerebrovascular accident, or recent trauma. Monitor hematocrit, platelets, PT, and PTT prior to and during continuous infusion therapy.

Occluded IV catheter:
Aspiration method: Use 5,000 U/ml conc. Instill 5,000 U in each lumen over 1–2 min, leave in place for 1–4 hr, then aspirate; may repeat with 10,000 U in each lumen if 5,000 U fails to clear.
For dialysis patients, 5,000 U in each lumen administered over 1–2 min; leave drug in for 1–2 days, then aspirate
IV infusion method: 200 U/kg/hr in each lumen for 12–48 hr at a rate of at least 20 ml/hr

Valproic acid (Depakene) [Depakote–See Divalproex sodium]	Caps: 250 mg Syrup: 250 mg/5 ml (473 ml)	*PO:* Initial: 10–15 mg/kg/24 hr ÷ QD-TID Increment: 5–10 mg/kg/24 hr at weekly intervals to **max dose** of 60 mg/kg/24 hr	GI, liver, blood, CNS toxicity; weight gain, transient alopecia, pancreatitis, nausea, sedation, vomiting, headache, platelet dysfunction, hypersalivation, rash. Drug

(Continued.)

Drug	How Supplied	Dose and Route	Remarks
Valproic acid (*continued*).		Maintenance: 30–60 mg/kg/24 hr ÷ QD-TID *PR*: syrup, diluted 1:1 with water, may be given PR using the same doses at those given for PO	interactions: affects phenytoin and phenobarbital levels. Can cause hyperammonemia. **Do not give syrup with carbonated beverages. Therapeutic levels: 50–100 mg/L.**
Vancomycin (Vancocin and others)	Inj: 500, 1000 mg Caps: 125, 250 mg Sol: 1, 10 gm (reconstitute to 500 mg/6 ml)	*Neonates:* <7 days: <1 kg: 10 mg/kg/dose Q24 hr IV 1–2 kg: 10 mg/kg/dose Q18 hr IV >2 kg: 10 mg/kg/dose Q12 hr IV ≥7 days: <1 kg: 10 mg/kg/dose Q18 hr IV 1–2 kg: 10 mg/kg/dose Q12 hr IV >2 kg: 10 mg/kg Q8 hr IV. Give 15 mg/kg dose if CNS involved.	Ototoxicity, nephrotoxicity, allergy may occur. "Red man syndrome" associated with rapid IV infusion. Infuse over 60 minutes (may infuse over 120 min if 60 min infusion is not tolerated). **Note:** diphenhydramine is used to reverse red man syndrome. **Therapeutic levels: peak: 25–40 mg/L; trough: <10 mg/L.**

Infants and children:
CNS: 15 mg/kg/dose Q8 hr IV
Other: 10 mg/kg/dose Q8 hr IV
Adults: 2 gm/24 hr ÷ Q6–12 hr IV
Colitis:
Children: 40–50 mg/kg/24 hr ÷ Q6 hr PO
Max dose: 500 mg/24 hr
Adults: 125 mg/dose PO Q6 hr

Varicella-zoster (Immune globulin, VZIG)	1 vial = 125 U	≤10 kg: 125 U IM 10.1–20 kg: 250 U IM 20.1–30 kg: 375 U IM 30.1–40 kg: 500 U IM >40 kg: 625 U IM (not > 2.5 ml per inj site)	See Immunoprophylaxis chapter for indications. Dose may be given up to 96 hr post-exposure. Some pain, redness, swelling at the injection site may occur.
Vasopressin (Pitressin)	Inj: 20 U/ml (aqueous); 5 U/ml (tannate in oil) (for IM use only)	*Children:* Aqueous: 2.5– 10 U SC/IM BID-QID; tannate: 1.25–2.5 U IM Q2–3d. *Adults:* Aqueous: 5– 10 U SC/IM BID-QID; tannate: 1.5–5 U IM Q2– 3 days.	Tannate **must not be given** IV or SC. Side effects include tremor, sweating, vertigo, abdominal discomfort, nausea, vomiting, urticaria, anaphylaxis, hypertension,

(Continued.)

Drug	How Supplied	Dose and Route	Remarks
Vasopressin *(continued.)*.		*GI hemorrhage:* Initiate continuous IV drip at 0.2–0.4 U/min and titrate to **max dose** of 0.9 U/min *Growth hormone and corticotropin provocative test:* 0.3 U/kg **Max dose:** 10 U *Diabetes insipidus:* Children: 2.5–5.0 U IM/SC BID-QID Adults: 5–10 U IM/SC BID-QID PRN. Continuous infusion: Start at 0.5 mU/kg/hr (0.0005 U/kg/hr); titrate up to 2 mU/kg/hr (0.0002 U/kg/hr); **max dose:** 10 mU/kg/hr	and bradycardia. Drug interactions: lithium, demeclocycline, and alcohol reduce activity; carbamazepine, tricydic antidepressants, fluorocortisone, and chlorpropramine increase activity.
Vecuronium bromide (Norcuron)	Inj: 10 mg	>7 wk-1 yr: Initial: 0.08–0.1 mg/kg/dose IV Maintenance: 0.05–0.1 mg/kg/hr PRN IV >1 yr-adults: Initial: 0.08–0.01 mg/kg/dose IV	Use with **caution** in patients with hepatic impairment and neuromuscular disease. Infants from 7 wk to 1 yr are more sensitive to the drug and may have a longer

	Maintenance: 0.05–0.1 mg/kg/hr PRN; may administer via continuous infusion at 0.1 mg/kg/hr IV	recovery time. Children (1–10 yr) may require higher doses and more frequent supplementation than adults. Enflurane, isoflurane, aminoglycoside, metronidazole, tetracyclines, bacitracin, and clindamycin may increase the potency and duration of neuromuscular blockade. Neostigmine, pyridostigmine, or edrophonium are antidotes.
Verapamil (Isoptin, Calan)	Tabs: 40, 80, 120 mg Sustained-release tabs: 240 mg Inj: 2.5 mg/ml	*IV:* Give over 2–3 min. May repeat once after 30 mins. 0–1 yr: 0.1–0.2 mg/kg 1–15 yr: 0.1–0.3 mg/kg; **max dose:** 5 mg Adult: 5–10 mg (0.15 mg/kg) *PO* Children: 4–10 mg/kg/24 hr ÷ TID Adults: 240–480 mg/24 hr ÷ TID	**Contraindicated** in CHF, hypotension, shock, 2nd and 3rd degree AV block and right-to-left shunt. Use only with **extreme caution** in infants; may cause apnea, severe bradycardia, or hypotension. IV beta blockers should not be given within a few hours of verapamil as both cause myocardial

(Continued.)

Drug	How Supplied	Dose and Route	Remarks
Verapamil *(continued.)*.		*Adult antianginal dose:* 80 mg/dose Q6–8 hr PO; **max dose:** 480 mg/24 hr	depression. Must monitor ECG continuously. Have calcium and isoproterenol ready to reverse hypotension and bradycardia.
Vidarabine (adenine arabinoside, ara-A) (Vira-A)	Ophthalmic ointment: 3% (3.5 gm)	*Keratoconjunctivitis:* Apply 1/2 in ribbon of ointment to lower conjunctival sac Q3 hr, 5 ×/24 hr. Discontinue if not improved in 7 days.	Ophthalmic product may cause burning, lacrimation, keratitis.
Vitamin K₁ (Aqua-Mephyton, Konakion, Phytonadione, Mephyton)	Tabs: 5 mg Inj: 2, 10 mg/ml	*Neonatal hemorrhagic disease:* Prophylaxis and treatment: 0.5–1.0 mg/dose IM, SC, or IV × 1 *Oral anticoagulant overdose:* Infants: 1–2 mg/dose Q4–8 hr IM or SC Children and adults: 5–10 mg/dose IM or SC *Liver disease or malabsorption:* 2.5–25 mg/24 hr PO, IV, IM, or SC *Vitamin K deficiency:* Infants and children: 1–2 mg/dose IV × 1 or 2–5 mg/24 hr PO Adults: 5–25 mg/24 hr PO	Follow PT/PTT. Use with **caution** in presence of severe hepatic disease. Large doses (>25 mg) in newborns may cause hyperbilirubinemia. IV injection rate not to exceed 3 mg/m²/min or 1 mg/min. IV doses may cause flushing, dizziness, hypotension, anaphylaxis. IV administration is indicated **only** when other routes of administration are not feasible.

Warfarin (Coumadin, Panwarfin, Sofarin)	Tabs: 2, 2.5, 5, 7.5, 10 mg	Infants and children: 0.1 mg/kg/24 hr PO QD. Adjust dose to the desired PT. Maintenance dose range 0.05–0.34 mg/kg/24 hr PO QD Adult: 10–15 mg PO QD for 2–5 days; adjust dose to the desired PT. Maintenance dose range: 2–10 mg/24 hr PO QD	Infants < 12 mo may require doses at the high end of the range. **Contraindicated** in severe liver or kidney disease, uncontrolled bleeding, GI ulcers, and malignant hypertension. Warfarin's anticoagulant effects increase with concomitant use of ethacrynic acid, indomethacin, mefenamic acid, phenylbutazone, or aspirin, whereas vitamin K decreases warfarin's effect; the antidote is vitamin K and fresh frozen plasma.
Zidovudine (Azidothymidine, AZT, Retrovir)	Caps: 100 mg Liq: 50 mg/5 ml Inj: 10 mg/ml	Dosages may differ depending on protocol used. *Symptomatic children:* PO: 90–180 mg/m²/dose Q6 hr; **max dose:** 200 mg Q6 hr. *>12 yr-adult:* PO: 100–200 mg/dose Q4–8 hr	Most common side effects include: anemia, granulocytopenia, nausea, and headache (dosage reduction or discontinuance may be required). Use with caution in patients with impaired renal or hepatic function. Interacting drugs

(Continued.)

Drug	How Supplied	Dose and Route	Remarks
Zidovudine *(continued.)*		IV: 1–2 mg/kg/dose Q4 hr	include: acyclovir (increased toxicity); ganciclovir (increased hematological toxicity); drugs which affect glucuronidation (increases granulocytopenia).
Zinc salts	Caps (sulfate): 110 mg (25 mg Zn), 220 mg (50 mg Zn) Tabs (sulfate): 66 mg (15 mg Zn), 200 mg (45 mg Zn) Tabs (gluconate): 10 mg (1.4 mg Zn), 15 mg (2 mg Zn), 50 mg (7 mg Zn), 78 mg (11 mg Zn) Liq*: acetate: 5,10 mg elemental Zn/ml Inj: Sulfate salt 1 mg elemental Zn/ml	*Zinc deficiency:* Infants and children: 0.5–1 mg elemental Zn/kg/24 hr PO Adults (Zn sulfate): 100–220 mg/dose TID PO	Nausea, vomiting, gastric ulcers may occur at high doses. Patients with excessive losses (burns) or impaired absorption require higher doses. Approximately 20–30% of oral dose is absorbed.

*Indicates suspensions not commercially available; need to be extemporaneously compounded by a pharmacist. See references 6 and 7 for specific formulations.

REFERENCES

1. Package insert for products.
2. Benitz WE, Tatro, DS: *The Pediatric Drug Handbook.* St Louis, Mosby–Year Book, IL, 1988.
3. Boyd, JR (editor-in-chief): *Facts and Comparisons: Loose-leaf Drug Information Service,* Philadelphia, JB Lippincott, updated monthly.
4. *Physicians' Desk Reference.* Oradell, NJ, Medical Economics 1993.
5. McEvey G. McQuarrie GM (eds): *Drug Information 92, American Hospital Formulary Service.*
6. Committee on Extemporaneous Formulation, American Society of Hospital Pharmacists, SIG on Pediatric Pharmacy Practice: *Handbook on Extemporaneous Formulations.*
7. Johns Hopkins Hospital Department of Pharmacy—Pediatric Division: Extemporaneous Formulation Files.
8. Nelson, JD: *Pocketbook of Pediatric Antimicrobial Therapy,* 1993.
9. *Handbook of Antimicrobial Therapy.* New Rochelle, NY, Medical Letter, 1990.
10. Taketomo CK, et al: *American Pharmaceutical Association Pediatric Dosage Handbook.* Hudson, Ohio, Lexi-Comp, 1992.
11. Seidel HM, Rosenstein BJ: *Primary Care of the Newborn.* St Louis, Mosby-Year Book, 1993.
12. *Red Book* (RCID), 1991.
13. Yaffe SJ, Aranda JV: *Pediatric Pharmacology: Therapeutic Principles in Practice.* Philadelphia, WB Saunders, 1992.
14. Knoben JE, Anderson PO: *Handbook of Clinical Drug Data.* Hamilton, Ill, Drug Intelligence Publications, 1993.

SPECIAL DRUG TOPICS   **26**

I.   **TOPICAL CORTICOSTEROIDS:** In general, use intermediate and low potency preparations (groups 4–7) in pediatric patients. Conditions responsive to these preparations include eczema, atopic or seborrheic dermatitis, pruritus, and localized neurodermatitis. Contraindicated in varicella, vaccinia.

Occlusive dressing (including waterproof diapers) increase the systemic absorption of topical steroids and should not be used with group 1 preparations.

Apply 1–2 times daily. Penetration of skin is greatest in ointments, with decreasing effectiveness in gels, creams, and lotions. Prolonged use may result in systemic side effects.

Most compounds are dispensed in 15-, 30-, and 60-gm tubes (except betamethasone valerate, which is dispensed in 45-gm tubes); 1 gm of topical cream or ointment covers a 10 cm × 10 cm area. A 30- to 60-gm tube will cover the entire body of an adult one time.

Drug	Preparations
A. Low potency	
Group 7	
Dexamethasone (Hexadrol)	0.04% topical
Dexamethasone	0.1% gel
Dexamethasone phosphate	0.1% cream
Hydrocortisone base or acetate	0.25–2.5% lotion, cream, ointment
Methylprednisolone acetate	0.25%, 1% ointment
Group 6	
Aclomethasone dipropionate (Aclovate)	0.05% cream, ointment
Desonide (Tridesilon)	0.05% cream, ointment
Fluocinolone acetonide (Fluonid)	0.01% solution
Fluocinolone acetonide (Synalar)	0.01% cream

(Continued.)

Drug	Preparations
B. Intermediate potency	
Group 5	
Betamethasone dipropionate (Diprosone)	0.05% lotion
Betamethasone valerate (Valisone)	0.1% cream, ointment, lotion
Fluocinolone acetonide (Synalar)	0.025% cream, ointment
Hydrocortisone valerate (Westcort)	0.2% cream ointment
Triamcinolone acetonide (Kenalog, Aristocort, and others)	0.1% cream ointment, lotion
Group 4	
Desoximetasone (Topicort)	0.05% gel
Flurandrenolide (Cordran)	0.05% cream, ointment, lotion
C. High potency	
Group 3	
Betamethasone dipropionate (Diprosone)	0.05% cream, ointment, lotion
Diflorasone diacetate (Florone)	0.05% cream, ointment
Triamcinolone acetonide (Kenalog, Aristocort, and others)	0.5% cream, ointment
Group 2	
Amcinonide (Cyclocort)	0.1% ointment
Betamethasone dipropionate (Diprosone)	0.05% cream, ointment, lotion
Desoximetasone (Topicort)	0.25% cream, ointment
Fluocinonide (Lidex)	0.05% cream, ointment, solution
Halcinomide (Halog)	0.1% cream, ointment, solution
D. Ultrahigh potency	
Group 1	
Betamethasone dipropionate (augmented)	0.05% cream, ointment
Clobetasol propionate	0.05% cream, ointment
Diflorasone diacetate (Florone)	0.05% ointment

II.   SYSTEMIC CORTICOSTEROIDS

A.   Dose Equivalence: The following doses give approximately equivalent clinical effects.

Drug	Glucocorticoid Anti-inflammatory	Mineralocorticoid
Cortisone	100 mg	100 mg
Hydrocortisone	80 mg	80 mg
Prednisone	20 mg	100 mg
Prednisolone	20 mg	100 mg
Methylprednisolone	16 mg	No effect
Triamcinolone	16 mg	No effect
9-α Fluorocortisol	5 mg	0.2 mg
Dexamethasone	2 mg	No effect

B. Common Indications and Doses of Systemic Corticosteroids

Physiologic replacement	Cortisone 0.5–0.75 mg/kg/24h PO ÷ Q8h 0.25–0.35 mg/kg IM QD Hydrocortisone 0.5–0.75 mg/kg/24h PO **or** 20–25 mg/M2/24h PO ÷ Q8h 0.25–0.35 mg/kg IM QD Dexamethasone 0.03–0.15 mg/kg/24h **or** 0.6–0.75 mg/M^2/24h PO/IV/IM ÷ Q6-12h
Stress dosing	Cortisone 50–62.5 mg/m^2/24h from 48h before until 48h after surgery
Acute asthma	Hydrocortisone 1–2 mg/kg/dose Q6h × 24h, then 2–4 mg/kg/24h ÷ Q6h Prednisone 1–2 mg/kg/24h ÷ QD-BID for 3-5 days; **Max:** 60 mg/24h Prednisolone 1–2 mg/kg/24h ÷ QD-BID for 3-5 days; **Max:** 60 mg/24h Methylprednisolone 2 mg/kg IV × 1, then 0.5–1 mg/kg/dose IV Q6h
Acute adrenal insufficiency	Hydrocortisone 1–2 mg/kg IV bolus, then 25–250 mg/day ÷ BID-TID
Congenital adrenal hyperplasia	Fludrocortisone acetate 0.05–0.1 mg/day PO Hydrocortisone Initial: 30–36 mg/m^2/24h PO (1/3 in AM, 2/3 evening, or 1/4 in AM, 1/4 midday, 1/2 evening) Maintenance: 20–25 mg/m^2/24h PO ÷ TID
Nephrotic syndrome	Prednisone 2 mg/kg/24h (**max** 80 mg/24h) ÷ TID-QID until urine is protein-free for 5 days (28 day max course). If proteinuria persists, give 4 mg/kg/dose QOD × 28 days. Maintenance: 2 mg/kg/dose QOD × 28 days, then taper over 4–6 wks.
Airway edema	Dexamethasone 0.5–1 mg/kg/24h PO/IV/IM ÷ Q6h (begin 24h prior to extubation.) Continue × 4–6 doses after extubation.

Cerebral edema/meningitis	Dexamethasone >2 mo: 0.6 mg/kg/24h ÷ Q6h × 4 days; begin prior to 1st dose of antibiotics for meningitis.

Immunosuppresive/ antiinflammatory	Cortisone
	  PO: 2.5–10 mg/kg/24h **or** 20–300 mg/m^2/24h ÷ Q6–8h.
	  IM: 1–5 mg/kg/24h **or** 14–375 mg/m^2/24h ÷ Q12–24h
	Hydrocortisone
	  PO: 2.5–10 mg/kg/24h **or** 75–300 mg/m^2/24h ÷ Q6–8h; IM, IV: 1–5 mg/kg/24h **or** 30–150 mg/m^2/24h ÷ Q12–24h
	Prednisone
	  PO 0.05–2 mg/kg/24h ÷ QD-QID
	Prednisolone
	  PO, IV: 0.1–2 mg/kg/24h ÷ QD-QID
	Methylprednisolone
	  PO, IV, IM: 0.16–0.8 mg/kg/24h **or** 5–25 mg/M^2/24h ÷ Q6-12h
	Triamcinolone
	  IM: 0.03–0.2 mg/kg Q1-7days.

III. **INHALED STEROIDS FOR REACTIVE AIRWAY DISEASE:** Please see Formulary (Chapter 25) for dosing guidelines.
A. **Beclomethasone**
B. **Dexamethasone**
C. **Flunisolide**
D. **Triamcinolone**

IV. **COMPLICATIONS OF PROLONGED USE OF SYSTEMIC CORTICOSTEROIDS**
A. **Hypothalamic-pituitary-adrenal axis suppression (up to 1 yr)**
B. **Growth retardation**
C. **Osteoporosis and osteonecrosis**
D. **Decreased glucose tolerance, increased serum triglycerides**
E. **Exacerbation of peptic ulcer disease with masking of symptoms**
F. **Hypertension**

G. **Hypokalemic acidosis**
H. **Behavioral effects ranging from euphoria to irritability to psychosis**
I. **Pseudotumor cerebri**
J. **Cushingoid habitus**
K. **Decreased resistance to infection**

V. **OXIDIZING AGENTS AND G6PD DEFICIENCY:** The following drugs and chemicals may cause hemolysis of "reacting" (primaquine sensitive) red blood cells, e.g., in patients with G6PD deficiency.

Antimalarials	
Primaquine	

Sulfonamides	
Sulfanilamide	Sulfisoxazole (Gantrisin)*
Salicylozosulfapyridine (Azulfidine)	Sulfacetamide (Sulamyd)
Trisulfapyrimidine (Sultrin)	

Nitrofurans	
Nitrofurantoin (Furadantin)	Furazolidone (Furoxone)

Antipyretics and Analgesics	
Acetylsalicylic acid	Acetophenetidin (Phenacetin)*
Antipyrine	p-Aminosalicylic acid

Others	
Sulfoxone*	Napthalene*
Methylene blue*	Probenecid
Fava bean	Vitamin K: water-soluble analogs only
Aniline dyes	Ascorbic acid†
Chloramphenicol‡	

*Only slightly hemolytic to G6PD A~ patients in very large doses
†Hemolytic in G6PD Mediterranean but not in G6PD A~ or Canton
‡In massive doses

Note: Many other compounds have been tested, but are free of hemolytic activity. Penicillin, the tetracyclines, and erythromycin, for example, will not cause hemolysis. Also, the incidence of allergic reaction in these individuals is not any greater than that observed in normals. Therefore, a patient may receive any drug that is not included in the list of those known to cause hemolysis.

VI. MATERNAL DRUGS AND BREASTFEEDING
A. Maternal Drugs Contraindicated in Breast-Feeding

Drug	Effect
Bromocriptine	Suppresses lactation
Cyclophosphamide	Possible immune suppression; unknown effect on growth or association with carcinogenesis; neutropenia
Cyclosporine	Possible immune suppression; unknown effect on growth or association with carcinogenesis
Diphenhydramine	Increased infant sensitivity to antihistamines
Doxorubicin	Possible immune suppression; unknown effect on growth or association with carcinogenesis
Ergotamine	Vomiting, diarrhea, convulsions (doses used in migraine medications)
Lithium	1/3-1/2 therapeutic blood concentration in infants
Methotrexate	Possible immune suppression; unknown effect on growth or association with carcinogenesis; neutropenia
Phenindione	Anticoagulant; increased prothrombin and partial thrombo plastin time in 1 infant (not used in USA)

B. Drugs of Abuse Contraindicated in Breast-Feeding

Drug	Effect
Amphetamine	Irritability, poor sleep pattern
Cocaine	Cocaine intoxication
Heroin	
Marijuana	Only one report in literature; no effect mentioned
Nicotine (smoking)	Shock, vomiting, diarrhea, rapid heart rate, restlessness, decreased milk production
Phencyclidine	Potent hallucinogen

C. **Radiopharmaceuticals and Breast-Feeding:** Breast-feeding must be stopped temporarily when these radioactive substances are given.

Drug	Duration Radioactivity Present in Milk
Gallium-67	2 wk
Indium-111	Small amount present at 20 hr
Iodine-125	12 days (risk of thyroid cancer)
Iodine-131	2–14 days (depending on study)
Radioactive sodium	96 hr
Technetium-99 m	15 hr-3 days

D. **Drugs With Unknown Effects:** The effects of these drugs are unknown, but use during the breast-feeding may be of concern.

Drug	Effect
Psychotropic	Special concern with prolonged use while nursing
Antianxiety	
Diazepam	None
Lorazepam	None
Prazepam	None
Quazepam	None
Antidepressant	
Amitriptyline	None
Amoxapine	None
Desipramine	None
Dothiepin	None
Imipramine	None
Trazodone	None
Antipsychotic	
Chlorpromazine	Galactorrhea in adult; drowsiness, lethargy in infant
Chlorprothixene	None
Haloperidol	None
Mesoridazine	None
Chloramphenicol	Possible idiosyncratic bone marrow suppression
Metoclopramide K	None desribed; potent CNS drug
Metronidazole	In vitro mutagen; may discontinue breast-feeding 12–24 hr to allow excretion of dose when single-dose therapy is given to mother
Tinidazole	See Metronidazole

E. **Drugs With Effects on Some Infants:** These drugs have been reported to cause adverse side effects in at least one infant and should be used cautiously.

Drug	Effect
Aspirin (salicylates)	Metabolic acidosis (dose related); may affect platelet function; rash
Chlorpromazine	Galactorrhea in adults; drowsiness, lethargy in infant
Clemastine	Drowsiness, irritability, refusal to feed, high-pitched cry, neck stiffness (1 case)
Metronidazole	In vitro mutagen; may discontinue breast-feeding 12–24 hr to allow excretion of dose when single-dose therapy is given to mother
Phenobarbital	Sedation; infantile spasms after weaning from milk containing phenobarbital, methemoglobinemia (1 case)
Salicylazosulfapyridine (sulfasalazine)	Bloody diarrhea in 1 infant

Ref: Adapted from report of Committee on Drugs, AAP, Pediatrics 1989; 84: 924-936.

VII. INSULIN: Insulin is currently available as human, purified pork, pork/beef, and beef preparations. The human and more purified preparations produce less subcutaneous atrophy and less insulin resistance. For management of DKA and subsequent insulin therapy, see Emergency Management, Chapter 3.

Type of Insulin	Time and Route of Administration	Time of Onset (hr)	Peak (hr)	Duration of Action (hr)	General Kinetic Category
Regular	IV (for ketoacidosis 0.1 units/kg bolus, then 0.1 units/kg/hr as continuous infusion; or SC, 15–20 min before meals.)	0.5–1	2–5	5–8	Rapid onset and short duration
Semi-lente (amorphous zinc)*	0.5–0.75 hr before breakfast; deep SC, never IV	0.5–1.5	5–10	12–16	Rapid onset and short duration
Lente (combination of 30% semi-lente and 170% ultra-lente)*	1 hr before breakfast; deep SC, never IV	1–2.5	7–15	24	Intermediate onset and intermediate duration
NPH (neutral-protamine-Hagedorn)	1 hr before breakfast; SC, never IV	1–2	6–12	18–24	Delayed onset and intermediate duration
Ultra-lente	1 hr before breakfast; deep SC, never IV	4–8	10–30	36+	Delayed onset and long duration

*Human NPH may have a slightly decreased duration of action as compared to pork-derived NPH and the dose conversion may not be one-to-one.

Note: Newly diagnosed patients with DKA may be relatively sensitive to insulin and should receive loading and initial maintenance doses that are half of those indicated above.

VIII. **PANCREATIC ENZYME REPLACEMENT:** For specific dosing information, see Formulary (Chapter 25).

Product	Dosage Form	Lipase USP Units	Amylase USP Units	Protease USP Units
Pancreatin				
Creon	Capsule, delayed-release	8,000	30,000	13,000
Creon 25	Capsule, enteric-coated	25,000	74,700	62,500
Pancreatin, single-strength	Tablet	650	8125	8125
Pancreatin 5X	Tablet	12,000	60,000	60,000
Pancreatin 8X	Tablet	22,500	180,000	180,000
Pancreatin Enseals	Tablet, enteric-coated	2,000	25,000	25,000
Pancrelipase				
Cotazym Ku-Zyme HP	Capsule	8,000	30,000	30,000
Cotazym-S	Capsule, enteric-coated spheres	5,000	20,000	20,000
Entolase				
Pancrease	Capsule, delayed-release	4,000	20,000	25,000
Pancrease MT25		25,000	75,000	75,000

Protilase	Tablet, delayed-release	6,000	30,000	20,000
Festal II	Tablet	11,000	30,000	30,000
Ilozyme				
Pancrease MT				
4	Capsule, enteric-coated microtablets	4,000	12,000	12,000
10		10,000	30,000	30,000
16		16,000	48,000	48,000
Ultrase MT				
	Capsule, enteric-coated minitabs	6,000	19,500	19,500
12		12,000	39,000	39,000
		18,000	58,500	58,500
20		20,000	65,000	65,000
24		24,000	78,000	78,000
		30,000	97,500	97,500
Viokase	Powder	16,800 per 0.7 gm	70,000 per 0.7 gm	70,000 per 0.7 gm
	Tablet	8,000	30,000	30,000
Zymase	Capsule, enteric-coated spheres	12,000	24,000	24,000

Ref: Adapted from: Taketomo CK, Pharm.D., Hodding JH, Pharm.D., and Kraus DM, Pharm.D., American Pharmaceutical Association Pediatric Dosage Handbook 1992; Ohio: Lexi-Comp, Inc. 343–344.

IX. CANCER CHEMOTHERAPEUTIC AGENTS

Drug Class and Name	Primary Clinical Use	Route	Toxicity (A=Acute, D=Delayed, *=Dose-Limiting Side Effects)
Alkylating agents			
Busulfan (Myleran)	CML, BMT	PO	A: N/V; diarrhea. D: myelosuppression (onset, 10–14 days)*; pulmonary infiltrates/fibrosis; hepatotoxicity; hyperpigmentation; cataracts; gynecomastia; ovarian failure; sterility.
Cisplatin (CDDP)	Brain, germ cell, neuroblastoma, osteosarcoma, Wilms'	IV	A: N/V; hypersensitivity; fever. D: renal toxicity*; hypomagnesemia; hypocalcemia; hypokalemia; myelosuppression (onset, 10–14 days)*; ototoxicity; hepatotoxicity; hemolysis; neurotoxicity (peripheral neuropathy); infertility.
Carboplatin (CBDCA)	Sarcomas, BMT	IV	Similar to cisplatin, but less renal and less ototoxicity.
Carmustine (BCNU)	Brain, Hodgkin's, NHL	IV	A: N/V; local phlebitis. D: myelosuppression (delayed onset, 3–5 wk)*; neurotoxicity (lethargy); renal toxicity; hepatotoxicity; pulmonary fibrosis; alopecia.
Cyclophosphamide (Cytoxan)	Leukemia, lymphoma, neuroblastoma, sarcoma, BMT	PO, IV	A: N/V; anaphylaxis. D: myelosuppression (onset 7–10 days)*; hemorrhagic cystitis; alopecia; SIADH; gonadal suppression; sterility; cardiotoxicity; pulmonary infiltrates/fibrosis; secondary malignancy.
Ifosfamide (Ifex)	Brain, lymphoma, sarcomas, testicular	IV	A: N/V; neurotoxicity (lethargy, seizures, coma)*. D: myelosuppression (onset, 7–10 days)*; hemorrhagic cystitis; cardiotoxicity.

Melphalan (Alkeran)	Myeloma, neuroblastoma, solid tumors, BMT	PO	A: N/V. D: myelosupression (onset, 2–4 wk); diarrhea; mucositis; alopecia; rash; pulmonary fibrosis; hepatotoxicity; SIADH; secondary malignancy; amenorrhea; sterility.
Nitrogen Mustard (Mechlorethamine)	Hodgkin's	IV	A: N/V; thrombophlebitis. D: myelosuppresion (onset, 10–14 days)*; rash; alopecia; secondary malignancy.
Antimetabolites			
Cytarabine HCl (ARA-C)	Leukemia, lymphoma	IV, IT	A: N/V; fever; diarrhea; anaphylaxis; flu-like syndrome; conjunctivitis. D: myelosuppression (onset, 7–10 days)*; mucositis; alopecia; hepatic damage; cerebellar toxicity; photosensitivity.
Fluorouracil (5-FU)	Solid tumors	IV	A: N/V; diarrhea, hypersensitivity reaction. D: stomatitis and mucositis*; myelosuppression (onset, 7–21 days)*; alopecia; neurotoxicity (cerebellar).
Methotrexate (MTX)	Leukemia (ALL), Non-Hodgkins Lymphoma brain, osteosarcoma, carcinomas	PO, IM, IV, IT	A: N/V; diarrhea; fever; anaphylaxis. D: mucositis*; myelosuppression (onset, 4–10 days)*; skin rash; hepatotoxicity; renal toxicity; pulmonary infiltrates/fibrosis; neurotoxicity (aseptic meningitis; seizures).
Mercaptopurine (6-MP)	Leukemia	PO, IV	A: N/V; diarrhea. D: myelosuppression (onset, 7–14 days); mucositis*; hepatotoxicity; cholestasis.
Thioguanine (6-TG)	AML, CML	PO, IV	A: N/V. D: bone marrow depression*; hepatotoxicity; stomatitis.
Antitumor antibiotics			
Bleomycin (Blenoxane)	Brain, germ cell, lymphoma, osteosarcoma	SC, IM, IV	A: N/V; fever; anaphylaxis; rash. D: pulmonary toxicity (fibrosis)*; erythema; stomatitis; alopecia; pruritus; hyperpigmentation; hyperkeratosis; Raynaud's.

(Continued.)

Drug Class and Name	Primary Clinical Use	Route	Toxicity (A=Acute, D=Delayed, *=Dose-Limiting Side Effects)
Dactinomycin (Actinomycin D)	Sarcomas, Wilms'	IV	A: N/V; diarrhea; phlebitis; anaphylaxis. D: stomatitis/mucositis*; myelosuppresion (onset, 7–14 days)*; erythroderma: hyperpigmentation; alopecia; radiation recall. **Note: Usual dosage expressed in micrograms!**
Daunorubicin (Daunomycin), doxorubicin (ADR, Adriamycin), idarubicin	ALL, AML, carcinomas, lymphoma, neuroblastoma, osteosarcoma, sarcomas	IV	A: N/V; fever; red urine (not hematuria); extravasation causes tissue necrosis; diarrhea; anaphylactoid reaction. D: myelosuppression (onset, 10–14 days)*; cardiotoxicity* [Pediatrics 89:942 (1992)]; stomatitis; hepatotoxicity; alopecia; radiation recall.
Tubulin-binding agents			
Etoposide (VP-16, Vepesid)	Brain, leukemia, lymphoma, neuroblastoma, sarcomas, BMT	IV, PO	A: N/V; diarrhea; abdominal cramping; fever; hypotension; anaphylaxis; rash. D: myelosuppresion (onset, 7–14 days)*; alopecia; peripheral neuropathy; secondary leukemia.
Teniposide (VM-26)	Lymphoma, neuroblastoma	IV	A: N/V; diarrhea; abdominal cramping; fever; phlebitis; anaphylaxis; rash. D: myelosuppresion (onset, 7–14 days)*; alopecia; peripheral neuropathy; secondary leukemia; hepatotoxicity.
Vinblastine (Velban)	Hodgkins, testicular	IV	A: N/V; extravasation causes skin necrosis. D: bone marrow depression*; mucositis (more than VCR); constipation; neurotoxicity (less than VCR: paresthesias, loss of DTRs); SIADH; jaw pain; headache.

Vincristine (VCR, Oncovin)	ALL, lymphoma, sarcomas	IV	A: N/V; extravasation causes skin necrosis. D: constipation; abdominal pain; jaw pain; bone pain; gradually reversible neurotoxicity (paresthesias, loss of DTRs, foot drop)*; jaw pain; alopecia; mild myelosuppresion; SIADH; hepatic damage.
Miscellaneous			
Asparaginase (L-ASP, Elspar)	ALL, AML, lymphomas	IM, IV	A: N/V; fever; chills; headache; hypersensitivity; anaphylaxis; abdominal pain; hyperglycemia leading to coma. D: pancreatitis; renal toxicity; hepatotoxicity; coagulopathy (bleeding/thrombosis); neurotoxicity.
Dacarbazine (DTIC)	Hodgkin's, melanoma, sarcomas	IV	A: N/V*; pain at injection site; facial flushing; flu-like syndrome. D: myelosuppression (onset, 10–14 days to 2–4 wk)*; alopecia; renal toxicity; hepatotoxicity; photosensitivity.
Hydroxyurea (Hydrea)	AML, CML, solid tumors	PO	A: N/V; hypersensitivity. D: bone marrow depression*; megaloblastosis; stomatitis; diarrhea; neurotoxicity.
Adjunctive agents			
Leucovorin	Reduces methotrexate toxicity	PO, IV/IM	Nontoxic in therapeutic doses.
Mesna	Reduces likelihood of hemorrhagic cystitis	IV	A: N/V; headache; limb pain; rarely, hypotension.

PAIN AND SEDATION

27

I. **ASSESSMENT:** Monitor at regular intervals and document information.

    Goal: Accurate information about intensity and location of pain and effectiveness of pain relief measures.

A. **Infant**
    1. **Physiologic response:** Monitor heart rate, blood pressure and respiratory rate. Neither sensitive nor specific.
    2. **Behavioral response:** Observe cry characteristics and duration, facial expression, visual tracking, body movement, and response time to stimuli.

B. **Preschooler:** In addition to physiologic and behavioral responses, can use either a self-report scale (0=no pain, 10=worst pain in life) or the "faces" diagram in Figure 27.1. Learn what word the child uses for pain.

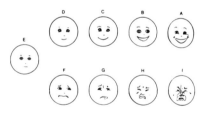

FIG 27.1.
Nine-Face Interval Scale

C. **School-Aged and Adolescents:** In addition to physiologic and behavioral responses, can use a self-report scale such as the linear analogue scale (Figure 27.2).

Ref: Beyer JE, Wells N, Pediatr Clin North Am 1989; 36:837. Used with permission.

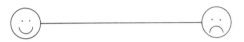

FIG 27.2.
The Linear Analogue Scale

II. PAIN MANAGEMENT DRUGS
A. Non-narcotic Analgesics
1. Acetaminophen: 10–15 mg/kg PO-PR Q4 hr. No anti-inflammatory activity.
2. Nonsteroidal anti-inflammatory drugs (NSAIDS): "ceiling effect" above which these drugs alone cannot relieve pain. Use with opioids to reduce opioid dose. See Formulary (Chapter 25) for details.
   a. Ibuprofen: 4–10 mg/kg Q6–8 hr (**max:** 3200 mg).
   b. Indomethacin: 0.3–1 mg/kg Q6 hr (**max:** 150 mg).
   c. Ketorolac: Load: 0.4–1 mg/kg IV; Maintenance: 0.2–0.5 mg/kg Q6 hr (**max:** 150 mg).
   d. Naproxen: 5–10 mg/kg Q12 hr (**max:** 1000 mg).
   e. Salicylic acid: 10–15 mg/kg Q4–6 hr (**max:** 4000 mg).

B. Opioids
Note: Please refer to cardiovascular monitoring guidelines, section V. The combination of opioids and sedatives produces more respiratory depression than either drug class given alone. Start with a lower dose in infants (e.g., 1/4–1/3 dose morphine in infants younger than 6 mo). Risk of respiratory depression increased in infants <2 mo, premature infants <48 wk postconceptual age, patients with an abnormal control of ventilation, and patients with an altered level of consciousness.

Opioids

Drug (Route)	Equianalgesic Dose (mg)*	Onset (min)	Duration (hr)	Conversion Factor (IV:PO)	Comments
Codeine (PO)	200 (PO)	10–30	3–4	—	Prescribe with acetaminophen.
Fentanyl (IV)	0.1–0.2 (IV)	3–8 (IV)	0.5–1.0	—	Bradycardia, minimal hemodynamic alterations. Treat chest wall rigidity (>5 µg/kg rapid IV bolus) with naloxone, succinylcholine, pancuronium.
Hydromorphone (IV, SC, PO)	1.5 (IV), 7.5 (PO)	5–10	3–4	1:5	Less sedating than morphine.
Meperidine (IV, PO)	100 (IV), 300 (PO)	5–10	3–4	1:2–3	Catastrophic interactions with MAO inhibitors. Produces seizures, tachycardia. A negative inotrope. Not recommended for chronic use.
Methadone (IV, PO)	10 (IV), 20 (PO)	5–10 (IV)	4–24	1:2	Can be given IV even though the package insert says SC or IM. **Max dose:** 10 mg/dose
Morphine (IV, SC, PO)	10 (IV), 60 (PO)	5–10 (IV)	3–4	1:1.5–6	Seizures in newborns, also in all patients at high doses. Histamine release, vasodilation. Avoid with asthma, circulatory compromise. May potentiate biliary colic.
Oxycodone (PO)	30 (PO)	30–60	3–4	—	Good oral bioavailability.

*For complete dosing information, please refer to the Formulary, Chapter 25.

Ref: Adapted from Yaster M, Nicholas E: Pain Management in Children. Current Practice in Anesthesiology, 2:245; Wong D, Whaley L: Clinical Manual of Pediatric Nursing, ed. 3. 1990. Mosby–Year Book; LA Childrens Housestaff Manual, ed 6. 1991; Ohio:Lexi-Comp, Inc.,460-461; Yaster M, et. al. Pain, Sedation, and Postoperative Anesthetic Management in the Pediatric Intensive Care Unit; in Rogers MC, Textbook of Pediatric Intensive Care, Williams & Wilkins:Baltimore. 1987.

C. Local Anesthetics: Contraindicated in infected sites, degenerative axonal disease, and in coagulation disorders.

Medication	Concentration	Dose (mg/kg)	Comments
Lidocaine	0.5–2.0%	5–7*	Mix 10:1 by volume with NaHCO$_3$ 1 mEq/ml
Bupivacaine	0.25–0.5%	1.5–2.5*	
Cocaine		1–2	Topical use only

*Higher dose recommended only when used with epinephrine.

Ref: Yaster M, et. al. The management of acute pain in children with local anesthetic: A primer for the non-anesthesiologist. Comprehensive Therapy. 1989; 15:14–26.

D. Patient-Controlled Analgesia (PCA): Device that allows patient to self-administer small doses of opioids (in addition to continuous infusion).
1. **Indication:** Acute pain (e.g., sickle cell disease, cancer) and postoperative pain.
2. **Dose:** Pain team members program basal infusion, bolus dose, number of boluses allowed per hour, and lock-out periods.

Suggested Doses: Morphine

Basal rate	0.01–0.02 mg/kg/hr
Bolus	0.01–0.03 mg/kg
Lock-out	6–10 min; 4–6 boluses/hr

3. Contraindications:
   a. Inability to push bolus button.
   b. Inability to understand how to use machine.
   c. Patient's desire not to assume responsibility for care.
   Ref: Yaster M, Deshpande JK. Management of pediatric pain with opioid analgesics. J Pediatr 1988; 113:421–429.

III. PAIN MANAGEMENT: NERVE BLOCKS
A. Digital Nerve Block
1. Indication: Laceration of fingers or toes, paronychia, tissue debridement.

2. Dose: 0.5–1.0 ml of **epinephrine-free** local anesthetic.
3. Technique
   a. Wash skin using aseptic technique.
   b. Insert 25-gauge needle between the heads of the meta-carpals on either side of the digit (Fig. 27.3).
   c. Keep needle perpendicular to plane of hand or foot and advance from dorsal to palmar surface, injecting continuously.

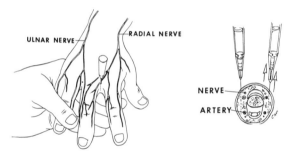

FIG 27.3.
Digital Nerve Block

B. Penile Nerve Block
1. Indication: circumcision.
2. Dose: Bupivacaine (0.25 %) 1-3 ml in older children, lidocaine (1%) 0.8 ml in newborn. **Do not use epinephrine-containing solutions.**
3. Technique
   a. Wash skin using aseptic technique.
   b. Identify location of dorsal nerve on either side of the dorsal artery and vein of the penis (Fig. 27.4).
   c. Using a 25- or 26-gauge needle, inject anesthetic at the 10:30 and 1:30 o'clock positions at penile base beneath Buck's fascia about 3–5 mm from surface.

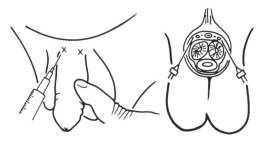

FIG 27.4.
Penile Nerve Block

Ref: Yaster M, Maxwell L, Nicholas E. Pediatrics 1991; 17(10): 1-12.

IV. MANAGEMENT OF SEDATED PATIENTS

1. Vital Signs: During procedure
   a. Blood pressure
   b. Pulse oximetry
   c. ECG
   d. Physical examination
2. Vital signs: After procedure—as above, plus
   a. Airway patency
   b. Pulse
   c. Mental status (talking, sitting unaided, ambulating)
3. IV Access: Have Ringer's lactate, D_5W with salt available.
4. Airway Management: Make sure that the following items are available:
   a. Suction
   b. Oxygen
   c. Oxygen delivery system
   d. Airway management equipment (oral airways, bag/mask, laryngoscope, blades, ET tubes, stylets)
5. Emergency Drugs: Have the following drugs available:
   a. Epinephrine
   b. Atropine
   c. Lidocaine
   d. Glucose
   e. Bretylium

    f. Naloxone
    g. Flumazenil

> Ref: American Academy of Pediatrics Committee on Drugs. Pediatrics 1985; 76:317. Modified with assistance from Yaster, M.

V. PEDIATRIC SEDATION: Contraindications to sedation: full stomach (solid foods within 8 hr, clear liquids 4–6 hr), impaired respiratory status and altered level of consciousness. See section V. for guidelines to monitor the sedated patient.

A. Benzodiazepines: Potent amnestic, anticonvulsant, sedative, hynotic, and skeletal muscle relaxants. Lower doses used concurrently with opiates.

1. Diazepam (Valium)
   a. 0.15–0.3 mg/kg/dose PO
   b. 0.05–0.1 mg/kg/dose IV
   c. IM ineffective, very painful
2. Lorazepam (Ativan): 0.05 mg/kg/dose IM, IV
3. Midazolam (Versed): 0.05–0.08 mg/kg/dose IV, PR, PO (**max:** 2.5 mg)

B. Barbiturates: Globally depress CNS causing sedation to general anesthesia. Not analgesic.

1. Pentobarbital (Nembutal)
   a. 2–6 mg/kg/dose PO, PR, IM
   b. 0.5–1.0 mg/kg/dose IV

C. Narcotics: Cause sedation and analgesia. See Opioids, section II.B.

D. Miscellaneous Drugs

Droperidol (Inapsine)	0.025–0.075 mg/kg/dose IV
Promethazine (Phenergan)	0.5–1.0 mg/kg/dose IM
Chlorpromazine (Thorazine)	0.5–1.0 mg/kg/dose IM, IV; **max dose**, 50 mg
Chloral hydrate	25–100 mg/kg/dose PO, PR; **max dose**, 2 gm
Ketamine*	3–5 mg/kg/dose IM (>5 mg/kg may cause general anesthesia)
	0.25–0.5 mg/kg/dose IV (>1.0–1.5 mg/kg may induce general anesthesia)
Hydroxyzine (Vistaril)	0.5–1.0 mg/kg/dose IM

*Combine with antisialagogue (e.g, atropine 0.01 mg/kg). Recommend Midazolam 0.05–0.1 mg/kg to reduce incidence of night terrors. Contraindicated in increased ICP, catecholamine depletion, profound shock.

E. Drug Combinations
1. Meperidine: 1.5 mg/kg PO
2. Diazepam: 0.2 mg/kg PO
3. Atropine: 0.02 mg/kg PO
4. Fentanyl: 0.001–0.002 mg/kg slow IV
5. Midazolam: 0.05–0.2 mg/kg slow IV (2.5 mg max)

Ref: Yaster M, et. al. Pain, Sedation and Postoperative Anesthetic Management in the Pediatric Intensive Care Unit. Snodgrass W, Dodge W. Ped Clin North Amer 1989, 36:1285.

DRUGS IN RENAL **28** FAILURE

I. DRUGS IN RENAL FAILURE
A. Dose Adjustment Methods

1. Maintenance dosage in patients with renal insufficiency may be adjusted using either of the following methods:

   a. "Interval extension" method: Lengthen the intervals between individual doses, keeping the dosage size normal.

   b. "Dose reduction" method: Reduce the amount of individual doses, keeping the interval between doses normal. This method is recommended particularly for drugs in which a relatively constant blood level is desired.

2. The tables on the following pages contain recommended dosage adjustments for antimicrobial and non-antimicrobial agents for various degrees of renal failure (estimated by glomerular filtration rate). The method of dosage adjustment is identified as either **D** for dose reduction, **I** for interval extension, or **DI** for both dose reduction and interval extension.

3. For the dose reduction method, the percentage of the usual dose is shown, which should be given at the normal dosing interval. For the interval extension method, the dosing interval is given at which the usual drug doses should be administered.

   Note: These dosage modifications are only approximations. Each patient *must* be followed closely for signs of drug toxicity and serum drug levels must be measured when available. Drug dosage and interval should be modified accordingly.

B. Dialysis: The quantitative effects of hemodialysis **(He)** and peritoneal dialysis **(P)** on drug removal are shown. **"Yes"** refers to removal of enough drug to warrant a supplemental dosage for maintenance of adequate therapeutic blood levels. **"No"** indicates no need for dosage adjustment with dialysis. **Note: The designation "no" does not preclude the use of dialysis or hemoperfusion for drug overdose.**

Ref: Trompeter RS, Pediatr Nephrol 1987:183; Bennett WM, Clinical Pharmacokinetics 1988; 15:326.

II. ANTIMICROBIALS REQUIRING ADJUSTMENT IN RENAL FAILURE

	Pharmacokinetics				Adjustments in Renal Failure			
					Creatinine Clearance (ml/min)			Supplemental Dose for Dialysis
Drug	Route of Excretion	Normal T$_{1/2}$ (hr)	Normal Dose Interval	Method	>50	10–50	<10	
Acyclovir	Renal	2.1–3.8	Q8h	I	Q8h	Q24h	Q48h	Yes (He)
Amikacin	Renal	2–3.0	Q8–12h	I	Q12h	Q12–18h	Q24h	Yes (He,P)
Amoxicillin	Renal (hepatic)	0.9–2.3	Q8h	D	60–90%	30–70%	20–30%	Yes (He) No (P)
Amphotericin B	Nonrenal	24	Q24h	I	Q24h	Q24h	24–36h	No (He,P)
Ampicillin	Renal (hepatic)	0.8–1.5	Q4–6h	I	Q6h	Q6–12h	Q12–16h	Yes (He) No (P)
Carbenicillin*	Renal (hepatic)	1.2–1.5	Q4–6h	I	Q8–12h	Q12–24h	Q24–48h	Yes (He) No (P)
Cefaclor	Renal (hepatic)	0.75	Q8h	D	100%	50–100%	33%	Yes (He,P)
Cefamandole	Renal	1.0	Q4–8h	I	Q6h	Q6–8h	Q8h	Yes (He)
Cefazolin	Renal	1.4–2.2	Q8h	I	Q8h	Q12h	Q24–48h	Yes (He) No (P)
Cefotaxime	Renal (hepatic)	1	Q6–8h	I	Q6–8h	Q8–12h	Q12–24h	Yes (He) No (P)
Cefoxitin	Renal	1.0	Q6–8h	I	Q8h	Q8–12h	Q24–48h	Yes (He) No (P)

(Continued.)

| | Pharmacokinetics | | | | Adjustments in Renal Failure | | | |
| | | | | | Creatinine Clearance (ml/min) | | | Supplemental Dose for Dialysis |
Drug	Route of Excretion	Normal $T_{1/2}$ (hr)	Normal Dose Interval	Method	>50	10–50	<10	
Ceftazidime	Renal (hepatic)	1.8	Q8–12h	I	Q12h	Q12–24h	Q24–48h	Yes (He) No (P)
Cefuroxime	Renal	1.6–2.2	Q6–8h	I	Q8–12h	Q24–48h	Q48–72h	Yes (He) No (P)
Cephalexin	Renal	0.9	Q6h	I	Q6h	Q6–8h	Q8–12h	Yes (He) No (P)
Cephalothin‡	Renal (hepatic)	0.5–1.0	Q6h	I	Q6h	Q6–8h	Q8–12h	Yes (He) No (P)
Ethambutol	Renal	4	Q24h	I	Q24h	Q24–36h	Q48h	Yes (He, P)
Fluconazole‡	Renal	20–50	Q24h	D	100%	25–50%	25%	Yes (He, P)
Flucytosine	Renal	3–6	Q6h	I	Q6h, 50%	Q12–24h, 30–50%	Q24–48h, 20–30%	Yes (He,P)
Ganciclovir	Renal	2.5–3.6	Q8–12h	DI	50–100% and Q8–12h	25–50% and Q24h	25% and Q24h	Yes (He)
Gentamicin‡	Renal	2.5–3.0	Q8–12h	D	60–90%	30–70%	20–30%	Yes (He, P)
				I	Q8–12h,	Q12h,	Q24h,	
Isoniazid	Hepatic (renal)	2–4 (slow)†, 0.5–1.5 (fast)	Q24h	D	100%	100%	66–75%	Yes (He,P)

Drug	Route of excretion	Half-life (h)	Normal interval	Method	GFR >50	GFR 10–50	GFR <10	Dialysis
Kanamycin	Renal	2–3	Q8h	I	Q8–12h, 60–90%	Q12h, 30–70%	Q24h, 20–30%	Yes (He,P)
Methicillin	Renal (hepatic)	0.5–1.0	Q4–6h	D	Q4–6h	Q6–8h	Q8–12h	No (He,P)
Metronidazole	Hepatic (renal)	6–14	Q8h	I	Q8h	Q8–12h	Q12–24h	Yes (He) No (P)
Nitrofurantoin	Nonrenal	1–1.7	Q8h	D	100%	Avoid	Avoid	Yes (He)
Penicillin G	Renal (hepatic)	0.5	Q4–6h	I	Q6–8h	Q8–12h	Q12–16h	Yes (He) No (P)
Piperacillin	Renal (hepatic)	0.8–1.5	Q6h	I	Q4–6h	Q6–8h	Q8h	Yes (He)
Sulfamethoxazole	Hepatic (renal)	9–11	Q12h	I	Q12h	Q18h	Q24h	Yes (He) No (P)
Ticarcillin*	Renal (hepatic)	1–1.5	Q4–6h	I	Q8–12h	Q12–24h	Q24–48h	Yes (He,P)
Tobramycin†	Renal	2.5–3	Q8h	D	Q8–12h, 60–90%	Q12h, 30–70%	Q24h, 20–30%	Yes (H) No (P)
Trimethoprim	Renal (hepatic)	8–15	Q12h	I	Q12h	Q18h	Q24h	Yes (He) No (P)
Vancomycin	Renal	6–10	Q6–8h	I	Q24–72h	Q72–240h	Q240h	Y/N (He)§ No (P)

*May inactivate aminoglycosides in patients with renal impairment.
†Rate of acetylation of isoniazid.
‡May add to peritoneal dialysate to obtain adequate serum levels.
§If using high-flux polysulfone hemodialysis, give supplemental dose following dialysis.

III. NON-ANTIMICROBIALS REQUIRING ADJUSTMENT IN RENAL FAILURE

	Pharmacokinetics				Adjustments in Renal Failure			
					Creatinine Clearance (ml/min)			Supplemental Dose for Dialysis
Drug	Route of Excretion	Normal $T_{1/2}$ (hr)	Normal Dose Interval	Method	>50	10–50	<10	
Acetaminophen	Hepatic	2	Q4h	I	Q4h	Q6h	Q8h	Yes (He) No (P)
Acetylsalicylic Acid*	Hepatic (renal)	2–19	Q4h	I	Q4h	Q4–6h	Avoid	Yes (He,P)
Adriamycin	Renal (hepatic)	16–30	Single treatment	D	100%	100%	75%	?
Allopurinol	Renal	0.7–1.6	Q24h	I D D	Q8h, 100%, Q24h	Q8–12h, 75%, Q24h	Q12–24h, 50% 75%, Q36h	Yes (He)
Azathioprine#	Hepatic	IV: 12.5 min; PO: 0.5–4h	Q24h	I				Yes (He)
Captopril	Renal (hepatic)	1.9	Q12h	D	100%	100%	50%	Yes (He)
Carbamazepine	Hepatic (renal)	20–36	Q8–12h	D	100%	100%	75%	No (He,P)
Chloral Hydrate	Hepatic	7–14	Q8h PRN	D	100%	Avoid	Avoid	Yes (He)

Cimetidine	Renal (hepatic)	1.5–2	Q12h	I	Q6h, 100%	Q8h, 75%	Q12h, 50%	No (He)
Digoxin†	Renal (GI)	36–44	Q24h	D	100%, Q24h	25–75%, Q36h	10–25%, Q48h	No (He,P)
Diphenhydramine	Hepatic	4–7	Q6h	I	Q6h	Q6–9h	Q9–12h 25%	?
Enalapril	Renal (hepatic)	7	Q12–24h	D	100%	50%	25%	Yes (He)
Famotidine	Renal (hepatic)	2.5–4	Q12–24h	I	Q20–40h, 100%	Q30–60h, 50%	Q68–136h, 25%	No (He,P)
Hydralazine‡	Hepatic (GI)	2–4.5	Q8h (fast),§ Q12h (slow)	I	Q8–12h	Q8–12h	Q8–16h (fast), Q12–24h (slow)	No (He,P)
Insulin (regular)	Hepatic (renal)	9 min	Variable	D	100%	75%	50%	?
Metoclopramide	Renal (hepatic)	4	Q6–8h	D	100%	75%	50%	No (He)
Methotrexate	Renal	Triphasic, 0.1, 2.3, 27	Single Treatment	D	100%	50%	Avoid	Yes (He) No (P)

(Continued.)

| Drug | Pharmacokinetics | | | Adjustments in Renal Failure | | | | Supplemental Dose for Dialysis |
| | Route of Excretion | Normal $T_{1/2}$ (hr) | Normal Dose Interval | Method | Creatinine Clearance (ml/min) | | | |
					>50	10–50	<10	
Phenobarbital	Hepatic (renal, 30%)	65–150	Q8–12h	I	Q8–12h	Q8–12h	Q12–16h	Yes (He,P)
Primidone	Hepatic (renal, 20%)	6–12	Q8–12h	I	Q8–12h	Q8–12h	Q12–24h	Yes (He)
Ranitidine	Renal (hepatic)	1.5–3	Q8–12h	D	100%	75%	50%	Yes (He)
Spironolactone	Renal (hepatic)	10–35	Q6h	I	Q6–12h	Q12–24h‖	Avoid	?
Thiazides	Renal	1–2	Q12h	D	100%	100%	Avoid	?

*With large doses $T_{1/2}$ prolonged up to 30 hr.
†Decrease loading dose 50% in end-stage renal disease because of decreased volume of distribution.
‡Dose interval varies for rapid and slow acetylators with normal and impaired renal function.
§Rate of acetylation of hydralazine.
‖Hyperkalemia common with GFR <30 ml/min.
#Azathioprine rapidly converted to mercaptopurine.

IV. DRUGS REQUIRING NO ADJUSTMENT

Drug	Extra Dose for Dialysis
Antibiotics	
Ceftriaxone	
Chloramphenicol	He
Clindamycin	
Cloxacillin	
Erythromycin	
Ketoconazole	
Miconazole	
Nafcillin	
Pyrimethamine	
Rifampin	
Non-antibiotics	
Amitriptyline	
Busulfan	
Chlorpheniramine	
Chlorpromazine	He
Clonidine	
Codeine	
Corticosteroids (any)	
Cytosine arabinoside	
Diazepam	
Diazoxide	
Diltiazem	He, P
Fentanyl	
5-Fluorouracil	
Flurazepam	He
Furosemide	
Haloperidol	
Heparin	
Ibuprofen	
Imipramine	
Indomethacin	
Lidocaine	
Meperidine	
Metolazone	
Midazolam	

(Continued.)

Drug	Extra Dose for Dialysis
Minoxidil	
Morphine	
Naloxone	
Nifedipine	
Nitroprusside	He
Pentazocine	He
Pentobarbital	
Phenytoin	
Prazosin	
Propoxyphene	
Propranolol	
Quinidine	He, P
Secobarbital	
Succinylcholine	
Theophylline	He, P
Valproic acid	
Verapamil	
Vincristine	
Warfarin	

INDEX

A

Look for these bestsellers in your local bookstores.

Or call toll-free 1-800-426-4545 and use your major credit card.